Natural Products and Disease Prevention, Relief and Treatment

Natural Products and Disease Prevention, Relief and Treatment

Editor

Md Soriful Islam

MDPI • Basel • Beijing • Wuhan • Barcelona • Belgrade • Manchester • Tokyo • Cluj • Tianjin

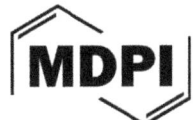

Editor
Md Soriful Islam
Johns Hopkins University
USA

Editorial Office
MDPI
St. Alban-Anlage 66
4052 Basel, Switzerland

This is a reprint of articles from the Special Issue published online in the open access journal *Nutrients* (ISSN 2072-6643) (available at: https://www.mdpi.com/journal/nutrients/special_issues/natural_products_and_disease_prevention_relief_and_treatment).

For citation purposes, cite each article independently as indicated on the article page online and as indicated below:

LastName, A.A.; LastName, B.B.; LastName, C.C. Article Title. *Journal Name* **Year**, *Volume Number*, Page Range.

ISBN 978-3-0365-6137-0 (Hbk)
ISBN 978-3-0365-6138-7 (PDF)

© 2022 by the authors. Articles in this book are Open Access and distributed under the Creative Commons Attribution (CC BY) license, which allows users to download, copy and build upon published articles, as long as the author and publisher are properly credited, which ensures maximum dissemination and a wider impact of our publications.
The book as a whole is distributed by MDPI under the terms and conditions of the Creative Commons license CC BY-NC-ND.

Contents

About the Editor vii

Md Soriful Islam
Natural Products and Disease Prevention, Relief and Treatment
Reprinted from: *Nutrients* **2022**, *14*, 2396, doi:10.3390/nu14122396 1

Natalia Nowacka-Jechalke, Renata Nowak, Marta Kinga Lemieszek, Wojciech Rzeski, Urszula Gawlik-Dziki, Nikola Szpakowska and Zbigniew Kaczyński
Promising Potential of Crude Polysaccharides from *Sparassis crispa* against Colon Cancer: An In Vitro Study
Reprinted from: *Nutrients* **2021**, *13*, 161, doi:10.3390/nu13010161 5

Hemavathy Subramaiam, Wan-Loy Chu, Ammu Kutty Radhakrishnan, Srikumar Chakravarthi, Kanga Rani Selvaduray and Yih-Yih Kok
Evaluating Anticancer and Immunomodulatory Effects of *Spirulina* (Arthrospira) *platensis* and Gamma-Tocotrienol Supplementation in a Syngeneic Mouse Model of Breast Cancer
Reprinted from: *Nutrients* **2021**, *13*, 2320, doi:10.3390/nu13072320 23

Hye-Yoom Kim, Jung-Joo Yoon, Dae-Sung Kim, Dae-Gill Kang and Ho-Sub Lee
YG-1 Extract Improves Acute Pulmonary Inflammation by Inducing Bronchodilation and Inhibiting Inflammatory Cytokines
Reprinted from: *Nutrients* **2021**, *13*, 3414, doi:10.3390/nu13103414 39

Ahyeon Kim, Jiwon Ha, Jeongeun Kim, Yongmin Cho, Jimyung Ahn, Chunhoo Cheon, Sung-Hoon Kim, Seong-Gyu Ko and Bonglee Kim
Natural Products for Pancreatic Cancer Treatment: From Traditional Medicine to Modern Drug Discovery
Reprinted from: *Nutrients* **2021**, *13*, 3801, doi:10.3390/nu13113801 57

Kyeong-Min Kim, So-Yeon Kim, Tamanna Jahan Mony, Ho Jung Bae, Sang-Deok Han, Eun-Seok Lee, Seung-Hyuk Choi, Sun Hee Hong, Sang-Deok Lee and Se Jin Park
Dracocephalum moldavica Ethanol Extract Suppresses LPS-Induced Inflammatory Responses through Inhibition of the JNK/ERK/NF-κB Signaling Pathway and IL-6 Production in RAW 264.7 Macrophages and in Endotoxic-Treated Mice
Reprinted from: *Nutrients* **2021**, *13*, 4501, doi:10.3390/nu13124501 95

Yoshinaga Aoyama, Aya Naiki-Ito, Kuang Xiaochen, Masayuki Komura, Hiroyuki Kato, Yuko Nagayasu, Shingo Inaguma, Hiroyuki Tsuda, Mamoru Tomita, Yoichi Matsuo, Shuji Takiguchi and Satoru Takahashi
Lactoferrin Prevents Hepatic Injury and Fibrosis via the Inhibition of NF-κB Signaling in a Rat Non-Alcoholic Steatohepatitis Model
Reprinted from: *Nutrients* **2022**, *14*, 42, doi:10.3390/nu14010042 107

Pissared Khuituan, Nawiya Huipao, Nilobon Jeanmard, Sitthiwach Thantongsakul, Warittha Promjun, Suwarat Chuthong, Chittipong Tipbunjong and Saranya Peerakietkhajorn
Sargassum plagiophyllum Extract Enhances Colonic Functions and Modulates Gut Microbiota in Constipated Mice
Reprinted from: *Nutrients* **2022**, *14*, 496, doi:10.3390/nu14030496 123

Ru Hui Sim, Srinivasa Rao Sirasanagandla, Srijit Das and Seong Lin Teoh
Treatment of Glaucoma with Natural Products and Their Mechanism of Action: An Update
Reprinted from: *Nutrients* **2022**, *14*, 534, doi:10.3390/nu14030534 137

Yu Toyoda, Tappei Takada, Hiroki Saito, Hiroshi Hirata, Ami Ota-Kontani, Youichi Tsuchiya and Hiroshi Suzuki
Identification of Inhibitory Activities of Dietary Flavonoids against URAT1, a Renal Urate Re-Absorber: In Vitro Screening and Fractional Approach Focused on Rooibos Leaves
Reprinted from: *Nutrients* **2022**, *14*, 575, doi:10.3390/nu14030575 . . . . **177**

Alaa Sirwi, Rasheed A. Shaik, Abdulmohsin J. Alamoudi, Basma G. Eid, Mahmoud A. Elfaky, Sabrin R. M. Ibrahim, Gamal A. Mohamed, Hossam M. Abdallah and Ashraf B. Abdel-Naim
Mokko Lactone Alleviates Doxorubicin-Induced Cardiotoxicity in Rats via Antioxidant, Anti-Inflammatory, and Antiapoptotic Activities
Reprinted from: *Nutrients* **2022**, *14*, 733, doi:10.3390/nu14040733 . . . . **197**

Do-Hoon Kim, Ji-Young Lee, Young-Jin Kim, Hyun-Ju Kim and Wansu Park
Rubi Fructus Water Extract Alleviates LPS-Stimulated Macrophage Activation via an ER Stress-Induced Calcium/CHOP Signaling Pathway
Reprinted from: *Nutrients* **2020**, *12*, 3577, doi:10.3390/nu12113577 . . . . **211**

About the Editor

Md Soriful Islam

Md Soriful Islam, a Senior Research Fellow, is currently working at the Johns Hopkins University, Baltimore, Maryland, USA. He holds a Ph.D. in Reproductive Sciences (Uterine Fibroid) from Università Politecnica delle Marche, Ancona, Italy. His research interests include the molecular basis of fibroid cellular function, Hippo signaling, mechanical signaling, hormone signaling, inflammation and fibrosis, selective progesterone receptor modulators, small molecule inhibitors, and natural compounds. He is the author of more than 35 scientific articles published in several prestigious journals. His work has been cited over 2500 times. He is a member of the American Society for Reproductive Medicine, the Society for Reproductive Investigation, and the European Society of Human Reproduction and Embryology. Recently, he received an SRI and Bayer Discovery/Innovation grant to conduct research in the field of women's health.

Editorial

Natural Products and Disease Prevention, Relief and Treatment

Md Soriful Islam

Department of Gynecology and Obstetrics, Johns Hopkins University School of Medicine, 720 Rutland Ave, Ross Research Building, Room 624, Baltimore, MD 21205, USA; soriful84@gmail.com; Tel.: +1-410-614-2000; Fax: +1-410-614-7060

Keywords: Rubi Fructus; Mokko lactone; YG-1 extract; *Dracocephalum moldavica* ethanol extract; lactoferrin; *Sparassis crispa*; fisetin and quercetin; *Sargassum plagiophyllum* extract; inflammation; fibrosis

This Special Issue focusses on the role of natural products in disease prevention, relief and treatment. Natural products are known to regulate key pathophysiological processes, such as inflammation, fibrosis, hypoxia, oxidative stress, cell proliferation, angiogenesis, migration, and metabolism, that are linked to human diseases. In this Special Issue, we have published a number of high-quality manuscripts that bring attention to the emerging role of natural products in a wide range of human diseases, including inflammatory and fibrotic diseases, as well as cancers. This editorial will discuss individual reports published in this Special Issue.

Rubi Fructus, the unripe fruits of *Rubus coreanus* Miquel., is well known for its different active biological properties. Kim et al. examined the effect of Rubi Fructus (RF) on inflammatory signaling pathways in RAW 264.7 macrophages [1]. The data showed that RF was effective as an anti-inflammatory product. RF exhibited anti-inflammatory activity on LPS-stimulated macrophages by regulating a series of inflammatory mediators, including IL6 (interleukin 6), MCP-1 (monocyte chemotactic activating factor 1), TNF-α (tumor necrosis factor-α), as well as their associated signaling pathways (such as STAT, JAK2, c-Jun, and CHOP) [1].

Mokko lactone (ML), a naturally occurring guaianolide sesquiterpene, is known for its antioxidant and anti-inflammatory properties. Sirwi et al. investigated the protective effect of ML in doxorubicin (DOX)-induced cardiotoxicity [2]. Rats were treated with ML for 10 days, followed by one IP injection of DOX. The results showed a significant protective effect of ML in DOX-induced cardiotoxicity in terms of amelioration of oxidative stress, apoptosis, and inflammation [2]. These findings suggest that ML can be used to alleviate DOX-induced cardiotoxicity in patients.

YG-1 extract is a mixture of three different plants, including Lonicera japonica, Arctii Fructus, and Scutel lariae radix. Kim and coworkers investigated the effect of different concentrations of YG-1 extract on bronchodilatation, as well as acute bronchial and pulmonary inflammation relief ex vivo and in vivo, respectively [3]. Ex vivo, YG-1 extract showed concentration-dependent bronchodilation effects in Sprague Dawley rats by upregulating cAMP (cyclic adenosine monophosphate) levels through the β2-AR (β2-adrenergic receptor)/PKA pathway [3]. In vivo, the effects of YG-1 extract on acute bronchial and pulmonary inflammation were investigated in C57BL/6 mice. The results showed that YG-1 extract treatment reduced the prevalence of respiratory symptoms and the incidence of non-specific lung diseases. YG-1 treatment also improved acute bronchial and pulmonary inflammation, at least in part, by regulating the inflammasome signaling pathways (such as NLRP3/caspase-1) [3]. These results support further exploration of YG-1 extract as an effective natural product in developing therapeutics for respiratory diseases.

DMEE is an ethanol extract from the herb *Dracocephalum moldavica*, which contains the active compound oleanolic acid. Kim et al. demonstrated the anti-inflammatory effect of

DMEE on LPS-induced inflammatory responses in 264.7 macrophages and murine model of sepsis. The data showed that that DMEE effectively reduced LPS-induced inflammatory responses in RAW 264.7 macrophages and LPS-induced septic shock mice. These effects were mediated, at least in part, by inhibiting MAPK and NF-κB signaling pathways (such as JNK, ERK and p65), as well as reducing the production of inflammatory cytokine IL6. These findings are interesting and significant for future research in the area of natural products for sepsis [4].

Lactoferrin (LF) is an iron-binding glycoprotein found in all exocrine fluids, including tears, sweat, and saliva. It is also abundant in milk. Aoyama et al. investigated the possible antioxidant, anti-inflammatory and antitumoral activities of lactoferrin in a combined high-fat diet/dimethylnitrosamine treated C×32 dominant negative transgenic (C×32ΔTg) rat model of NASH (non-alcoholic steatohepatitis). Lactoferrin showed a selective chemopreventive effect against liver tissue injury and progression via regulating the NF-κB /TGF-β1 signaling pathways [5].

Sparassis (also known as cauliflower mushroom), a genus of parasitic and saprobic mushrooms, is characterized by its unique shape and appearance. Nowacka-Jechalke et al. investigated the chemical composition and potential biologic activity of crude polysaccharides isolated from *Sparassis crispa* (CPS). CPS mainly consists of carbohydrates and exerts cytotoxic effects on colon cancer cells. Interestingly, CPS was found to be non-toxic to normal human colon epithelial cells. CPS showed moderate antioxidant activity and inhibited inflammatory molecules, such as COX-2 [6]. These results suggest that CPS may be important as a part of the regular human diet. Further study is needed to explore its potentiality as a chemopreventive and therapeutic agent in colon cancers.

Circulating uric acid is thought to be effective against loss of bone mineral density and oxidative damage. However, excess serum uric acid is associated with diseases such as gout, hypertension, and cardiovascular disease. URAT1, a member of the OAT (organic anion transporter) family, is an anion-exchanging uptake transporter localized to the apical membrane of renal proximal tubular cells. URAT1 regulates most urate reabsorption into blood; therefore, the inhibition of URAT1 may help decrease serum urate levels by increasing the net renal urate excretion. Toyoda et al. brings to attention the beneficial effect of natural compounds on the inhibition of URAT1. This group used cell-based urate transport assay to investigate the inhibitory effects of 162 extracts of plant materials on URAT1. They found that fisetin and quercetin showed significant inhibitory effects on URAT1 cell-based urate transport assay [7]. Overall, this study pointed out that some selective phytochemicals should be investigated further in human studies, and may provide new clues for using nutraceuticals to promote human health.

Seaweed is widely known for its beneficial role for human health. Khuituan et al. examined the effects of *Sargassum plagiophyllum* extract (SPE) on constipated mice, particularly the functions of the gastrointestinal tract and gut microbiota [8]. SPE contains phenolic compounds and carotenoids (such as fucoxanthin), as well as long-chain-sulfated polysaccharides (such as fucoidan). This study showed that SPE pretreatment increased the frequency of gut contraction, leading to reduced gut transit time. The beneficial effect of SPE may be due to the presence of bioactive compounds. Overall, SPE might be useful for the development of human food supplements to prevent constipation.

Subramaiam et al. examined the immunomodulatory, anti-metastatic, gene expression analysis and anticancer effects of combined Spirulina and γT3 against breast cancer using a syngeneic mouse model [9]. They found that the combination of Spirulina and γT3 does not appear to have any synergistic anticancer or immunomodulatory effects in this tumor-bearing mouse [9]. This negative study would be a resource for future study in this area, particularly for Spirulina.

This Special Issue also published two review articles that outlined the benefits of natural products for the treatment of pancreatic cancer and glaucoma. Kim et al. reviewed and analyzed 68 natural products that have anti-pancreatic cancer effects reported during the past five years. They divided this large number of natural products into four categories based on their mechanisms of actions, and presented a summary of their findings [10]. Most of the natural products have been reported to induce apoptosis in pancreatic cancer cells. There are some natural products, including Moringa, Coix seed, etc., that showed multi-functional properties. Overall, this review suggests that some selective natural products can be useful for human pancreatic cancer.

Sim and colleagues provided a comprehensive review of the effects of various dietary supplements in the protection of retinal ganglion cells (RGCs) and in the preservation of the function of the anterior chamber outflow pathways that enable better regulation of intraocular pressure (IOP) [11]. The available data suggest that IOP can be suppressed by natural compounds, including baicalein, forskolin, marijuana, ginsenoside, resveratrol and hesperidin. There are some other plant and plant derived products, including Ginkgo biloba, Lycium barbarum, Diospyros kaki, Tripterygium wilfordii, saffron, curcumin, caffeine, anthocyanin, coenzyme Q10 and vitamins B3 and D that have shown neuroprotective effects on retinal ganglion cells. These data are encouraging but require further extensive investigations in the future to ensure the efficacy and safety of natural products as an alternative therapy for glaucoma.

In conclusion, this Special Issue has highlighted the recent preclinical studies on various natural products with their anti-inflammatory, antioxidative, neuroprotective, cardioprotective, antifibrotic, and anticancer effects, as well as other health benefit effects. Overall, this Special Issue has been a good source of some promising natural products. These include Rubi Fructus, Mokko lactone, YG-1 extract, *D. moldavica* ethanol extract (DMEE), lactoferrin, *S. crispa*, fisetin and quercetin, as well as *S. plagiophyllum* extract. Further clinical studies are needed to validate these encouraging findings.

Funding: This research received no external funding.

Conflicts of Interest: The author declares no conflict of interest.

References

1. Kim, D.-H.; Lee, J.-Y.; Kim, Y.-J.; Kim, H.-J.; Park, W. Rubi Fructus water extract alleviates lps-stimulated macrophage activation via an er stress-induced calcium/CHOP signaling pathway. *Nutrients* **2020**, *12*, 3577. [CrossRef]
2. Sirwi, A.; Shaik, R.A.; Alamoudi, A.J.; Eid, B.G.; Elfaky, M.A.; Ibrahim, S.R.; Mohamed, G.A.; Abdallah, H.M.; Abdel-Naim, A.B. Mokko lactone alleviates doxorubicin-induced cardiotoxicity in rats via antioxidant, anti-Inflammatory, and antiapoptotic activities. *Nutrients* **2022**, *14*, 733. [CrossRef] [PubMed]
3. Kim, H.-Y.; Yoon, J.-J.; Kim, D.-S.; Kang, D.-G.; Lee, H.-S. YG-1 Extract Improves Acute Pulmonary Inflammation by Inducing Bronchodilation and Inhibiting Inflammatory Cytokines. *Nutrients* **2021**, *13*, 3414. [CrossRef] [PubMed]
4. Kim, K.-M.; Kim, S.-Y.; Mony, T.J.; Bae, H.J.; Han, S.-D.; Lee, E.-S.; Choi, S.-H.; Hong, S.H.; Lee, S.-D.; Park, S.J. Dracocephalum moldavica Ethanol Extract Suppresses LPS-Induced Inflammatory Responses through Inhibition of the JNK/ERK/NF-κB Signaling Pathway and IL-6 Production in RAW 264.7 Macrophages and in Endotoxic-Treated Mice. *Nutrients* **2021**, *13*, 4501. [CrossRef] [PubMed]
5. Aoyama, Y.; Naiki-Ito, A.; Xiaochen, K.; Komura, M.; Kato, H.; Nagayasu, Y.; Inaguma, S.; Tsuda, H.; Tomita, M.; Matsuo, Y. Lactoferrin Prevents Hepatic Injury and Fibrosis via the Inhibition of NF-κB Signaling in a Rat Non-Alcoholic Steatohepatitis Model. *Nutrients* **2021**, *14*, 42. [CrossRef] [PubMed]
6. Nowacka-Jechalke, N.; Nowak, R.; Lemieszek, M.K.; Rzeski, W.; Gawlik-Dziki, U.; Szpakowska, N.; Kaczyński, Z. Promising potential of crude polysaccharides from Sparassis crispa against colon cancer: An in vitro study. *Nutrients* **2021**, *13*, 161. [CrossRef] [PubMed]
7. Toyoda, Y.; Takada, T.; Saito, H.; Hirata, H.; Ota-Kontani, A.; Tsuchiya, Y.; Suzuki, H. Identification of Inhibitory Activities of Dietary Flavonoids against URAT1, a Renal Urate Re-Absorber: In Vitro Screening and Fractional Approach Focused on Rooibos Leaves. *Nutrients* **2022**, *14*, 575. [CrossRef] [PubMed]
8. Khuituan, P.; Huipao, N.; Jeanmard, N.; Thantongsakul, S.; Promjun, W.; Chuthong, S.; Tipbunjong, C.; Peerakietkhajorn, S. Sargassum plagiophyllum Extract Enhances Colonic Functions and Modulates Gut Microbiota in Constipated Mice. *Nutrients* **2022**, *14*, 496. [CrossRef] [PubMed]
9. Subramaiam, H.; Chu, W.-L.; Radhakrishnan, A.K.; Chakravarthi, S.; Selvaduray, K.R.; Kok, Y.-Y. Evaluating Anticancer and Immunomodulatory Effects of Spirulina (Arthrospira) platensis and Gamma-Tocotrienol Supplementation in a Syngeneic Mouse Model of Breast Cancer. *Nutrients* **2021**, *13*, 2320. [CrossRef] [PubMed]

10. Kim, A.; Ha, J.; Kim, J.; Cho, Y.; Ahn, J.; Cheon, C.; Kim, S.-H.; Ko, S.-G.; Kim, B. Natural Products for Pancreatic Cancer Treatment: From Traditional Medicine to Modern Drug Discovery. *Nutrients* **2021**, *13*, 3801. [CrossRef] [PubMed]
11. Sim, R.H.; Sirasanagandla, S.R.; Das, S.; Teoh, S.L. Treatment of Glaucoma with Natural Products and Their Mechanism of Action: An Update. *Nutrients* **2022**, *14*, 534. [CrossRef] [PubMed]

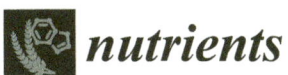

Article

Promising Potential of Crude Polysaccharides from *Sparassis crispa* against Colon Cancer: An In Vitro Study

Natalia Nowacka-Jechalke [1,*], Renata Nowak [1], Marta Kinga Lemieszek [2], Wojciech Rzeski [2,3], Urszula Gawlik-Dziki [4], Nikola Szpakowska [5] and Zbigniew Kaczyński [5]

[1] Department of Pharmaceutical Botany, Medical University of Lublin, 1 Chodźki Street, 20-093 Lublin, Poland; renata.nowak@umlub.pl
[2] Department of Medical Biology, Institute of Rural Health, 2 Jaczewskiego Street, 20-090 Lublin, Poland; martalemieszek@gmail.com (M.K.L.); rzeski.wojciech@imw.lublin.pl (W.R.)
[3] Department of Functional Anatomy and Cytobiology, Maria Curie Skłodowska University, 19 Akademicka Street, 20-033 Lublin, Poland
[4] Department of Biochemistry and Food Chemistry, University of Life Sciences in Lublin, 8 Skromna Street, 20-704 Lublin, Poland; urszula.gawlik@up.lublin.pl
[5] Faculty of Chemistry, University of Gdańsk, 63 Wita Stwosza Street, 80-308 Gdańsk, Poland; nikola.szpakowska@ug.edu.pl (N.S.); zbigniew.kaczynski@ug.edu.pl (Z.K.)
* Correspondence: natalia.nowacka@umlub.pl; Tel.: +48-814-487-060

Abstract: The aim of the present study was to evaluate in vitro the beneficial potential of crude polysaccharides from *S. crispa* (CPS) in one of the most common cancer types—colon cancer. The determination of the chemical composition of CPS has revealed that it contains mostly carbohydrates, while proteins or phenolics are present only in trace amounts. ^{1}H NMR and GC–MS methods were used for the structural analysis of CPS. Biological activity including anticancer, anti-inflammatory and antioxidant properties of CPS was investigated. CPS was found to be non-toxic to normal human colon epithelial CCD841 CoN cells. Simultaneously, they destroyed membrane integrity as well as inhibited the proliferation of human colon cancer cell lines: Caco-2, LS180 and HT-29. Antioxidant activity was determined by various methods and revealed the moderate potential of CPS. The enzymatic assays revealed no influence of CPS on xanthine oxidase and the inhibition of catalase activity. Moreover, pro-inflammatory enzymes such as cyclooxygenase-2 or lipoxygenase were inhibited by CPS. Therefore, it may be suggested that *S. crispa* is a valuable part of the regular human diet, which may contribute to a reduction in the risk of colon cancer, and possess promising activities encouraging further studies regarding its potential use as chemopreventive and therapeutic agent in more invasive stages of this type of cancer.

Keywords: β-glucan; anticancer activity; antioxidant; anti-inflammatory; cyclooxygenase; lipoxygenase; cauliflower mushroom

1. Introduction

Polysaccharides constitute an abundant group of macromolecules present in fungal cell walls. Due to their wide structural variability, they have been shown to have great potential to be biological response modifiers (BRMs). The composition of monosaccharide residues, including their sequence and placement as well as their connections and position of glycosidic linkages, affect polysaccharide activities [1]. One of the mushroom polysaccharides—chitin—is a water-insoluble and indigestible compound in the human gastrointestinal tract acting as dietary fiber [2]. In turn, most polysaccharides present in mushrooms are water-soluble glucans with different types of glycosidic linkages, e.g., (1→3)-α-glucans and (1→3), (1→6)-β-glucans [3].

Mushrooms constitute an inexpensive and abundant source of glucans with health-promoting potential. Nowadays, when the number of health-conscious consumers is growing, there is a need for developing new strategies for the acquisition of beneficial glucans. According to the latest data, the global market of β-glucans is expected to grow significantly and reach over 1 billion dollars in 2020 [4].

Mushroom polysaccharides, especially glucans, are known to exert anticancer activity through immunostimulatory potential, which involves the activation of the innate immune system as well as the acceleration of the host's defense mechanisms [1,5]. In addition to the anticancer potential, mushroom polysaccharides possess a vast spectrum of biological activities, including antimicrobial, antiviral, antioxidant, anti-inflammatory, or prebiotic properties [6–10]. The major glucans isolated from the fungal species used in the treatment of cancer in Asian countries are β-glucans, e.g., lentinan from *Lentinus edodes*, schizophyllan from *Schizophyllum commune*, krestin from *Trametes versicolor*, and grifolan from *Grifola frondosa* [11–14]. Colon cancer is believed to be preventable with the use of natural chemopreventive agents. The strategy of chemoprevention assumes reversing, suppressing, or preventing carcinogenic progression [15]. With their multidirectional activity, mushroom polysaccharides are able to act at different steps in the carcinogenic process, with the overall goal of reducing cancer incidence. Moreover, there are some already known strategies based on the use of mushroom β-glucans not only to inhibit tumor growth but also induce synergistic effects with chemotherapeutic agents or other immune stimulators. An innovative approach assumes that β-glucans may be used to deliver nanoparticles containing chemotherapeutic agents to the colon cancer site to improve their therapeutic efficacy [16].

Moreover, there are many applications of β-glucans in food products related to their ability to form a gel and enhance the viscosity of aqueous solutions. The use of β-glucans allows the replacement of fat to develop calorie-reduced food products or enhance their appearance and texture [17]. Therefore, they can be considered functional food ingredients providing consumers with health benefits and bringing significant technological advantages.

Sparassis crispa, also known as cauliflower mushroom in English or Hanabiratake in Japanese and Ggoksongee (meaning a blossom) in Korean, is an edible and medicinal mushroom growing in the temperate regions of Europe and North America [18]. It is also a very popular cultivable species in Asian countries, especially in Japan [19]. Despite its popularity, bioactive polysaccharides from *S. crispa* have not been exactly defined and studied to date. The present study is an attempt to extend this knowledge. The aim of the present study was to evaluate the content of α- and β-glucans and determine the chemical composition and structure of the crude polysaccharides from *S. crispa* collected from the natural environment in Poland. Furthermore, the anticancer, anti-inflammatory and antioxidant activity of *S. crispa* crude polysaccharides were examined in vitro to determine their chemopreventive potential.

2. Materials and Methods

2.1. Materials

The wild-growing fruiting bodies of *Sparassis crispa* (Wulf.: Fr.). were collected in the forests of Puszcza Solska (Lublin Voivodeship, Poland) in September 2018. Mushroom specimens were authenticated by Prof. Renata Nowak from the Chair and Department of Pharmaceutical Botany, Medical University of Lublin, Poland (voucher specimen No. MSH-076). After collection, the mushrooms were immediately lyophilized, pulverized and kept in a freezer ($-30\ °C$) until further analysis.

2.2. Chemicals and Apparatus

The COX (ovine) Colorimetric Inhibitor Screening Assay Kit was obtained from Cayman Chemical Company, Ann Arbor, MI, USA. The Megazyme Mushroom and Yeast Beta-Glucan Assay Kit was purchased from Megazyme International Ireland Ltd., Wicklow, UK. The in vitro Toxicology Assay Kit Lactate Dehydrogenase Based, thiazolyl blue tetrazolium bromide (MTT), Dulbecco's modified Eagle's medium (DMEM), DMEM/Nutrient Mixture F-12 Ham (DMEM/F12 Ham), fetal bovine serum (FBS), penicillin and streptomycin were obtained from Sigma Aldrich (St. Louis, MO, USA). Cell Proliferation ELISA BrdU (bromodeoxyuridine) was obtained from Roche Diagnostics GmbH (Penzberg, Germany). Eagle's Minimum Essential Medium (EMEM) was obtained from the American Type Culture Collection (ATCC, Manassas, VA, USA). Redistilled phenol, Bradford reagent, 2,2′-azinobis-(3-ethylbenzothiazoline-6-sulfonic acid) (ABTS$^{\bullet+}$), bovine serum albumin (BSA), and gallic acid were purchased from Sigma-Aldrich Fine Chemicals (St. Louis, MO, USA). Soybean 15-lipooxygenase, xanthine oxidase, catalase, Trolox, 2,2′-azobis (2-methylpropionamide) dihydrochloride (AAPH), and linoleic acid were provided by Sigma-Aldrich Chemical Co. (St. Louis, MO, USA). Fluorescein sodium salt was purchased from Roth (Karlsruhe, Germany). D_2O was obtained from Deutero GmbH (Kastellaun, Germany).

All other chemicals and solvents were of analytical grade and were purchased from Avantor Performance Materials Poland (Gliwice, Poland).

Colorimetric and fluorescence measurements were performed on a 96-well transparent and black microplates (both from Nunclon, Nunc; Roskilde, Denmark), respectively, using an Infinite Pro 200F microplate reader from Tecan Group Ltd. (Männedorf, Switzerland). The evaporation of extracts was conducted using a Heidolph Basis Hei-VAP Value evaporator (Schwabach, Germany). Lyophilization was performed in the Free Zone 1 apparatus (Labcono, Kansas City, KS, USA).

2.3. Extraction of Crude Polysaccharides (CPS)

Freeze-dried and milled fruiting bodies of *S. crispa* (10 g) were macerated with 99.8% ethanol (100 mL) for 24 h at room temperature and then extracted two times with 99.8% ethanol using ultrasonic-assisted extraction (UAE) to remove low molecular weight compounds. Then, the supernatant was removed, and the residue was extracted two times for 30 min with distilled water (200 mL) by UAE at 80 °C. The combined aqueous extracts were concentrated under vacuum to 20 mL. The concentrated extracts were further purified by deproteinization using the Sevage reagent (chloroform/isoamyl alcohol, 4:1, v/v) [20]. Subsequently, polysaccharides were precipitated with cold 99.8% ethanol (1:4, v/v) and kept overnight in the refrigerator at 4 °C. The resulting precipitates of crude polysaccharides were collected by centrifugation (9055 G, 15 min) and lyophilized (Figure 1). The polysaccharide yields (%) were calculated as described below:

$$\text{Yield } (\%, w/w) = \text{Weight of extracted polysaccharides} / \text{Weight of dried material} \times 100 \quad (1)$$

2.4. Chemical Composition of Crude Polysaccharides

2.4.1. Sugar Content Determination

The total sugar content was determined with the phenol–sulphuric acid method [21] using glucose as a standard. One microliter of the sample was mixed with 25 µL of an 80% (w/v) aqueous phenol solution in a test-tube and 2.5 mL of concentrated H_2SO_4 was added. The absorbance was measured at $\lambda = 485$ nm. The results were converted into mg of glucose equivalents and expressed as % of CPS.

2.4.2. Protein Content Determination

The protein concentration in CPS was determined with the Bradford method as previously described [22] using bovine serum albumin as a standard. The reaction mixture consisted of 1 mL of Bradford Reagent and 0.1 mL of the sample. Absorbance at $\lambda = 595$ nm was measured. The results were expressed as % of CPS.

2.4.3. Total Phenolic Content Determination

The content of phenolic compounds was assayed using the method described in detail by [23] using gallic acid as a standard. Twenty microliters of the sample was added to 20 µL of the diluted Folin–Ciocalteu reagent (with water 1:4, v/v) followed by the addition of 160 µL of sodium carbonate (75 g/L). The absorbance was measured at $\lambda = 680$ nm after 20 min of incubation. The results were expressed as % of CPS.

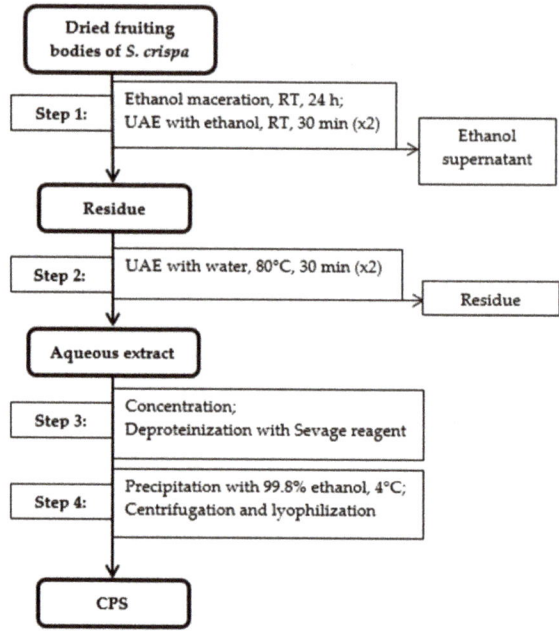

Figure 1. Schematic diagram of extraction of crude polysaccharides from fruiting bodies of *S. crispa* (CPS). Abbreviations: RT—room temperature; UAE—ultrasonic-assisted extraction.

2.5. Structural Analysis

2.5.1. Sugar Composition

The sugar composition of CPS was determined using sugar analysis. The polysaccharide fraction (~0.5 mg) was hydrolyzed with trifluoroacetic acid (2 M TFA, 2 h at 120 °C), reduced with sodium borohydride, and acetylated with acetic anhydride in the presence of sodium acetate (120 °C for 2 h). The alditol acetate derivatives obtained were analyzed by GC–MS using a Shimadzu GC–MS QP2010SE system equipped with a Rtx-5 (30 m) capillary column [24].

2.5.2. NMR Spectroscopy

CPS (~5 mg) was dissolved in 1 mL of 99% D_2O to replace all exchangeable protons, freeze-dried, and dissolved in 0.75 mL of 99.9% D_2O for measurements. The ^1H NMR spectrum was recorded at 40 °C using a Bruker Avance III 500 MHz spectrometer. ^1H chemical shifts were referenced to acetone (δH 2.225).

2.6. α- and β-Glucan Determination

The content of glucans in *S. crispa* was determined using the Megazyme Mushroom and Yeast Beta-Glucan Assay Kit according to the manufacturer's instructions. To determine the total glucan content, milled *S. crispa* was hydrolyzed with concentrated hydrochloric acid and neutralized with 2 M potassium hydroxide. Then, the digestion with exo-1,3-β-glucanase (20 U/mL) plus β-glucosidase (4 U/mL) in 200 mM sodium acetate buffer (pH 5.0) was performed. To measure the glucan content, glucose oxidase/peroxidase and 4-aminoantipyrine in p-hydroxybenzoic acid and sodium azide (GOPOD) reagent was added. The absorbance was measured at λ = 510 nm against the GOPOD reagent blank. For measuring the content of α-glucans, a milled mushroom sample was hydrolyzed in 2 M KOH and neutralized with 1.2 M sodium acetate buffer (pH 3.8). Then, amyloglucosidase

(1630 U/mL) and invertase (500 U/mL) were added into the hydrolysate and incubated at 40 °C for 30 min. After enzymatic hydrolysis, the GOPOD reagent was added and incubated at 40 °C for 20 min. The absorbance was measured at $\lambda = 510$ nm against the reagent blank including the sodium acetate buffer instead the sample tested. The total glucan and α-glucan contents were calculated by comparison to the D-glucose standard. The β-glucan content was determined by subtracting the α-glucan from the total glucan content. All measurements were taken a minimum of three times. The results were expressed as g/100 g of dry weight and are expressed as the mean ± standard deviation (SD).

2.7. Anticancer Potential—In Vitro Studies

2.7.1. Cell Lines

The human colon epithelial cell line CCD 841 CoN and the human colon adenocarcinoma cell line Caco-2 were purchased from the American Type Culture Collection (ATCC, Manassas, VA, USA). The human colon adenocarcinoma cell lines HT-29 and LS180 were obtained from the European Collection of Cell Cultures (ECACC, Centre for Applied Microbiology and Research, Salisbury, UK). The CCD 841 CoN cells were grown in DMEM. The Caco-2 cells were grown in EMEM. The HT-29, and LS180 cells were grown in DMEM/F12 Ham. All media were supplemented with penicillin (100 U/mL), streptomycin (100 mg/mL), and FBS in the amount 10% (CCD841 CoN, LS180, HT-29) or 20% FBS (Caco-2). The cells were maintained in a humidified atmosphere of 95% air and 5% CO_2 at 37 °C.

2.7.2. MTT Assay

The cells were seeded on 96-well microplates at a density of 3×10^4 cells/mL (cancer cells) and 5×10^4 cells/mL (normal cells). On the following day, the culture medium was removed, and the cells were exposed to serial dilutions (10, 25, 50, and 100 µg/mL) of the crude polysaccharide extract from *S. crispa* prepared in the fresh medium with the standard content of FBS. The cell metabolic activity was assessed after 96 h of incubation in standard conditions (5% CO_2, 37 °C) by means of the MTT assay, in which the yellow tetrazolium salt (MTT) was metabolized by viable cells to purple formazan crystals. After the incubation period, MTT solution (5 mg/mL in PBS) was added into the cells for 3 h. The resultant crystals were solubilized overnight in SDS buffer at pH 7.4 (10% SDS in 0.01 M HCl), and the product was quantified spectrophotometrically by measuring the absorbance at a wavelength of $\lambda = 570$ nm using the microplate reader (BioTek ELx800, Highland Park, Winooski, VT, USA). The results were presented as a percentage of metabolic activity of cells treated with the investigated compound versus cells grown in the control medium (indicated as 100%).

2.7.3. BrdU Assay

Cells were seeded on 96-well microplates at a density of 3×10^4 cells/mL (cancer cells) and 5×10^4 cells/mL (normal cells). On the following day, the culture medium was removed, and the cells were exposed to serial dilutions (10, 25, 50, and 100 µg/mL) of the crude polysaccharide extract from *S. crispa* prepared in the fresh medium with a standard content of FBS. After 48 h of incubation in standard conditions (5% CO_2, 37 °C), the impact of CPS on DNA synthesis was measured by a colorimetric immunoassay, namely the Cell Proliferation ELISA BrdU according to the manufacturer's instructions. The test measures cell proliferation by quantitating BrdU (analog of thymidine, 5-bromo-20-deoxyuridine) incorporated into the newly synthesized DNA in proliferating cells. Absorbance was measured at a $\lambda = 450$ nm wavelength using the microplate reader (BioTek ELx800, Highland Park, Winooski, VT, USA). The results were presented as a percentage of the BrdU incorporation to DNA in cells treated with the investigated compound versus the cells grown in the control medium (indicated as 100%).

2.7.4. LDH Assay

Cells were seeded on 96-well microplates at a density of 5×10^4 cells/mL (cancer cells) and 1×10^5 cells/mL (normal cells). On the following day, the culture medium was removed, and the cells were exposed to serial dilutions (10, 25, 50, and 100 µg/mL) of the crude polysaccharide extract from *S. crispa* prepared in the fresh medium supplemented with 2% FBS. After 24 h of incubation in standard conditions (5% CO_2, 37 °C) the culture supernatants were collected in new 96-well microplates, which were used to perform the lactate dehydrogenase (LDH) assay following the manufacturer's instruction. The test was based on the measurement of lactate dehydrogenase (LDH) released into the culture medium upon damage to the cell plasma membrane. The absorbance was recorded on a microplate reader (BioTek ELx800, Highland Park, Winooski, VT, USA) at a wavelength of $\lambda = 450$ nm. The results were presented as the percentage of LDH released from cells treated with the tested compound versus the cells grown in the control medium (indicated as 100%).

2.8. Anti-Inflammatory Activity

2.8.1. Inhibition of COX Activity

The ability of crude polysaccharides from *S. crispa* to inhibit cyclooxygenase activity was determined in vitro with the use of the COX (ovine) Colorimetric Inhibitor Screening Assay Kit. Briefly, 10 µL of the polysaccharide sample (1 mg/mL, in 5% DMSO) were added to the reaction mixture containing 150 µL of assay buffer, 10 µL of heme, and 10 µL of the enzyme (either COX-1 or COX-2). Peroxidase activity can be assayed colorimetrically by monitoring the appearance of oxidized N,N,N',N'-tetramethyl-*p*-phenylenediamine (TMPD) at $\lambda = 590$ nm. Acetylsalicylic acid (1 mM) was used as a control. The percent COX inhibition was calculated as shown below:

COX inhibition activity (%) = 1 − Absorbance of the inhibitor well at $\lambda = 590$ nm/ Absorbance of the 100% initial activity without the inhibitor at $\lambda = 590$ nm × 100

2.8.2. Inhibition of LOX Activity

Inhibition of 15-lipoxygenase (LOX) was determined as previously described with some modifications using soybean 15-LO, generally regarded as predictive for the inhibition of the mammalian enzyme [25]. The LOX inhibition was determined spectrophotometrically at 20 °C by measuring the increase in absorbance at $\lambda = 234$ nm over a 2 min period. The reaction mixture consisted of 0.2 M borate buffer (pH 9.00), the CPS sample (1 mg/mL, in water), the enzyme (167 U/mL), and linoleic acid (134 µM) as a substrate. Acetylsalicylic acid (1 mM) was used as a control. All measurements were carried out in triplicate. The LOX inhibitory activity was expressed as the percentage inhibition of LOX in the above assay mixture system in relation to the control without the inhibitor (indicated as 100%). The mode of inhibition on the enzyme was shown using the Lineweaver–Burk plot.

2.9. Antioxidant Activity

2.9.1. Antiradical Activity against $ABTS^{\bullet+}$

Antiradical activity against $ABTS^{\bullet+}$ was determined with the method described by [26]. Twenty microliters of the sample was mixed with 180 µL of the $ABTS^{\bullet+}$ solution (0.096 mg/mL). The mixture was shaken and incubated for 6 min. The absorbance was measured at $\lambda = 734$ nm. The scavenging activity of the extracts was determined using the following formula:

$$\% \text{ Reduction} = [(AB - AA)/AB] \times 100 \quad (2)$$

where AB is the absorption of the control sample ($ABTS^{\bullet+}$ solution and solvent instead of the sample), and AA is the absorption of the sample with $ABTS^{\bullet+}$ reagent. Six dilutions of CPS were examined to plot a dose–response curve and determine the EC_{50} value (concentration of CPS providing 50% of activity).

2.9.2. Reducing Power

Reducing power (RP) was determined using the method described by [27], in which 2.5 mL of the sample was mixed with 2.5 mL of phosphate buffer (200 mM, pH 6.6) and 2.5 mL of 1% aqueous solution of $K_3[Fe(CN)_6]$. After 20 min of incubation at 50 °C, 0.5 mL of 10% trichloroacetic acid was added. The mixture was centrifuged at $25 \times g$ for 10 min. 2.5 mL pf the upper layer of solution was mixed with 2.5 mL of distilled water and 0.5 mL of $FeCl_3$. The absorbance was measured at $\lambda = 700$ nm. Six dilutions of CPS were examined to plot a dose–response curve. The result was expressed as the concentration of polysaccharides providing 50% of activity based on a dose-dependent mode of action (EC_{50}).

2.9.3. Inhibition of Lipid Peroxidation

The degree of inhibition of linoleic acid peroxidation (LPO) was performed according to [28] described in detail by [29]. Absorbances of reaction mixtures were measured at $\lambda = 480$ nm. Six dilution of CPS were examined to plot a dose–response curve. The result was expressed as the concentration of polysaccharides providing 50% of activity based on a dose-dependent mode of action (EC_{50}).

2.9.4. Metal Chelating Activity

Chelating power (CHP) was determined with the method described by [30]. The reaction mixture consisted of 5 mL of CPS, 0.1 mL of $FeCl_2$ (2mM) and 0.2 mL of ferrozine (5 mM). Absorbance was measured at $\lambda = 562$ nm after 10 min of incubation at room temperature. Six dilutions of CPS were examined to plot a dose–response curve. The result was expressed as the concentration of polysaccharides providing 50% of activity based on the dose-dependent mode of action (EC_{50}).

2.9.5. Oxygen Radical Absorbance Capacity (ORAC) Assay

The analysis was performed according to the slightly modified method proposed by [31] and described in detail by [26]. The sample activity was expressed as µM of Trolox/mg of crude polysaccharides. All determinations were carried out in triplicate.

2.9.6. Catalase Activity Assay

The influence of *S. crispa* crude polysaccharides on catalase (CAT) activity was assayed with the method developed by [32] with some modification. The assay mixture consisted of phosphate buffer (0.05 M, pH 7.0), the CPS sample (1 mg/mL, in water), the enzyme solution (60 U/mL), and H_2O_2 (0.019 M). The decomposition of H_2O_2 was determined directly by the extinction at $\lambda = 240$ nm per unit time (3 min) was used as a measure of catalase activity.

2.9.7. Inhibition of Xanthine Oxidase Activity

Inhibition of xantine oxidase (XO) was determined as previously described with some modifications [33]. The assay mixture consisted of phosphate buffer (1/15 M, pH 7.5), the CPS sample (1 mg/mL, in water), the enzyme solution, and xanthine as a substrate. The assay mixture was incubated at 30 °C with the absorbance ($\lambda = 295$ nm) measured spectrophotometrically over a 2 min period. The XO inhibitory activity was expressed as the percentage inhibition of XO in the assay mixture system.

2.10. Statistical Analysis

All results were expressed as the mean ± standard deviation (SD) from three replications. Calculations were performed in STATISTICA 10.0 (StatSoft Poland, Cracow, Poland). The data from the anticancer activity determination were presented as the mean value and standard error of the mean (SEM). Statistical analysis was performed using one way-ANOVA with the Tukey post hoc test and column statistics used for comparisons. Significance was accepted at $p < 0.05$. The IC_{50} value (concentration causing proliferation inhibition by 50% compared to the control) was calculated according to the Litchfield and Wilcoxon method [34].

3. Results

3.1. Chemical Composition of S. crispa Crude Polysaccharides and Contents of α- and β-Glucans

Crude polysaccharides (CPS) were precipitated with cold ethanol from the aqueous extract of *S. crispa* with an efficiency of 9.5% of d.w. In the first stage, the chemical composition of CPS was investigated by total sugar, protein, and total phenolic content analysis. The results (Table 1) indicate that CPS consists mainly of sugars (60.5%). Proteins and phenolics are only present in trace amounts.

Table 1. Chemical composition of *S. crispa* crude polysaccharides (CPS). Abbreviations: TPC–total phenolic content.

Sugar Content (% of CPS)	Protein Content (% of CPS)	TPC (% of CPS)
60.5 ± 0.98	0.48 ± 0.01	0.15 ± 0.00

Sugar analysis of CPS revealed the presence of three different hexoses and one 6-deoxyhexose in the molar ratio ~1.0:0.4:0.2:0.1. Monosaccharides were identified as glucose, galactose, mannose, and fucose, respectively, by the comparison of the retention times with the authentic standards.

The profile of the ^{1}H NMR spectrum (Figure 2) is characteristic of polysaccharides. It contains some anomeric proton signals in the region of 4.5–5.3 ppm and the remaining proton signals in the region of 3.0–4.3 ppm.

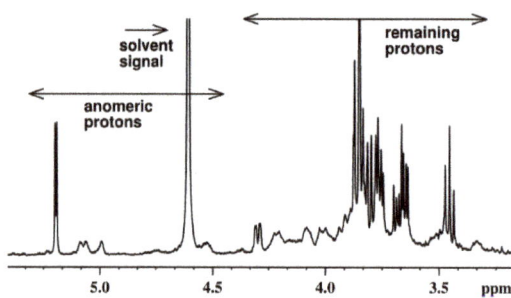

Figure 2. ^{1}H NMR spectrum of the polysaccharide fraction isolated from *S. crispa*.

The amounts of total as well as α- and β-glucans in *S. crispa* were determined with the enzymatic method. The results are presented in Table 2. The total content of glucans in the cauliflower mushroom was 29.96 g/100 g of dry weight. It was found that the amount of β-glucans was higher than that of α-glucans. β-glucans accounted for 91.86% of the total glucans in *S. crispa*.

Table 2. Total glucan, α-glucan, and β-glucan content in *S. crispa* fruiting bodies expressed in g per 100 g of dry weight.

Total Glucan (g/100 g d.w.)	α-Glucan (g/100 g d.w.)	β-Glucan (g/100 g d.w.)
29.96 ± 0.59	2.44 ± 0.03	27.52 ± 0.32

3.2. Biological Activity of CPS

3.2.1. Anticancer Potential—In Vitro Studies

The crude polysaccharides from the cauliflower mushroom were subjected to both antiproliferative activity determination (MTT and BrdU assay) and cytotoxicity examination

(LDH assay) using human colon epithelial cell line CCD841 CoN and three human colon adenocarcinoma cell lines: Caco-2, LS180, and HT-29. The results are presented in Figure 3.

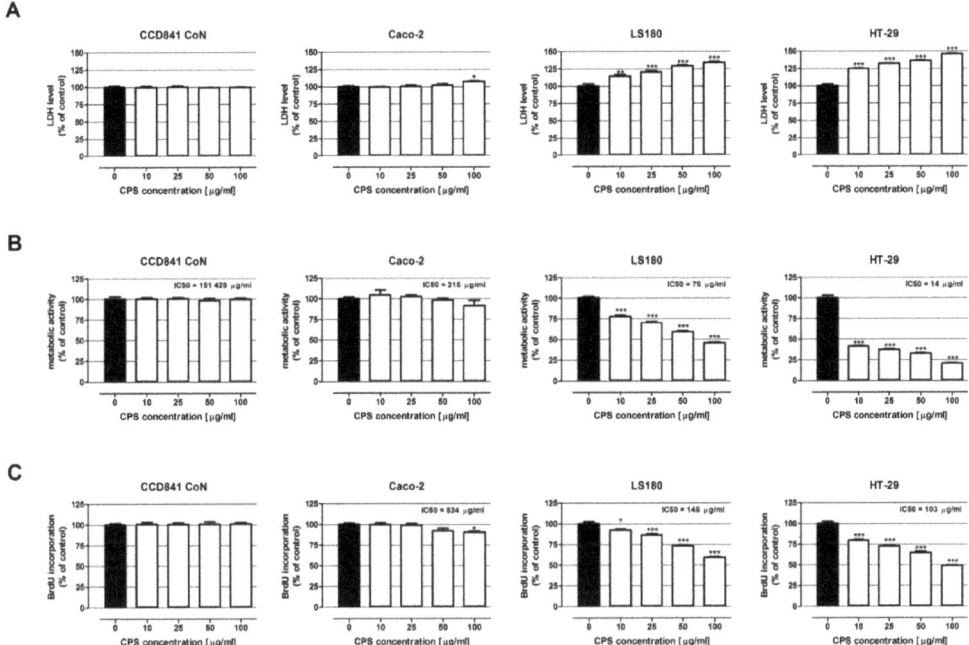

Figure 3. Antiproliferative and cytotoxic effect of crude polysaccharides isolated from *S. crispa* on human colon epithelial cell line CCD841 CoN and human colon adenocarcinoma cell lines: Caco-2, LS180, and HT-29. The cells were exposed to the culture medium alone (control) or the crude polysaccharides from *S. crispa* (CPS) at concentrations of 10, 25, 50, and 100 µg/mL for 24 h (LDH assay), for 48 h (BrdU assay) and for 96 h (MTT assay). CSP cytotoxicity was measured photometrically by means of the LDH assay (**A**), while the antiproliferative impact of CSP was examined photometrically by means of the MTT assay (**B**) and BrdU assay (**C**). Results are presented as mean ± SEM of at least 4 measurements. * $p < 0.05$ versus control, ** $p < 0.01$ versus control, *** $p < 0.001$ versus control, one-way ANOVA test; post-test: Tukey.

The results of the LDH assay have shown that the crude polysaccharides isolated from *S. crispa* were not cytotoxic to the human colon epithelial CCD841 CoN cells. On the contrary, CPS damaged the cell membranes of all investigated colon cancer cell lines. The most significant changes were observed in the HT-29 cells, wherein the LDH level in response to CPS increased from 124.7% (10 µg/mL) to 146.1% (100 µg/mL). A slightly weaker cytotoxic effect was induced by the tested polysaccharides in the LS180 cells; 10 µg/mL CPS increased LDH release by 14.3%, while 100 µg/mL CPS accelerated the cell membrane damage by 33.8%. In the case of the Caco-2 cells, only the highest concentration of *S. crispa* polysaccharides elevated the LDH level by 7.2%.

The MTT test demonstrated no impact of the CPS on the metabolic activity of both CCD841 CoN and Caco-2 cells. At the same time, the polysaccharides exerted a significant antiproliferative effect on the LS180 and HT-29 cells (IC50 LS180 = 78 µg/mL; IC50 HT-29 = 14 µg/mL). The strongest inhibition of proliferation was observed in the HT-29 cells, wherein the lowest and the highest investigated concentrations of CPS caused a decrease in cancer cell proliferation by 58.6% and 79.1%, respectively. The LS180 cells were less sensitive to the CPS; nevertheless, even the lowest dose of *S. crispa* polysaccharides reduced the cancer cell proliferation by 22.6%.

The BrdU assay (more sensitive and specific antiproliferative assay) revealed no influence of CPS on DNA synthesis in human colon epithelial CCD841 CoN cells. Simultaneously, S. crispa polysaccharides decreased the proliferation of all investigated human colon cancer cells in a dose-dependent manner (IC50 Caco-2 = 834 µg/mL; IC50 LS180 = 145 µg/mL; IC50 HT-29 = 103 µg/mL). Among the examined colon cancer cell lines, Caco-2 was the most resistant to the antiproliferative abilities of CPS. The significant inhibition of DNA synthesis (9.4%) was noted only after the treatment with polysaccharides at a concentration of 100 µg/mL. On the contrary, the strongest anticancer effect was observed in HT-29 cells, wherein even 10 µg/mL of CPS inhibited the cell proliferation by 20.1%, while 100 µg/mL of CPS caused a 50.8% reduction in DNA synthesis. LS180 cells were more resistant to CPS treatment than HT-29, and the decrease in BrdU incorporation was in the range from 7.3% (10 µg/mL) to 40.6% (100 µg/mL).

3.2.2. Antioxidant Activity

We determined the antioxidant activity of CPS using different methods involving different modes of antioxidant action. The results are presented in Table 3. They revealed that the crude polysaccharide from S. crispa exhibited moderate potential in antiradical activity against ABTS$^{\bullet+}$ with the EC_{50} level of 16.27 mg/mL CPS. CPS was found to have the highest antioxidant potential in the determination of reducing properties (EC_{50} = 0.82 mg/mL) and chelating activity (EC_{50} = 0.76 mg/mL). Our study also included an evaluation of the ability of CPS to inhibit lipid peroxidation. The EC_{50} value obtained indicates a high activity of CPS (2.76 mg/mL). The antioxidant activity of CPS was then evaluated with the ORAC assay, giving the result 168.51 ± 0.21 µM Trolox/g CPS.

Table 3. Antioxidant activity of crude polysaccharides from S. crispa determined with different methods expressed as EC_{50} values (mg/mL). The results are presented as the mean ± standard deviation of 3 measurements. Abbreviations: ABTS—antiradical activity against ABTS$^{\bullet+}$, RP—reducing power, LPO—inhibition of lipid peroxidation, CHP—metal chelating activity, EC_{50}—the polysaccharides concentration providing 50% of activity based on dose-dependent mode of action.

Antioxidant Assay	CPS Antioxidant Activity EC_{50} ± SD [mg/mL]
ABTS$^{\bullet+}$	16.27 ± 3.42
RP	0.82 ± 0.01
LPO	2.76 ± 0.02
CHP	0.76 ± 0.19

The antioxidant activity of CPS was also evaluated using enzymatic assays with xanthine oxidase (XO) and catalase (CAT). The results are presented in Table 4. CPS was found to have no influence on XO activity, as neither the activation nor inhibition of this enzyme was observed. The catalase activity assay revealed that CPS did not activate this enzyme, which suggests an absence of antioxidant activity. On the contrary, our study revealed that catalase activity was inhibited by CPS in 32.74% at the CPS concentration of 5 mg/mL.

Table 4. Antioxidant activity of crude polysaccharides from S. crispa determined by enzymatic assays. Abbreviations: XO—xanthine oxidase, CAT—catalase.

Enzymatic Assay	CPS Activity
XO	not detected
CAT	32.74 ± 0.49% of inhibition

3.2.3. Anti-Inflammatory Activity

In our study, the crude polysaccharides from S. crispa were tested for their ability to inhibit the activity of cyclooxygenase and lipooxygenase. The results are presented in

Figure 4. CPS was found to inhibit COX-1 activity at a level similar to that of acetylsalicylic acid, i.e., a commonly known nonsteroidal anti-inflammatory drug. In the case of COX-2, the CPS activity, estimated at 32.95%, was lower than that of acetylsalicylic acid. The LOX enzyme, which is involved in the development of inflammation in the human organism, was inhibited by 23.8%. This result was higher than that obtained for acetylsalicylic acid (18.73%).

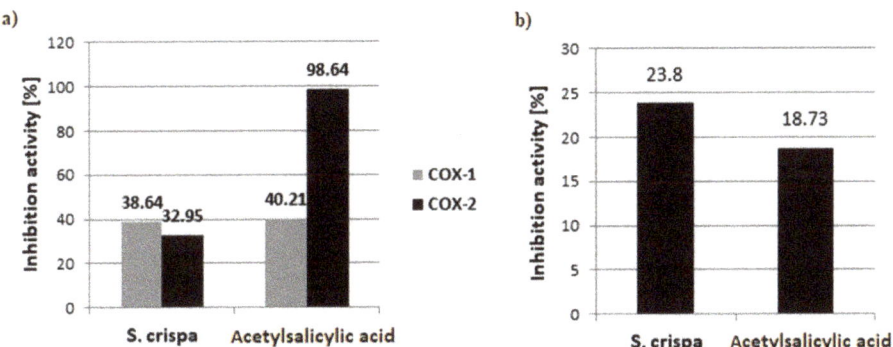

Figure 4. Inhibition of: (**a**) cyclooxygenase-1, cyclooxygenase-2 and (**b**) lipooxygenase activity by crude polysaccharides from *S. crispa* (5 mg/mL) expressed in %. Acetylsalicylic acid (1 mM) was used as a control.

The mode of LOX inhibition by CPS was determined using the Lineweaver–Burk plot presented in Figure 5. The y-intercept and the slope of a Lineweaver–Burk plot indicate that CPS caused the noncompetitive inhibition of LOX, in which the inhibitor binds to an allosteric site, resulting in the decreased efficacy of the enzyme. In this mode of inhibition, CPS shares the same affinity for both the enzyme and the enzyme–substrate complex and the enzyme is prevented from forming its product [35].

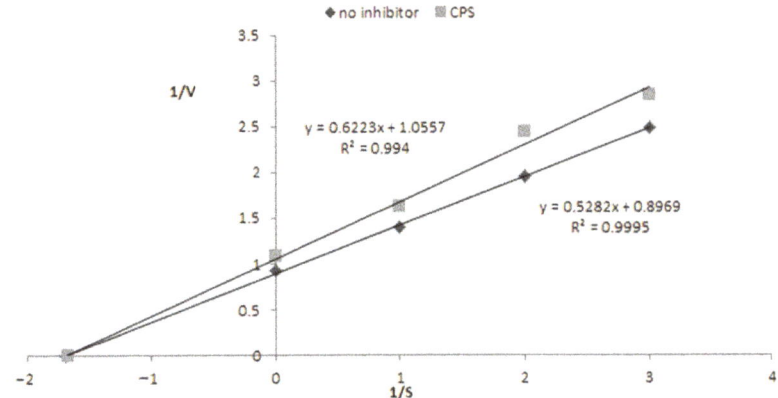

Figure 5. Mode of 15-lipoxygenase (LOX) inhibition by CPS determined by the Lineweaver–Burk plot.

4. Discussion

4.1. Chemical Composition of CPS

S. crispa is a medicinal mushroom with a long history of use in traditional Asian therapies. The fruiting body of *S. crispa* contains approximately 13.4 g of protein, 21.5 g of carbohydrates, and 2.0 g of fat per 100 g of dry weight [19]. Ultrasonic-assisted extraction (with water as an eluent) was used to obtain polysaccharides, since the ultrasonic enhancement of the process causes the disruption of cell walls, reduces particle size, and enhances transfer of cell components resulting in better extraction efficiency than traditional techniques [36]. The isolation of the crude polysaccharides was preceded by preliminary extraction with ethanol (to remove small molecules) and involved the deproteinization method (with Sevage reagent). Therefore, proteins and phenolics were finally present in CPS only in trace amounts. Sugars constituted the main group of compounds in crude polysaccharides (Table 1). They were identified as glucose, galactose, mannose, and fucose with the GC–MS method. Structural analysis based on the ^{1}H NMR spectrum of CPS confirmed that it contained polysaccharides (Figure 2). The ^{1}H NMR spectrum contains some anomeric proton signals in the region of 4.5–5.3 ppm and the remaining proton signals in the region of 3.0–4.3 ppm. The signals in the region of 4.5–4.6 ppm are characteristic for β-monosaccharides and confirmed the presence of β-glucan, which was determined with the enzymatic method and described in Table 2.

According to our knowledge, previous structural studies of polysaccharides isolated from S. crispa revealed the presence of a glucan, namely of a β-(1-3)-D-glucan backbone with a single β-(1-6)-D-glucosyl side branching units at every three residues [37].

Various medicinal properties of S. crispa are mostly attributed to the presence of β-glucans. According to Japan Food Research Laboratories (Tokyo, Japan), the β-glucan content in S. crispa is more than 40% of the dry weight [38]. Our results revealed a lower amount of β-glucans (Table 2). This discrepancy may result from the origin of the mushrooms, since the S. crispa used in this study was collected from the natural environment in Poland, while Asian species are mostly cultivated. Moreover, the taxonomy and systematics of Sparassis Fr. species have been refined according to phylogenetic relationships and placement. It was proposed that Sparassis should be classified into three groups: S. crispa from Europe and eastern North America, S. radicata from western North America, and S. latifolia from Asia [39,40]. There are no available data showing possible differences in the chemical composition of each species from the different regions.

4.2. Biological Activity of CPS

The antitumor activity of S. crispa β-glucan has been previously examined alone or in combination with some chemotherapeutics. As demonstrated by [41], polysaccharide fractions from S. crispa exhibited anticancer activity to the solid form of Sarcoma 180 in mice and showed a hematopoietic response to cyclophosphamide-induced leukopenia in mice. Moreover, β-glucan from S. crispa suppressed the number and growth of lung metastatic colonies in B16-BL6-bearing mice [42].

To the best of our knowledge, there is no information about the chemopreventive properties of polysaccharide fractions from S. crispa against colon cancer. Therefore, crude polysaccharides from the wild growing cauliflower mushroom were subjected to both antiproliferative activity determination and cytotoxicity examination. The studies were performed on human colon epithelial cell line CCD841 CoN and on three different human colon adenocarcinoma cell lines, which represent the successive stages of colon cancer development according to Dukes classification (Caco-2: Dukes B, LS180: Dukes B, HT-29: Dukes C).

The present study revealed in vitro the great bioactive properties of crude polysaccharides isolated from the wild growing cauliflower mushroom. They were found to be non-toxic to normal human colon epithelial cells; simultaneously, they significantly inhibited the proliferation of the human colon cancer cells and destroyed their cell membrane integrity. It needs to be highlighted that CPS had the lowest efficiency in the elimination of the Caco-2 cancer cells, which are the most differentiated but the least invasive cell line among the investigated ones. On the contrary, the HT-29 cells representing the advanced stage of colon cancer development were the most sensitive to the anticancer effect of CPS [43,44]. There was a positive correlation between the CPS anticancer activity and the colon cancer invasiveness and undifferentiation. The S. crispa polysaccharides had better activity in the more destruction-resistant colon cancer cells. Obviously, this observation is worth further verification in more advanced studies, e.g., in in vivo models.

Inflammation is a host response to infections or tissue injury that occurs throughout a complex set of interactions among soluble factors and cells. In normal conditions, the inflammatory response is self-limiting. However, prolonged inflammation can cause many diseases [45]. There was a strong relationship between long-term inflammation and the development of colon cancer. Colitis-associated cancer (CAC) is a subtype of colorectal cancer linked to inflammatory bowel disease (IBD). Chronic inflammation in CAC is responsible for oxidative damage to DNA, resulting in p53 mutations observed in tumor cells and the inflamed but nondysplastic epithelium [46]. Therefore, searching for natural anti-inflammatory agents without or with low toxic effects seems necessary. There are numerous studies indicating that mushroom polysaccharides, including β-glucans, possess immunomodulatory or anti-inflammatory activities [47]. Inducible cyclooxygenase-2 (COX-2) and 5-lipooxygenase (5-LOX) are among the best known inflammatory biomarkers produced in the human body. Previous research revealed that a non-aqueous fraction from S. crispa extract inhibited the production of PGE_2 via the downregulation of the expression of COX-2 [48]. A study conducted by [49] revealed that the water extract of S. crispa suppressed mast cell-mediated allergic inflammation by regulating calcium, MAPK, and NF-κB. Moreover, several phthalides from cauliflower mushroom exerted an inhibitory effect on LPS-stimulated NO and PGE_2 production by RAW264 cells [50]. It was demonstrated that a branched β-glucan from S. crispa induced macrophages to produce several mediators, including the inflammatory cytokines interleukin-1 (IL-1), IL-6, tumor necrosis factor-a (TNF-a), and nitric oxide (NO) [51]. Our study demonstrates the anti-inflammatory potential of CPS in the direct inhibition of pro-inflammatory enzymes such as COX-2 and LOX. Further studies are necessary to establish whether there are any additional mechanisms of the anti-inflammatory activity of S. crispa polysaccharides.

The overproduction of reactive oxygen species (ROS) in the human body leads to oxidative stress, causing numerous pathological conditions, including development of colon cancer. It occurs through high susceptibility to the influence of pro-oxidative and toxic factors and the following increase in the proliferation of cancer cells [52]. Therefore, it seems reasonable to introduce antioxidants to everyday diet as chemopreventive agents. Mushroom polysaccharides from edible species are interesting candidates for this purpose. The present study has revealed that the crude polysaccharides from S. crispa possess moderate antiradical activity and strong reducing properties and chelating activity as well as high potential in inhibition of lipid peroxidation. It has already been found that the mechanism of the antioxidant activity of polysaccharides from mushrooms depends on their chemical structure. Molecular weight, monosaccharide composition, chain conformation, and structural configuration may affect the antioxidant capacity of this group of compounds [53]. In the case of free radical scavenging, polysaccharides are believed to have greater potential than monosaccharides. This activity may be determined by the size of molecules and the type of binding in the side branches of the main chain of the polysaccharides; nevertheless, their antioxidative activity is still rather moderate [36]. A previous study reported the antioxidant activity of polysaccharides from S. crispa revealed in the $ABTS^{\bullet+}$ assay. The authors found that the scavenging effect of two polysaccharides at the concentration of 5.0 mg/mL reached 84.02 and 80.70%, while the activity of the standard compound (vitamin C) was 97.48% [53]. Researchers demonstrated the antioxidant activity of crude polysaccharides from Cordyceps miltaris, i.e., one of the most famous functional and medicinal mushrooms, using methods similar to those employed in our study. The reducing power (expressed as the EC_{50} value) of various polysaccharides from C. militaris ranged from 1.06 to 6.07 mg/mL, and the chelating activity ranged from 3.09 to 7.74 mg/mL [54]. In comparison with our study, this implies that the polysaccharide fraction from S. crispa has significantly higher antioxidant properties (Table 3) than the polysaccharides from C. militaris. CPS was found to be able to inhibit lipid peroxidation on the hemoglobin-catalyzed the peroxidation of linoleic acid. Moreover, the ORAC assay, which relies on the utilization of the AAPH-derived peroxyl radical imitating lipid peroxyl radicals, was involved in the lipid peroxidation chain reaction in vivo [55], confirmed the antioxidant properties of polysaccharides from the cauliflower mushroom. The antioxidant activity of crude natural polysaccharides may be attributed to the presence of various compounds in mushroom extracts, e.g., phenolic compounds [56]. However, our current research shows that crude polysaccharides also exhibit moderate or even high antioxidant potential, which is not related to the total phenolic content. Antioxidant properties may be related especially to the presence of β-glucans in the polysaccharide fraction from mushrooms [54]. Certainly, further studies of the function–structure relationship are necessary.

Overproduction of ROS in vivo can also occur through some enzyme-mediated reactions. Xanthine oxidase constitutes one of the main enzymatic sources of ROS in vivo due to its participation in the oxidative damage resulting from the reperfusion of ischemic tissues, brain edema and injury, or vascular permeability changes [57]. The inhibition of XO by CPS was studied in our study. However, the results indicate no influence of CPS on the XO activity.

We also used another enzymatic method for testing antioxidant activity, i.e., the catalase assay. Catalase protects cells from oxidative stress through the decomposition of hydrogen peroxide to water and oxygen [32]. Therefore, the promotion of catalase activity is one of the indirect mechanisms of antioxidant activity that is beneficial from the point of view of normal cell physiology. On the other hand, it was shown that catalase contributed to the increased resistance of cancer cells to pro-oxidant drugs (especially in H_2O_2-mediated processes). The inhibition of catalase expression and activity results in increased oxidative stress in cancerous cells. This provides new insight into understanding the possible anticancer properties of some compounds [58,59]. Therefore, searching for catalase inhibitors seems reasonable in order to design synergistic agents for anti-cancer drugs, which may help to sensitize drug-resistant cancer cells [60]. Our study revealed that the *S. crispa* polysaccharides inhibited catalase activity. Therefore, their ability seems to be suitable to be applied for the enhancement of anti-cancer chemotherapy.

5. Conclusions

S. crispa is a popular edible and medicinal mushroom and a rich source of polysaccharides, including β-glucans. Our in vitro study revealed the promising chemopreventive potential of its crude polysaccharide (CPS) based on several different mechanisms of action. CPS was found to inhibit the proliferation of colon cancer cells significantly without a concurrent harmful effect on normal cells. Moreover, antioxidant and anti-inflammatory activities fitting into the strategy of colon cancer prevention were proved. Since colon cancer was found to be related to food and lifestyle, searching for natural chemopreventive agents administered as part of the daily diet seems crucial. Polysaccharides from *S. crispa* can be a valuable addition to human diet as nutraceuticals or functional food ingredients. The fruiting bodies of cauliflower mushroom may be consumed as a part of habitual regular diet. Moreover, CPS might be used as bioactive additives incorporated in various food products accessible for consumers. The potential use of polysaccharides from *S. crispa* in supporting colon cancer prevention and treatment in relation to their chemical structure will be addressed in further research.

Author Contributions: Conceptualization, N.N.-J. and R.N.; data curation, N.N.-J.; funding acquisition, R.N.; investigation, N.N.-J., M.K.L., U.G.-D., N.S. and Z.K.; methodology, N.N.-J., R.N., M.K.L., W.R., U.G.-D. and Z.K.; project administration, N.N.-J. and R.N.; resources, N.N.-J.; writing—original draft, N.N.-J.; writing—review and editing, R.N., M.K.L. and U.G.-D. All authors have read and agreed to the published version of the manuscript.

Funding: This research received no external funding.

Institutional Review Board Statement: Not applicable.

Informed Consent Statement: Not applicable.

Data Availability Statement: Data available on request.

Conflicts of Interest: The authors declare no conflict of interest.

References

1. Meng, X.; Liang, H.; Luo, L. Antitumor polysaccharides from mushrooms: A review on the structural characteristics, antitumor mechanisms and immunomodulating activities. *Carbohydr. Res.* **2016**, *424*, 30–41. [CrossRef] [PubMed]
2. Kalač, P. Chemical composition and nutritional value of European species of wild growing mushrooms: A review. *Food Chem.* **2009**, *113*, 9–16. [CrossRef]
3. Wasser, S.P. Medicinal mushrooms as a source of antitumor and immunomodulating polysaccharides. *Appl. Microbiol. Biotechnol.* **2003**, *60*, 258–274.
4. Global Beta Glucan Market-Growth, Trends and Forecasts (2017–2022). Available online: https://www.orbisresearch.com/reports/index/global-beta-glucan-market-growth-trends-and-forecasts-2017-2022 (accessed on 15 September 2020).
5. Rathore, H.; Prasad, S.; Sharma, S. Mushroom nutraceuticals for improved nutrition and better hu1man health: A review. *PharmaNutrition* **2017**, *5*, 35–46. [CrossRef]
6. Kothari, D.; Patel, S.; Kim, S.K. Anticancer and other therapeutic relevance of mushroom polysaccharides: A holistic appraisal. *Biomed. Pharmacother.* **2018**, *105*, 377–394. [CrossRef]
7. Nowak, R.; Nowacka-Jechalke, N.; Juda, M.; Malm, A. The preliminary study of prebiotic potential of Polish wild mushroom polysaccharides: The stimulation effect on Lactobacillus strains growth. *Eur. J. Nutr.* **2018**, *57*, 1511–1521. [CrossRef]
8. Singdevsachan, S.K.; Auroshree, P.; Mishra, J.; Baliyarsingh, B.; Tayung, K.; Thatoi, H. Mushroom polysaccharides as potential prebiotics with their antitumor and immunomodulating properties: A review. *Bioact. Carbohydr. Diet. Fibre* **2016**, *7*, 1–14. [CrossRef]
9. Wasser, S.P. Medicinal mushroom science: Current perspectives, advances, evidences, and challenges. *Biomed. J.* **2014**, *37*, 345–356. [CrossRef]
10. Nowacka-Jechalke, N.; Nowak, R.; Juda, M.; Malm, A.; Lemieszek, M.; Rzeski, W.; Kaczyński, Z. New biological activity of the polysaccharide fraction from Cantharellus cibarius and its structural characterization. *Food Chem.* **2018**, *268*, 355–361. [CrossRef]
11. Chihara, G.; Hamuro, J.; Maeda, Y.Y.; Arai, Y.; Fukuoka, F. Fractionation and Purification of the Polysaccharides with Marked Antitumor Activity, Especially Lentinan, from Lentinus edodes (Berk.) Sing. (an Edible Mushroom). *Cancer Res.* **1970**, *30*, 2776–2781.
12. Fang, J.; Wang, Y.; Lv, X.; Shen, X.; Ni, X.; Ding, K. Structure of a β-glucan from Grifola frondosa and its antitumor effect by activating Dectin-1/Syk/NF-κB signaling. *Glycoconj. J.* **2012**, *29*, 365–377. [CrossRef] [PubMed]
13. Kobayashi, H.; Matsunaga, K.; Oguchi, Y. Antimetastatic Effects of PSK (Krestin), a Protein-bound Polysaccharide Obtained from Basidiomycetes: An Overview. *Cancer Epidemiol. Biomark. Prev.* **1995**, *4*, 275–281.
14. Zhu, F.; Du, B.; Bian, Z.; Xu, B. β-Glucans from edible and medicinal mushrooms: Characteristics, physicochemical and biological activities. *J. Food Compos. Anal.* **2016**, *41*, 165–173. [CrossRef]
15. Nowak, R.; Olech, M.; Nowacka, N. Plant Polyphenols as Chemopreventive Agents. In *Polyphenols in Human Health and Disease*; Watson, R.R., Preedy, V.R., Zibadi, S., Eds.; Elsevier: New York, NY, USA, 2013; Volume 2, pp. 1289–1307. ISBN 9780123984562.
16. Chen, J.; Zhang, X.D.; Jiang, Z. The Application of Fungal Beta-glucans for the Treatment of Colon Cancer. *Anticancer Agents Med. Chem.* **2013**, *13*, 725–730. [CrossRef]
17. Du, B.; Meenu, M.; Liu, H.; Xu, B. A concise review on the molecular structure and function relationship of β-glucan. *Int. J. Mol. Sci.* **2019**, *20*. [CrossRef]
18. Chandrasekaran, G.; Oh, D.S.; Shin, H.J. Properties and potential applications of the culinary-medicinal cauliflower mushroom, Sparassis crispa Wulf.:Fr. (Aphyllophoromycetideae): A review. *Int. J. Med. Mushrooms* **2011**, *13*, 177–183. [CrossRef]
19. Kimura, T. Natural products and biological activity of the pharmacologically active cauliflower mushroom Sparassis crispa. *Biomed. Res. Int.* **2013**, *2013*, 982317. [CrossRef]
20. Staub, A.M. Removal of protein-Sevag method. *Methods Carbohydr. Chem.* **1965**, *5*, 5–6.
21. Dubois, M.; Gilles, K.A.; Hamilton, J.K.; Rebers, P.A.; Smith, F. Colorimetric method for determination of sugars and related substances. *Anal. Chem.* **1956**, *28*, 350–356. [CrossRef]
22. Bradford, M.M. A rapid and sensitive method for the quantitation of microgram quantities of protein utilizing the principle of protein-dye binding. *Anal. Biochem.* **1976**, *72*, 248–254. [CrossRef]
23. Olech, M.; Nowak, R. Influence of different extraction procedures on the antiradical activity and phenolic profile of Rosa rugosa petals. *Acta Pol. Pharm. Drug Res.* **2012**, *69*, 501–507.
24. Szpakowska, N.; Kowalczyk, A.; Jafra, S.; Kaczyński, Z. The chemical structure of polysaccharides isolated from the Ochrobactrum rhizosphaerae PR17T. *Carbohydr. Res.* **2020**, *497*, 15–18. [CrossRef] [PubMed]
25. Maiga, A.; Malterud, K.E.; Diallo, D.; Paulsen, B.S. Antioxidant and 15-lipoxygenase inhibitory activities of the Malian medicinal plants Diospyros abyssinica (Hiern) F. White (Ebenaceae), Lannea velutina A. Rich (Anacardiaceae) and Crossopteryx febrifuga (Afzel) Benth. (Rubiaceae). *J. Ethnopharmacol.* **2006**, *104*, 132–137. [CrossRef] [PubMed]
26. Olech, M.; Łyko, L.; Nowak, R. Influence of accelerated solvent extraction conditions on the LC-ESI-MS/MS polyphenolic profile, triterpenoid content, and antioxidant and anti-lipoxygenase activity of rhododendron luteum sweet leaves. *Antioxidants* **2020**, *9*, 822. [CrossRef]

27. Oyaizu, M. Studies on Products of Browning Reactions: Antioxidative Activities of Product of Browning Reaction Prepared from Glucosamine. *Jpn. J. Nutr.* **1986**, *44*, 307–315. [CrossRef]
28. Kuo, J.M.; Yeh, D.B.; Pan, B.S. Rapid photometric assay evaluating antioxidative activity in edible plant material. *J. Agric. Food Chem.* **1999**, *47*, 3206–3209. [CrossRef]
29. Gawlik-Dziki, U.; Dziki, D.; Baraniak, B.; Lin, R. The effect of simulated digestion in vitro on bioactivity of wheat bread with Tartary buckwheat flavones addition. *LWT Food Sci. Technol.* **2009**, *42*, 137–143. [CrossRef]
30. Guo, J.T.; Lee, H.L.; Chiang, S.H.; Lin, F.I.; Chang, C.Y. Antioxidant Properties of the Extracts from Different Parts of Broccoli in Taiwan. *J. Food Drug Anal.* **2001**, *9*, 96–101. [CrossRef]
31. Dienaitė, L.; Pukalskas, A.; Pukalskienė, M.; Pereira, C.V.; Matias, A.A.; Venskutonis, P.R. Phytochemical composition, antioxidant and antiproliferative activities of defatted sea buckthorn (Hippophaë rhamnoides L.) berry pomace fractions consecutively recovered by pressurized ethanol and water. *Antioxidants* **2020**, *9*, 274. [CrossRef]
32. Claiborne, A. Catalase activity. In *CRC Handbook of Methods for Oxygen Radical Research*; Greenwald, R.A., Ed.; CRC Press: Boca Raton, FL, USA, 1985; pp. 283–284.
33. Sweeney, A.P.; Wyllie, S.G.; Shalliker, R.A.; Markham, J.L. Xanthine oxidase inhibitory activity of selected Australian native plants. *J. Ethnopharmacol.* **2001**, *75*, 273–277. [CrossRef]
34. Litchfield, J.T., Jr.; Wilcoxon, F. A simplified method of evaluating does-effect experiments. *J. Pharmacol. Exp. Ther.* **1949**, *96*, 99–113.
35. Blat, Y. Non-competitive inhibition by active site binders. *Chem. Biol. Drug Des.* **2010**, *75*, 535–540. [CrossRef] [PubMed]
36. Gong, P.; Wang, S.; Liu, M.; Chen, F.; Yang, W.; Chang, X.; Liu, N.; Zhao, Y.; Wang, J.; Chen, X. Extraction methods, chemical characterizations and biological activities of mushroom polysaccharides: A mini-review. *Carbohydr. Res.* **2020**, *494*, 108037. [CrossRef] [PubMed]
37. Tada, R.; Harada, T.; Nagi-Miura, N.; Adachi, Y.; Nakajima, M.; Yadomae, T.; Ohno, N. NMR characterization of the structure of a β-(1→3)-D-glucan isolate from cultured fruit bodies of Sparassis crispa. *Carbohydr. Res.* **2007**, *342*, 2611–2618. [CrossRef] [PubMed]
38. Kimura, T.; Dombo, M. Sparassis crispa. In *Biological Activities and Functions of Mushrooms*; Kawagishi, H., Ed.; CMC Press: Tokyo, Japan, 2005; pp. 167–178.
39. Dai, Y.C.; Wang, Z.; Binder, M.; Hibbett, D.S. Phylogeny and a new species of Sparassis (Polyporales, Basidiomycota): Evidence from mitochondrial atp6, nuclear rDNA and rpb2 genes. *Mycologia* **2006**, *98*, 584–592. [CrossRef]
40. Ryoo, R.; Sou, H.D.; Ka, K.H.; Park, H. Phylogenetic relationships of Korean Sparassis latifolia based on morphological and ITS rDNA characteristics. *J. Microbiol.* **2013**, *51*, 43–48. [CrossRef]
41. Ohno, N.; Nagi-Miura, N.; Nakajima, M.; Yadomae, T. Antitumor 1, 3-β-Glucan from Cultured Fruit Body of Sparassis crispa. *Biol. Pharm. Bull.* **2000**, *23*, 866–872. [CrossRef]
42. Yamamoto, K.; Kimura, T.; Sugitachi, A.; Matsuura, N. Anti-angiogenic and anti-metastatic effects of β-1,3-D-glucan purified from hanabiratake, Sparassis crispa. *Biol. Pharm. Bull.* **2009**, *32*, 259–263. [CrossRef]
43. Ahmed, D.; Eide, P.W.; Eilertsen, I.A.; Danielsen, S.A.; Eknæs, M.; Hektoen, M.; Lind, G.E.; Lothe, R.A. Epigenetic and genetic features of 24 colon cancer cell lines. *Oncogenesis* **2013**, *2*, e71. [CrossRef]
44. Shabahang, M.; Buras, R.R.; Davoodi, F.; Schumaker, L.M.; Nauta, R.J.; Evans, S.R.T. 1,25-Dihydroxyvitamin D3 Receptor as a Marker of Human Colon Carcinoma Cell Line Differentiation and Growth Inhibition. *Cancer Res.* **1993**, *53*, 3712–3718.
45. Elsayed, E.A.; El Enshasy, H.; Wadaan, M.A.M.; Aziz, R. Mushrooms: A potential natural source of anti-inflammatory compounds for medical applications. *Mediat. Inflamm.* **2014**, *2014*, 805841. [CrossRef] [PubMed]
46. Terzić, J.; Grivennikov, S.; Karin, E.; Karin, M. Inflammation and Colon Cancer. *Gastroenterology* **2010**, *138*, 2101–2114. [CrossRef] [PubMed]
47. Taofiq, O.; Martins, A.; Barreiro, M.F.; Ferreira, I.C.F.R. Anti-inflammatory potential of mushroom extracts and isolated metabolites. *Trends Food Sci. Technol.* **2016**, *50*, 193–210. [CrossRef]
48. Han, J.M.; Lee, E.K.; Gong, S.Y.; Sohng, J.K.; Kang, Y.J.; Jung, H.J. Sparassis crispa exerts anti-inflammatory activity via suppression of TLR-mediated NF-κB and MAPK signaling pathways in LPS-induced RAW264.7 macrophage cells. *J. Ethnopharmacol.* **2019**, *231*, 10–18. [CrossRef] [PubMed]
49. Kim, H.H.; Lee, S.; Singh, T.S.K.; Choi, J.K.; Shin, T.Y.; Kim, S.H. Sparassis crispa suppresses mast cell-mediated allergic inflammation: Role of calcium, mitogen-activated protein kinase and nuclear factor-κB. *Int. J. Mol. Med.* **2012**, *30*, 344–350. [CrossRef]
50. Yoshikawa, K.; Kokudo, N.; Hashimoto, T.; Yamamoto, K.; Inose, T.; Kimura, T. Novel phthalide compounds from Sparassis crispa (Hanabiratake), Hanabiratakelide A-C, exhibiting anti-cancer related activity. *Biol. Pharm. Bull.* **2010**, *33*, 1355–1359. [CrossRef]
51. Harada, T.; Ohno, N. Contribution of dectin-1 and granulocyte macrophage-colony stimulating factor (GM-CSF) to immunomodulating actions of β-glucan. *Int. Immunopharmacol.* **2008**, *8*, 556–566. [CrossRef]
52. Migliore, L.; Coppedé, F. Environmental-induced oxidative stress in neurodegenerative disorders and aging. *Mutat. Res.* **2009**, *674*, 73–84. [CrossRef]
53. Zhang, W.; Guo, Y.; Cheng, Y.; Zhao, W.; Zheng, Y.; Qian, H. Ultrasonic-assisted enzymatic extraction of Sparassis crispa polysaccharides possessing protective ability against H_2O_2-induced oxidative damage in mouse hippocampal HT22 cells. *RSC Adv.* **2020**, *10*, 22164–22175. [CrossRef]

54. Liu, Y.; Li, Y.; Zhang, H.; Li, C.; Zhang, Z.; Liu, A.; Chen, H.; Hu, B.; Luo, Q.; Lin, B.; et al. Polysaccharides from Cordyceps miltaris cultured at different pH: Sugar composition and antioxidant activity. *Int. J. Biol. Macromol.* **2020**, *162*, 349–358. [CrossRef]
55. Tai, A.; Sawano, T.; Yazama, F.; Ito, H. Evaluation of antioxidant activity of vanillin by using multiple antioxidant assays. *Biochim. Biophys. Acta Gen. Subj.* **2011**, *1810*, 170–177. [CrossRef] [PubMed]
56. Olech, M.; Nowacka-Jechalke, N.; Maslyk, M.; Martyna, A.; Pietrzak, W.; Kubínski, K.; Zaluski, D.; Nowak, R. Polysaccharide-rich fractions from rosa rugosa thunb.-composition and chemopreventive potential. *Molecules* **2019**, *24*, 1354. [CrossRef] [PubMed]
57. Lavelli, V. Antioxidant activity of minimally processed red chicory (Cichorium intybus L.) evaluated in xanthine oxidase-, myeloperoxidase-, and diaphorase-catalyzed reactions. *J. Agric. Food Chem.* **2008**, *56*, 7194–7200. [CrossRef] [PubMed]
58. Shahraki, S.; Samareh Delarami, H.; Saeidifar, M. Catalase inhibition by two Schiff base derivatives. Kinetics, thermodynamic and molecular docking studies. *J. Mol. Liq.* **2019**, *287*, 111003. [CrossRef]
59. Smith, P.S.; Zhao, W.; Spitz, D.R.; Robbins, M.E. Inhibiting catalase activity sensitizes 36B10 rat glioma cells to oxidative stress. *Free Radic. Biol. Med.* **2007**, *42*, 787–797. [CrossRef]
60. Yekta, R.; Dehghan, G.; Rashtbari, S.; Ghadari, R.; Moosavi-Movahedi, A.A. The inhibitory effect of farnesiferol C against catalase; Kinetics, interaction mechanism and molecular docking simulation. *Int. J. Biol. Macromol.* **2018**, *113*, 1258–1265. [CrossRef] [PubMed]

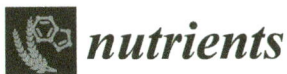

Article

Evaluating Anticancer and Immunomodulatory Effects of *Spirulina* (Arthrospira) *platensis* and Gamma-Tocotrienol Supplementation in a Syngeneic Mouse Model of Breast Cancer

Hemavathy Subramaiam [1,*], Wan-Loy Chu [2], Ammu Kutty Radhakrishnan [3], Srikumar Chakravarthi [4], Kanga Rani Selvaduray [5] and Yih-Yih Kok [6]

[1] School of Medicine, International Medical University, Kuala Lumpur 57000, Malaysia
[2] School of Postgraduate Studies, International Medical University, Kuala Lumpur 57000, Malaysia; wanloy_chu@imu.edu.my
[3] Jeffrey Cheah School of Medicine and Health Sciences, Monash University Malaysia, Bandar Sunway 47500, Malaysia; Ammu.Radhakrishnan@monash.edu
[4] Faculty of Medicine, Bioscience and Nursing, MAHSA University, Bandar Saujana Putra 42610, Malaysia; Srikumar@mahsa.edu.my
[5] Product Development and Advisory Services Division, Malaysian Palm Oil Board, Bandar Baru Bangi 43000, Malaysia; krani@mpob.gov.my
[6] School of Health Sciences, International Medical University, Kuala Lumpur 57000, Malaysia; yihyih_kok@imu.edu.my
* Correspondence: hemavathy@imu.edu.my; Tel.: +603-2731-7482

Citation: Subramaiam, H.; Chu, W.-L.; Radhakrishnan, A.K.; Chakravarthi, S.; Selvaduray, K.R.; Kok, Y.-Y. Evaluating Anticancer and Immunomodulatory Effects of *Spirulina* (Arthrospira) *platensis* and Gamma-Tocotrienol Supplementation in a Syngeneic Mouse Model of Breast Cancer. *Nutrients* 2021, 13, 2320. https://doi.org/10.3390/nu13072320

Academic Editor: Md Soriful Islam

Received: 11 May 2021
Accepted: 23 June 2021
Published: 6 July 2021

Publisher's Note: MDPI stays neutral with regard to jurisdictional claims in published maps and institutional affiliations.

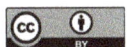

Copyright: © 2021 by the authors. Licensee MDPI, Basel, Switzerland. This article is an open access article distributed under the terms and conditions of the Creative Commons Attribution (CC BY) license (https://creativecommons.org/licenses/by/4.0/).

Abstract: Nutrition can modulate host immune responses as well as promote anticancer effects. In this study, two nutritional supplements, namely gamma-tocotrienol (γT3) and *Spirulina*, were evaluated for their immune-enhancing and anticancer effects in a syngeneic mouse model of breast cancer (BC). Five-week-old female BALB/c mice were fed *Spirulina*, γT3, or a combination of *Spirulina* and γT3 (*Spirulina* + γT3) for 56 days. The mice were inoculated with 4T1 cells into their mammary fat pad on day 28 to induce BC. The animals were culled on day 56 for various analyses. A significant reduction ($p < 0.05$) in tumor volume was only observed on day 37 and 49 in animals fed with the combination of γT3 + *Spirulina*. There was a marked increase ($p < 0.05$) of CD4/CD127$^+$ T-cells and decrease ($p < 0.05$) of T-regulatory cells in peripheral blood from mice fed with either γT3 or *Spirulina*. The breast tissue of the combined group showed abundant areas of necrosis, but did not prevent metastasis to the liver. Although there was a significant increase ($p < 0.05$) of MIG-6 and Cadherin 13 expression in tumors from γT3-fed animals, there were no significant ($p > 0.05$) differences in the expression of MIG-6, Cadherin 13, BIRC5, and Serpine1 upon combined feeding. This showed that combined γT3 + *Spirulina* treatment did not show any synergistic anticancer effects in this study model.

Keywords: breast cancer; *Spirulina*; tocotrienol; immunomodulatory; synergistic; metastasis

1. Introduction

Breast cancer (BC) is the most common cancer among women. It is estimated that 627,000 women worldwide died from this disease in 2018 alone [1]. Breast carcinoma can be stratified into different entities based on clinical behavior, histological features, and biological properties [2]. Some of the risk factors associated with BC include genetics [3], obesity [4], hormone replacement therapy [4], and having no children or having them after the age of 30 [5]. Symptoms of BC include swelling, redness or other visible differences in one or both breasts such as an increase in size or change in the shape of the breast, presence of lumps, and nipple discharge other than breast milk [6]. The BC can metastasize to distant organs such as bone [7], the lungs [8], liver [9], and brain [10]. In fact, most BC deaths are not due to the primary tumor itself, but are the result of metastasis [11].

Metastasis of cancer results from a sequential molecular cascade through which the cancer cells spread from the primary tumor site to distant anatomical sites, where they proliferate and create secondary neoplastic foci [12]. The cadherin family plays a crucial role in mediating cell-to-cell adhesion, and also exert a dominant role in metastasis of BC [13].

The initiation and progression of tumor cells elicit strong inflammatory responses. Inflammation and immunity are inherent characteristics of cancer [14]. According to the current literature, immune cells that are crucial in the fight against cancers include T-helper-1 (Th1) cells, which are $CD4^+$ T-cells that produce IFN-γ, $CD8^+$ cytotoxic T-lymphocytes (CTL), mature dendritic cells (DC), NK cells, and macrophages [15–17]. These cells can generate anti-tumor responses, which are useful in eliminating tumors. In contrast, $CD4^+$ Th2 cells and $CD4^+$ T-regulatory (Treg) cells can promote tolerance to tumors and induce immunosuppression, supporting tumor growth and progression [15–18]. Treatment options for BC includes surgery [19], radiation therapy [20], endocrine therapy [20], and chemotherapy [21]. However, many of these treatment options are associated with side-effects, such as decreased sensation in breast tissue, soreness, itching, peeling or redness in the treated area [22], hair loss, gastrointestinal disturbances, depressed immunity, and neutropenia [23]. As such, treatments with no or lesser side-effects or cytotoxic effects would be more beneficial for cancer patients. One such therapy that is rapidly gaining recognition as a potential treatment option for cancer is combination therapies that also use plant-based chemical compounds known as nutraceuticals, which have lower side-effects and toxicity. Amongst these nutraceuticals, tocotrienols (T3) were reported to possess strong anticancer effects. Tocotrienols are unsaturated vitamin E analogues found in several natural sources, such as palm oil, rice bran, and annatto seeds [24]. There are two major types of vitamin E, i.e., tocopherol (Toc) and T3, which exist naturally in four isoforms, which are alpha (α), beta (β), delta (δ), or gamma (γ). T3 can suppress the proliferation of cancer cells as well as induce apoptosis [25]. Furthermore, various studies have shown that T3 exerts anticancer effects by causing cell cycle arrest through inducing the expression of cell cycle inhibitory proteins and decreasing some cyclin-dependent kinases (CDK) [25–27]. T3 also induces apoptosis through the TGFβ-Fas-JNK-signaling pathways in human fibroblast T-cells [28]. Cyclin-dependent kinases (e.g., CDK2, CDK4, and CDK6) and their inhibitors, such as p21, p27, and p53 [26,29], also inhibit the proliferation of cancers cells. Another nutraceutical that is readily available on the market, and reported to have less cytotoxic effects following human consumption, is *Spirulina*, a microscopic and filamentous cyanobacterium (blue-green alga) [30]. *Spirulina* was reported to have anticancer, anti-inflammatory, antioxidant, and immunomodulatory properties [30]. The anticancer effects of *Spirulina* were reported to induce mitochondrial dysfunction through the up-regulation of Bax (Bcl2-associated X-protein) and BAD (Bcl-2 related family member). The latter promotes cell death, and its function is regulated by phosphorylation [31]. As for immune protection, *Spirulina* was shown to increase the proliferation of spleen cells without affecting thymic-derived T-cells [32]. *Spirulina* was shown to enhance the production of IL-1 by murine peritoneal macrophages [32], increase phagocytic activity of macrophages in chickens [33], and increase the production of IFN-γ by human NK cells [34]. Combination therapy with nutraceuticals could be beneficial as nutraceuticals generally have no or minimal side-effects. Combined *Spirulina* and tocotrienol (T3) supplementation may be used as a potential treatment option for BC as both nutraceuticals exhibit anticancer and immunomodulatory properties. To date, there are no reports evaluating the anticancer and immunomodulatory effects of combinatory treatment using both *Spirulina* and T3 supplementation. This study was undertaken to investigate the anticancer and immunomodulatory effects of combined *Spirulina* and T3 against BC using a BC syngeneic mouse model.

2. Materials and Methods

2.1. Spirulina

Food grade *Spirulina* (*Arthrospira*) *platensis* (hereafter referred to as *Spirulina*) powder was obtained as a gift from Earthrise Natural, USA. The major constituents of the *Spirulina* powder, as stated in the product sheet, include total carotenoids (≥ 370 (mg%)), β-carotene (≥ 120 (mg%)), phycocyanin ($\geq 10\%$), crude protein ($\geq 55\%$), and chlorophyll ($\geq 0.9\%$).

2.2. Tocotrienol

The gamma-tocotrienol (γT3) (97%, oil form) was obtained as a gift from Davos Pharmaceuticals Pte Ltd., Singapore.

2.3. Breast Cancer Cell Line

The 4T1 mouse mammary cancer cell line was purchased from the American Type Culture Collection (ATCC) (ATCC, Rockville, MD, USA). The cells were cultured in the medium recommended by the ATCC (RPMI 1640 supplemented with 10% fetal bovine serum (FBS) (GIBCO/Invitrogen)).

2.4. Animals

Five-week-old female BALB/c mice were purchased from a local supplier (Chenneur Suppliers, Kuala Lumpur, Malaysia). The animals were housed in the animal holding facility (AHF) at the International Medical University (IMU, Kuala Lumpur, Malaysia). The animals were allowed to acclimatize for 7 days before experimental procedures began. All animals appeared healthy and exhibited normal eating patterns before the experimental procedures. All experiments with animals were performed in accordance with the international animal use guidelines approved by the Joint Committee on Research and Ethics, IMU (IMU 258/2012).

2.5. Experimental Design

After the acclimatization period, the mice were randomly assigned into four groups. The mice were fed daily through oral gavage with 50 μL of soy-oil (i) vehicle (control); (ii) 50 mg/kg body weight of *Spirulina*; (iii) 1 mg/day of γT3; or (iv) 50 mg/kg body weight of *Spirulina* and 1 mg/day of γT3 for 56 days (Table 1). On day 28, all the animals received a single injection of 100 μL of 4T1 cells (1×10^5 cells/mL) into their mammary fat pad to induce BC [35]. The animals were culled on day 56, and various tissues were taken for analyses.

Table 1. Experimental groups.

Treatment Groups	Supplementation (50 μL/Day)	Number of Animals	Tumor Induction
Control	Vehicle (soy oil)	6	Yes
Spirulina alone	*Spirulina* (50 mg/kg body weight)	6	Yes
γT3 alone	γT3 (1 mg/day)	6	Yes
Spirulina + γT3	*Spirulina* (50 mg/kg body weight) + γT3 (1 mg/day)	6	Yes
	γT3: gamma-tocotrienol		

2.6. Body Weight and Tumor Volume

Animal weight and tumor size were recorded every three days until the animals were sacrificed. Tumor volume was calculated using a formula that was previously described (V = 0.52 × width × length; V refers to tumor volume (mm^3), width and length refers to the short and long diameter of tumor (mm)) [36]. At autopsy, the tumor, lungs, liver, kidneys, and heart were collected and preserved in 10% formalin solution for histopathology studies. A portion of the tumor was snap-frozen and stored at -80 °C for gene expression studies.

2.7. Processing and Storage of Blood Samples

A cardiac puncture was performed on the sacrificed mice to withdraw peripheral blood. The blood was collected into a heparin-tube for immunophenotyping analysis. Plasma was isolated using centrifugation ($2795 \times g$ for 10 min at 4 °C) for various biochemical analyses.

2.8. Immunophenotyping

The expression of various cell surface markers (CD4, CD8, CD25, CD127, and CD73) on the peripheral blood leukocytes were analyzed using flow cytometry. Briefly, 500 µL of blood collected via cardiac puncture was transferred into appropriately labelled tubes. Then, 2 mL of red blood cell lysis solution (eBioscience, San Diego, CA, USA) was added to each tube. The tubes were gently vortexed and incubated in the dark at room temperature for 3–10 min. The lysis activity was stopped by adding $1\times$ cold phosphate-buffered saline (PBS). The cells were recovered by centrifugation ($350 \times g$ for 5 min). The supernatant was aspirated and discarded. The remaining pellet was re-suspended in 200 µL of sheath fluid (eBioscience, San Diego, CA, USA). Then, 1.0 µL of appropriate fluorochrome-conjugated monoclonal antibody was added to the sample, and the tube was incubated in the dark at room temperature for 20–40 min. Following this, the samples were washed with 300 µL of wash buffer (PBS), and the cells were recovered by centrifugation ($350 \times g$ for 5 min). The supernatant was discarded, 500 µL of sheath fluid was added to each tube, and the sample was analyzed using a flow cytometer (FACS Calibur, Becton-Dickinson, Franklin Lakes, NJ, USA). Data from 10,000 cells were acquired from each sample for analysis. The data collected was analyzed using Cell-Quest software. Dot-plots for the respective fluorochromes were obtained from the gated population for each sample.

2.9. Histopathological Analysis

The primary tumor, the lungs, liver, heart, and kidneys, stored in 10% formalin, were processed for histopathological studies. Briefly, the organs were transferred into appropriately labelled small cassettes. The cassettes were placed in an automatic tissue processer (Leica TP1020 automatic tissue processor, Leica, Wetzlar, Germany) and processed for histopathological studies. The paraffin-impregnated tissues were embedded into paraffin embedding media and cast into tissue blocks using a tissue embedding machine (Leica tissue embedding machine, Wetzlar, Germany). The tissue sections were deparaffinized by placing the slides in xylene solution and rehydrated through descending ethanol concentrations to water before staining with hematoxylin and eosin (H&E) stains. After removing excess stains, the tissue sections were dehydrated via ascending concentrations of ethanol and cleared in xylene substitute-X solution. The slides were then mounted with distyrene plasticizer xylene (DPX) and covered with coverslips. The slides were examined using a bright-field microscope (Nikon Eclipse 80i (CF160), Kanagawa, Japan), with a 12.0-megapixel resolution camera, at various magnifications ($100\times$, $200\times$ and $400\times$) and the relevant images were captured.

2.10. Gene Expression Analysis

For RNA extraction from the tumor tissue, 1 mL of Tripure isolation reagent (Roche Diagnostics, Mannheim, Germany) was added to the frozen tumor tissue (50 mg), and the tube was mixed thoroughly. The sample was centrifuged, and the quality of the RNA obtained was evaluated based on an optical density (OD) ratio of 260 nm: 280 nm, which should be between 1.8 and 2 [37], as well as an OD ratio of 260 nm:230 nm, which should be ≥ 1.8 [37] for real-time PCR amplification. The RNA concentration was determined by measuring absorbance at 260 nm, 280 nm, and 230 nm using a NanoQuant plate (Tecan). The target gene sequences for murine mitogen-inducible gene 6 (MIG-6), Cadherin 13 (Cdh13), Baculoviral IAP repeat containing 5 (BIRC5), serpin family E member 1 (Serpine1), as well as the reference genes, phosphoglycerate kinase-1 (Pgk1) and proteasome subunit beta type-2 (Psmb2), were downloaded from the gene bank to facilitate the designing of primers to carry out the two-step reverse-transcription quantitative PCR (RT-qPCR). A commercial primer design software (PREMIER Biosoft International, Palo Alto, CA, USA) was used to screen potential primer sets to ensure that they had similar annealing temperatures (≤ 60 °C) and did not produce dimers and hairpins. Primer pairs were also tested for specificity using the BLASTN (NCBI) program. All the primers were synthesized commercially (IDT Integrated DNA Technologies, Singapore). The melting curve analysis for (A) BIRC5, (B) Cadherin 13, (C) MIG6, (D) Serpine1, (E) pgk1, and (F) psmb2 are provided as Figure S1. Quantitative PCR was performed to compare mRNA expression levels from tumor tissues from the non-treated (control) versus the three treated groups (*Spirulina* alone, γT3 alone, or combined *Spirulina* + γT3). The RNA from all samples were amplified using two-step RT-qPCR using a thermocycler (LightCycler® 480 Real-Time Detection System, Roche Diagnostics). The qPCR PCR was performed using the LightCycler 480 SYBR Green I Mastermix (Roche Diagnostics, Mannheim, Germany).

2.11. Statistical Analysis

All data were analyzed using SPSS Statistics version 20. All the values were presented as the mean $\pm$ SEM of the six mice per group. The results were analyzed using the analysis of variance (ANOVA) statistical test followed by Tukey's post-hoc test in the SPSS (version 20). A *p*-value of less than 0.5 ($p < 0.05$) was considered significant (95% confidence interval) compared to the control group.

3. Results

3.1. Body Weight and Tumor Volume

There were no differences ($p > 0.05$) in the body weight at day 56 amongst all the study groups (*Spirulina* (23.4 $\pm$ 0.74 g); γT3 (23.02 $\pm$ 0.74 g); and combined treatment (23.65 $\pm$ 0.33 g)) compared to the control group (25.28 $\pm$ 0.33 g) (Figure 1). The animals were induced with BC at day 28 and a tumor was palpable 9 days' post-inoculation. The effects of supplementation of *Spirulina*, γT3 or combined treatment appeared to be quite varied. For instance, there were marked differences in tumor volume ($p < 0.05$) observed in the treated mice on day 37 (*Spirulina* (12.49 $\pm$ 0.51 mm^3); γT3 (11.67 $\pm$ 0.33 mm^3); and combined treatment (13.5 $\pm$ 0.38 mm^3) and day 49 (*Spirulina* (63.5 $\pm$ 1.46 mm^3); γT3 (59.86 $\pm$ 1.6 mm^3); and combined treatment (58.31 $\pm$ 1.91 mm^3) when compared to the control group (day 37: 15.83 $\pm$ 0.75 mm^3; and day 49: 70.35 $\pm$ 0.9 mm^3) (Figure 2). However, on day 43, a significant reduction in tumor volume was only observed in mice fed with *Spirulina* alone (24.4 $\pm$ 1 mm^3) compared to the control group (28.17 $\pm$ 0.72 mm^3). In contrast, on day 46, supplementation with *Spirulina* or γT3 alone significantly reduced tumor volumes ($p < 0.05$) compared to the control (Figure 2). On day 56, only γT3 supplementation showed a significant reduction ($p < 0.05$) in tumor volume compared to the control group (Figure 2).

3.2. Immunophenotypic Expression

There were no differences ($p > 0.05$) in the percentage of CD4$^+$ or CD8$^+$ T-cell populations amongst all the treated groups (*Spirulina*, γT3, or combined treatment) compared to the control (Figure 3). However, the percentage of Th cells that secrete IL-7 (CD4$^+$/CD127$^+$) were higher ($p < 0.05$) in mice fed with just γT3 (21.9 $\pm$ 1.55%) or *Spirulina* (24.9 $\pm$ 1.69%) compared to mice from the control group (9.45 $\pm$ 0.61%). There was a ten-fold reduction in the percentage of Treg cells (CD4$^+$/CD25$^+$) in mice that were fed with either γT3 or *Spirulina* alone when compared to the control or combined treatment groups (Figure 3). There was also a marked reduction ($p < 0.05$) of a subset of Treg population, which expresses the CD73 enzyme (CD4$^+$/CD25$^+$/CD73) in mice fed with either γT3 or *Spirulina*, but there was a marked increase of this Treg subset in mice from the control or combined treatment groups (Figure 3). Representation of dot plot distribution attached as Figure S2.

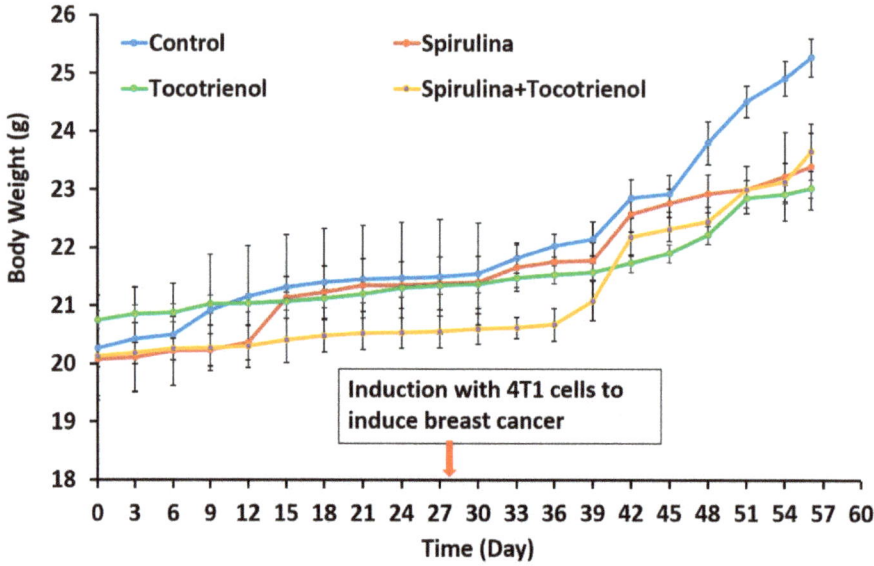

Figure 1. Changes in body weight before and after tumor induction in mice fed *Spirulina*, tocotrienol, and a combination of tocotrienol and *Spirulina*. Body weight of each mouse was recorded every three days from day 0 to day 56. Data expressed as mean ± standard error min (SEM) of six mice per group ($n = 6$). There were no significant differences in the body weight of animals from the control and treatment groups. Control: vehicle (soy oil); *Spirulina* (50 mg/kg body weight); γT3 (1 mg/day); and combination of γT3 (1 mg/day) and *Spirulina* (50 mg/kg body weight).

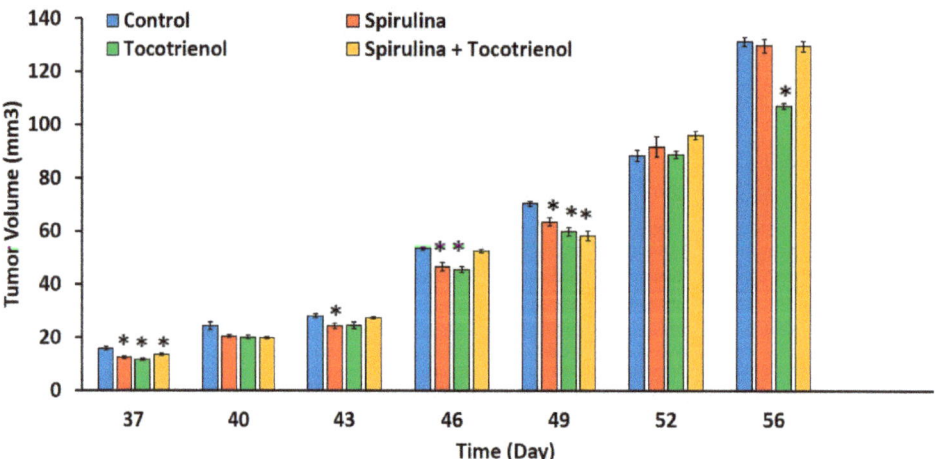

Figure 2. Tumor volume in mice fed *Spirulina*, γT3, and a combination of *Spirulina* and γT3. Diameter of tumor volume was measured every three days from day 37 to day 56. Data expressed as mean ± standard error mean (SEM) of six mice per group ($n = 6$). * $p < 0.05$: control versus treated group. Control: vehicle (soy oil); *Spirulina* (50 mg/kg body weight); γT3 (1 mg/day); and combination of γT3 (1 mg/day) and *Spirulina* (50 mg/kg body weight).

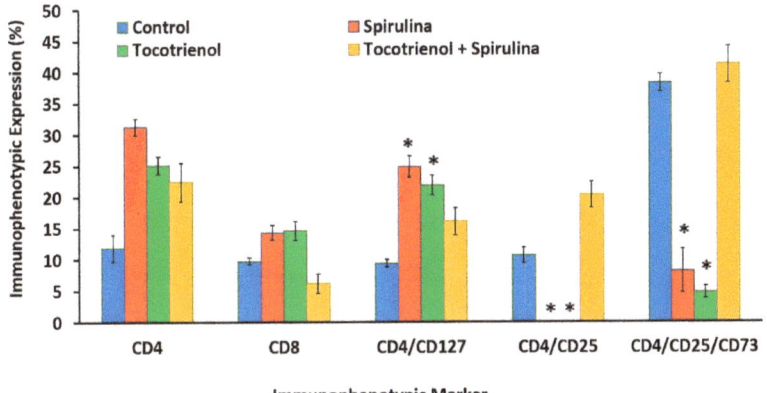

Figure 3. Flow cytometry analysis showing levels of Th cells (CD4$^+$), CTL (CD8$^+$), Th cells that secrete IL-7 (CD4$^+$/CD127$^+$), Treg cells (CD4$^+$/CD25$^+$), and Treg cells that expressed CD73 enzyme (CD4$^+$/CD25$^+$/CD73). Mice in the control group were fed the vehicle for 56 days while mice in the experimental group were supplemented with tocotrienol and *Spirulina*. Data expressed as mean ± standard error mean (SEM). (n = 6 for control, *Spirulina*, γT3 + *Spirulina*, and n = 5 for γT3) (* $p < 0.05$ compared to the control group).

3.3. Histopathology

There were large and pleomorphic cells with hyperchromatic nuclei and dense cytoplasm arranged in clusters and sheets in tumor sections from control mice. These sections also showed a large primary breast adenocarcinoma (shown by arrow), which was poorly differentiated (Figure 4a). Tumor sections from the *Spirulina*-fed group displayed poorly differentiated adenocarcinoma with abundant necrosis areas (shown by arrow) in the central areas (Figure 4b). In the γT3 treated group, the breast tissues showed predominantly tumor necrosis (shown by arrow) with sheets and islands of homogenous eosinophilic necrotic cells and little proliferating tumor tissue (Figure 4c). The breast tissue from mice fed a combination of γT3 and *Spirulina* showed abundant necrosis areas (shown by arrow) (Figure 4d). Clusters of tumor cells could be seen around the central vein and in the parenchyma (shown by arrow) in the liver section from animals in the control group (Figure 5a). Metastasis to the liver was also seen in sections from *Spirulina*-fed mice (Figure 5b). Liver sections from γT3-fed mice showed metastatic deposits around the blood vessels and in the parenchyma (Figure 5c). A similar finding was observed in the liver of mice fed a combination of γT3 and *Spirulina* (Figure 5d). There was no metastasis seen in the heart, lung, or kidney sections from mice in any of the study groups.

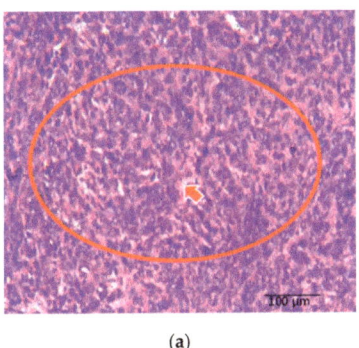

(a)

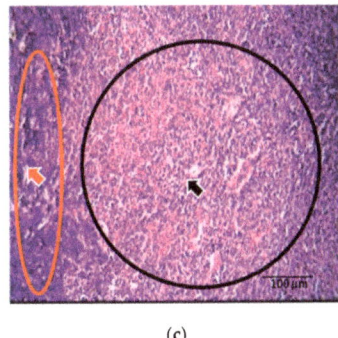

(c)

Figure 4. *Cont.*

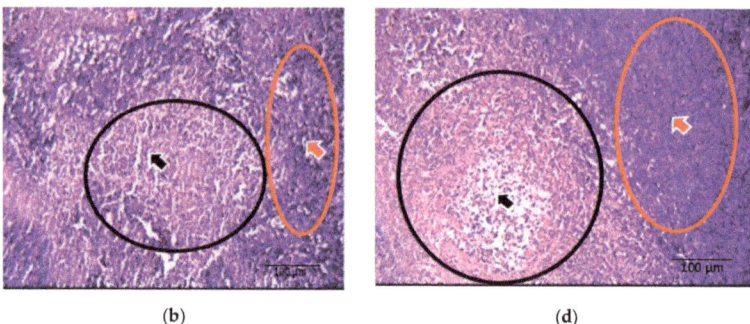

(b)   (d)

Figure 4. Comparison of tumor necrosis in breast tissue upon tocotrienol and *Spirulina* treatment. Photomicrographs (H&E, 200×) of breast tumor tissue from mice from the different treatment groups. The (**a**) control (non-treated), (**b**) *Spirulina* (50 mg/kg body weight), (**c**) γT3 (1 mg/day), and (**d**) combination of γT3 and *Spirulina* treated mice. Red colored arrow and circle indicate viable tumor cells, while the black colored arrow and circle indicate necrotic tumor cells.

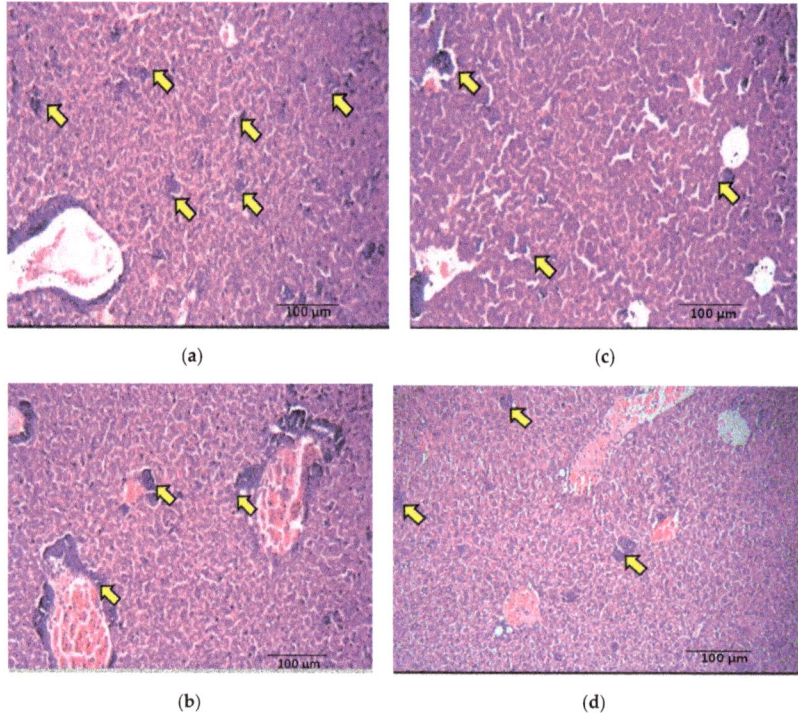

Figure 5. Comparison of metastasis from primary tumor site to the liver tissue upon γT3 and *Spirulina* treatment. Photomicrograph (H&E, 200×) comparing liver tissue (**a–d**) between (**a**) control (non-treated), (**b**) *Spirulina* (50 mg/kg body weight), (**c**) γT3 (1 mg/day), and (**d**) combination of γT3 and *Spirulina* treated mice. Arrow indicates metastasized tumor cells.

3.4. Gene Expression

The expression of the MIG6 (>two-fold) and Cadherin 13 (three-fold) genes were up-regulated ($p < 0.05$) in tumor tissue from γT3-fed mice (Figure 6). In contrast, there was no change ($p > 0.05$) in the expression of BIRC5 and Serpine-1 genes in tumor tissues from all treated groups when compared to the control group (Figure 6).

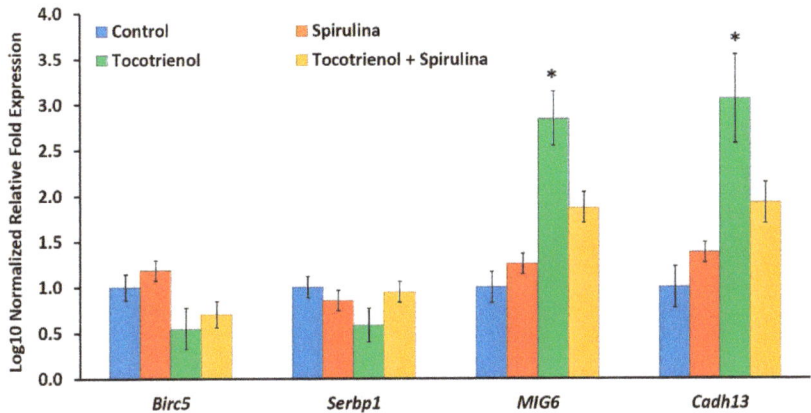

Figure 6. Comparison of BIRC5, Serpine1, MIG6 and Cadherin13 gene expression levels between the control (untreated), *Spirulina*, γT3, and combined *Spirulina* and γT3 treatment groups based on quantitative PCR analysis. Error bars represent standard error (SE) value, $n = 3$. (* $p < 0.05$ compared to control).

4. Discussion

There was no significant difference in mouse body weight from treatment groups compared to the control group. The tumor was palpable one week after tumor induction (day 37) in mice from all four groups. The tumor volume was significantly lower in animals fed daily with γT3, *Spirulina*, or a combination treatment in the early stages compared to the control. This might be because of the effectiveness of γT3, *Spirulina*, or combination treatment in suppressing tumor growth in the early stage of cancer development, especially as the mice were fed with the test compounds 28 days before tumor induction. It is also possible that the supplements may have helped enhance the animals' immune system to help them eliminate the tumor cells, which can result in reduced tumor mass. Similar observations have been reported previously with *Spirulina* [32,33,38] and T3 [39–41], possibly due to their immunomodulatory activities. On days 40, 43, 46, and 49, there was a reduction in tumor volume in all the treated groups with a significant reduction in mice from the *Spirulina*-treated group on days 43, 46, and 49. Mice from the γT3-fed group showed a significant reduction in tumor volumes on days 37, 46, and 56. The reduction in tumor volume indicates that the test nutraceutical could inhibit tumor growth. Among the three treatments, γT3 showed the most consistent reduction in tumor growth in comparison to the control group.

Cell-mediated immunity is an important adaptive immune response to combat tumors in the cancer microenvironment [42], which includes the actions of Th cells (CD4$^+$), CTL (CD8$^+$), and Treg cells (CD4$^+$/CD25$^+$). The CD8$^+$ T-cell and CD4$^+$ T-cell are the principal weapons of immunity against cancer [43], but prolonged immune responses can result in extended tissue damage, resulting in fatal immunopathology [44]. The balance between pro- and anti-inflammatory states of immune response could be regulated by Treg cells, which serve as gate-keepers of the immune system. Treg cells often accumulate in the tumor microenvironment [45]. Increased Treg cells in the tumor microenvironment can suppress anti-tumor T-cell responses, which can be associated with tumor progression [46–48]. Immunophenotyping showed that Th cells expressing the IL-7 receptor (CD4$^+$/CD127$^+$)

were significantly higher in peripheral blood from *Spirulina*-fed mice. These mice also showed a significant reduction of Treg cells ($CD4^+/CD25^+$) and Treg cells that express CD73 enzyme compared to the control group. These findings indicate that *Spirulina* supplementation may have induced immune protective effects against BC as there was an increase in IL-7 secreting Th cells, promoting the production of pro-inflammatory and lymphocyte growth cytokines to enhance immune activity [49,50]. In addition, the Treg populations were found to be reduced, which could have beneficial effects on the host immune system. The results indicate that *Spirulina* may modulate the T-cell populations and enhance anticancer effects in this mouse model. A study using a mouse BC model reported that phycocyanin from *Spirulina* promoted proliferation of thymocytes and splenocytes from BC-induced mice compared to the control group [51]. These findings also suggest that *Spirulina* had immune-enhancing effects by increasing the populations of immune cells involved in combatting cancer. A similar enhancement of immune response was also observed in mice fed with γT3 in the present study. There was a significant increase in Th cells ($CD4^+/CD127^+$) as well as a significant decrease in Treg cells ($CD4^+/CD25^+$ and $CD4^+/CD25^+CD73^+$) compared to the control group. These results suggested that, in this study model, γT3 enhanced immune-protection mediated by T-cells against BC. Such results are in accordance with other reports on the immunomodulatory effects of T3. For instance, in a study using athymic mice with BC, it was reported that supplementation with tocotrienol-rich fraction (TRF) up-regulated the expression of CD74/li and CD59 genes and down-regulated the expression of the IgG Fc receptor gene [39]. The CD4/li gene was reported to play a central role in the biological functions of major histocompatibility complex (MHC) class 1 proteins [52], while the IFITM-1 gene was shown to be involved in transduction of anti-proliferative and adhesion signals [53]. The binding of CD59 host cell membrane inhibited the action of the membrane attack complex (MAC) formed following activation of the complement system [54], which protects host cells [39]. These findings indicate that T3 might enhance anti-tumor effects by improving host immune responses. Combination treatment with γT3 and *Spirulina* did not show any significant difference in the T-cell populations. This may be due to a lack of synergy between γT3 and *Spirulina*. Furthermore, no previous studies reported on immunomodulatory effects when γT3 and *Spirulina* were used in combination.

Metastasis results from the dissemination of tumor cells from the primary neoplasm to a distant organ and the subsequent adaptation to a foreign tissue microenvironment [12,55]. The development of metastasis disease often signals poor prognosis, giving rise to increased morbidity and mortality [12]. In this study, tumor sections from the control group were large and pleomorphic with hyperchromatic nuclei and dense cytoplasm arranged in clusters and sheets, while tumor sections from *Spirulina*-treated groups showed primarily poorly differentiated adenocarcinoma with some areas of necrosis, indicating that there could be killing off of some of these tumor cells. Previous studies showed that phycocyanin from *Spirulina*-induced apoptosis reduced colony formation in the BC cell line [56]. There was marked necrosis in the tumor section from γT3-fed mice, which suggested that γT3 may induce tumor cell death.

In the current study, the metastasis of tumor cells from the primary site to liver tissues was observed even in mice fed with γT3, *Spirulina*, or the combination treatment. The findings suggest that supplementation with γT3, *Spirulina*, or combined treatment could not inhibit metastasis in this experimental model. However, there were no metastases to the lung, heart, and kidneys, which might be due to the limitation of the tumor cells' invasive capacity from the primary tumor to these organs compared to the liver. In previous studies using the same mouse model of BC, it was reported that VEGF expression was significantly reduced in mice fed with TRF compared to the control group [57]. This shows that palm tocotrienols exhibit anti-angiogenic properties that may assist in tumor regression. However, in the current study, γT3 did not appear to inhibit metastasis to the liver.

Combination treatment using γT3 and *Spirulina* was found to be ineffective in producing anticancer or immunomodulatory effects. In fact, the response seems to negate the positive effects when each nutraceutical was used on its own. Although combined treatment of γT3 with *Spirulina* was not reported on previously, combination of T3 with other bioactive compounds were tested in several tumor models. For instance, combination of T3 and gemcitabine was reported to down-regulate NF-Kβ activity along with NF-Kβ regulated gene products, such as cyclin D1, c-Myc, VEGF, MMP-9, and CXCR4 in pancreatic cancer [58]. This combination also potentiated the anti-tumor activity of gemcitabine by inhibiting NF-Kβ and NF-Kβ regulated gene products, leading to the inhibition of proliferation, angiogenesis, and invasion [58]. However, it should be noted that the concentration of T3 used in the pancreatic cancer model was higher than what was used in the present study. This may account for the differences observed. *Spirulina* used in combination with other natural compounds was reported to exert anti-invasive effects against BC. For instance, combination of phycocyanin from *Spirulina* with indol-3-carbinol, resveratrol, isoflavone, curcumin, and quercetin was shown to downregulate CD44, and reduce migration (wound healing assay) and invasion (matrigel assay) of human BC cell lines [59].

BIRC5/Survivin is known as an apoptosis inhibitor [60], while Serbp1/Serpine-1/PAI-1 is associated with tumor invasion [61], and MIG6 [62] and Cadherin 13 [63] are known as tumor suppressors. Further studies using more genes associated with specific pathways would help in understanding the anticancer effects of combined γT3 and *Spirulina* against BC. BIRC5/Survivin is an inhibitor of apoptosis protein (IAP) and is overexpressed in a wide spectrum of tumors, including breast cancer [64,65]. Its main function includes inhibiting apoptosis and regulating mitosis, which is associated with carcinogenesis [60]. Apoptosis, or programmed cell death, involves caspases responsible for proteolytic cleavages that lead to cell death. Two mechanisms are involved in apoptosis, namely death receptor (a subgroup of tumor necrosis factor (TNF) superfamily activation) and mitochondrial stress apoptotic signaling pathways [61]. This indicates that BIRC5/Survivin modification could be therapeutic against cancer. In the current study, there were no significant ($p > 0.05$) changes in BIRC5 gene expression upon treatment with *Spirulina*, γT3, or combined treatment with *Spirulina* and γT3.

Another gene analyzed in this study was Serbp1/Serpine-1/PAI-1, a multifaceted proteolytic factor that functions as an inhibitor of the serine protease and plays an important role in signal transduction, cell adhesion, and migration [66]. High levels of Serbp1/Serpine-1/PAI-1 have also been consistently reported to predict poor prognosis in several types of human cancers [67,68] and are associated with tumor aggressiveness and poor patient outcomes [69]. In the current study, there were no significant ($p > 0.05$) changes in Serbp1/Serpine-1/PAI-1 gene expression upon treatment with *Spirulina*, γT3, and combined treatment with *Spirulina* and γT3.

MIG6 is a negative feedback regulator of receptors for tyrosine kinases, and the expression of this gene was down-regulated in human breast carcinomas, correlating with reduced overall survival of breast cancer patients [70,71]. Previous studies showed that MIG6 expression is reduced in skin, breast, pancreatic, and ovarian carcinomas [72]. In this study, MIG6 gene expression was significantly ($p < 0.05$) up-regulated upon treatment with γT3 as compared to the control. Previous studies showed that α-T$_3$, γ-T$_3$, and δ-T$_3$ can up-regulate the expression of the MIG6 gene in a breast cancer cell line (MCF-7) [73]. Although the present study was based on the in vivo model, γT3 was still able to enhance tumor suppressor gene expression. In *Spirulina* and combined treatment, there were no significant ($p > 0.05$) differences in this gene expression.

Cadherin 13, also referred to as T- or H-cadherin, is expressed in multiple cell types in the breast gland, including myoepithelial, epithelial, and endothelial cells [74]. Characterization of Cadherin 13 suggests that it is not necessarily involved in adhesion, but instead is an adiponectin receptor [75] and adiponectin is secreted by adipocytes, which can sequester growth factors. Cadherin 13 is frequently silenced in different cancers, and it has long been considered a tumor suppressor [63]. In this study, γT3 significantly ($p < 0.05$) up-regulated the expression of Cadherin 13 compared to the control, which indicates that it enhanced the tumor suppressing effects and, thus, could inhibit tumor development. In the current study, there were no significant ($p > 0.05$) changes in Cadherin 13 gene expression upon treatment with *Spirulina* and combined treatment with *Spirulina* and γT3. On the whole, upon the combination of γT3 and *Spirulina*, there were no significant ($p > 0.05$) differences in the expression of the genes analyzed in this study compared to the control group.

5. Conclusions

The primary aim of the current research was to assess the immunomodulatory, antimetastatic, gene expression analysis, and anticancer effects of combined γT3 and *Spirulina* treatment against BC using a syngeneic mouse model of BC. Combination of γT3 and *Spirulina* did not cause any significant differences in body weight, and there was no consistent suppression of tumor volume observed. Moreover, there were no significant differences in the T-cell population upon combined treatment with γT3 and *Spirulina* as compared to the control group. In contrast, γT3 or *Spirulina* treatment on its own caused a significant increase in the Th population and a significant decrease in Treg populations compared to the control. Metastasis to the liver was present in sections from the control and all treatment groups, suggesting that these nutraceuticals could not inhibit metastasis to the liver. There were more necrotic cells in sections from γT3-supplemented mice compared to combined treatment (γT3 + *Spirulina*), which suggested that the necrotic effect upon combination is most likely from the γT3. In conclusion, the combination of γT3 + *Spirulina* did not appear to have any synergistic anti-cancer or immunomodulatory effects in this mouse model of BC.

Supplementary Materials: The following are available online at https://www.mdpi.com/article/10.3390/nu13072320/s1, Figure S1: The melting curve analysis of the target and reference genes, Figure S2: Dot plot distribution.

Author Contributions: Investigation, H.S.; project design and administration, W.-L.C., A.K.R., H.S., S.C., K.R.S. and Y.-Y.K.; draft preparation, H.S., W.-L.C. and A.K.R.; data curation, H.S.; formal analysis, H.S., W.-L.C., A.K.R. and S.C.; writing—review and editing, H.S., W.-L.C., A.K.R., S.C. and K.R.S.; supervision, W.-L.C., A.K.R. and S.C. All authors have read and agreed to the published version of the manuscript.

Funding: This research was funded by Internal Grant (IMU 258/2012) from the International Medical University (IMU).

Institutional Review Board Statement: The study was approved by the IMU Joint Committee (IMU 258/2012) on Research and Ethics.

Acknowledgments: The authors would like to acknowledge Earthrise Natural, USA and Davos Life Science, Malaysia for providing the food-grade *Spirulina* powder and the DavosLife γ-T3, respectively.

Conflicts of Interest: The authors declared no conflict of interest with respect to the research authorship, and/or publications of this article.

References

1. World Health Organisation (WHO). Available online: https://www.who.int/cancer/prevention/diagnosis-screening/breast-cancer/en/ (accessed on 27 October 2020).
2. Russnes, H.G.; Lingjaerde, O.C.; Borresen-Dale, A.L.; Caldas, C. Breast Cancer Molecular Stratification: From Intrinsic Subtypes to Integrative Clusters. *Am. J. Pathol.* **2017**, *187*, 2152–2162. [CrossRef]
3. Haber, D. Prophylactic oophorectomy to reduce the risk of ovarian and breast cancer in carriers of BRCA mutations. *N. Engl. J. Med.* **2002**, *346*, 1660–1662. [CrossRef]
4. Byrne, C.; Brinton, L.A.; Haile, R.W.; Schairer, C. Heterogeneity of the Effect of Family History on Breast Cancer Risk. *Epidemiology* **1991**, *2*, 276–284. [CrossRef]
5. Carey, L.A. Through a Glass Darkly: Advances in Understanding Breast Cancer Biology, 2000–2010. *Clin. Breast Cancer* **2010**, *10*, 188–195. [CrossRef]
6. Ruder, E.H.; Dorgan, J.F.; Kranz, S.; Kris-Etherton, P.M.; Hartman, T.J. Examining Breast Cancer Growth and Lifestyle Risk Factors: Early Life, Childhood, and Adolescence. *Clin. Breast Cancer* **2008**, *8*, 334–342. [CrossRef]

7. Kingsley, L.A.; Fournier, P.G.; Chirgwin, J.M.; Guise, T.A. Molecular biology of bone metastasis. *Mol. Cancer Ther.* **2007**, *6*, 2609–2617. [CrossRef]
8. Minn, A.J.; Gupta, G.P.; Siegel, P.M.; Bos, P.D.; Shu, W.; Giri, D.D.; Viale, A.; Olshen, A.B.; Gerald, W.L.; Massagué, J. Genes that mediate breast cancer metastasis to lung. *Nat. Cell Biol.* **2005**, *436*, 518–524. [CrossRef]
9. Vlastos, G.; Smith, D.L.; Singletary, S.E.; Mirza, N.Q.; Tuttle, T.M.; Popat, R.J. Long-term survival after an aggressive surgical approach in patients with breast cancer hepatic metastases. *Ann. Surg. Oncol.* **2004**, *11*, 869–874. [CrossRef] [PubMed]
10. Yau, T.; Swanton, C.; Chua, S.; Sue, A.; Walsh, G.; Rostom, A.; Johnston, S.R.; O'Brien, M.E.; Smith, I.E. Incidence, pattern and timing of brain metastases among patients with advanced breast cancer treated with trastuzumab. *Acta. Oncol.* **2006**, *45*, 196–201. [CrossRef] [PubMed]
11. Weigelt, B.; Peterse, J.L.; van't Veer, L.J. Breast cancer metastasis: Markers and models. *Nat. Rev. Cancer* **2005**, *5*, 591–602. [CrossRef] [PubMed]
12. Steeg, P.S. Tumor metastasis: Mechanistic insights and clinical challenges. *Nat. Med.* **2006**, *12*, 895–904. [CrossRef]
13. Li, D.-M.; Feng, Y.-M. Signaling mechanism of cell adhesion molecules in breast cancer metastasis: Potential therapeutic targets. *Breast Cancer Res. Treat.* **2011**, *128*, 7–21. [CrossRef]
14. Hanahan, D.; Weinberg, R.A. Hallmarks of Cancer: The Next Generation. *Cell* **2011**, *144*, 646–674. [CrossRef]
15. Gobert, M.; Treilleux, I.; Bendriss-Vermare, N.; Bachelot, T.; Goddard-Leon, S.; Arfi, V.; Biota, C.; Doffin, A.C.; Durand, I.; Olive, D.; et al. Regulatory T Cells Recruited through CCL22/CCR4 Are Selectively Activated in Lymphoid Infiltrates Surrounding Primary Breast Tumors and Lead to an Adverse Clinical Outcome. *Cancer Res.* **2009**, *69*, 2000–2009. [CrossRef]
16. Ruffell, B.; DeNardo, D.G.; Affara, N.I.; Coussens, L.M. Lymphocytes in cancer development: Polarization towards pro-tumor immunity. *Cytokine Growth Factor Rev.* **2010**, *21*, 3–10. [CrossRef]
17. Zamarron, B.; Chen, W. Dual Roles of Immune Cells and Their Factors in Cancer Development and Progression. *Int. J. Biol. Sci.* **2011**, *7*, 651–658. [CrossRef]
18. Emens, L.A. Breast cancer immunobiology driving immunotherapy: Vaccines and immune checkpoint blockade. *Expert Rev. Anticancer Ther.* **2012**, *12*, 1597–1611. [CrossRef]
19. Matsen, C.B.; Neumayer, L.A. Breast cancer: A review for the general surgeon. *JAMA Surg.* **2013**, *148*, 971–979. [CrossRef]
20. Dhankhar, R.; Vyas, S.P.; Jain, A.; Arora, S.; Rath, G.; Goyal, A.K. Advances in Novel Drug Delivery Strategies for Breast Cancer Therapy. *Artif. Cells Blood Substit. Biotechnol.* **2010**, *38*, 230–249. [CrossRef]
21. Early Breast Cancer Trialists' Collaborative Group (EBCTCG); Peto, R.; Davies, C.; Godwin, J.; Gray, R.; Pan, H.C.; Clarke, M.; Cutter, D.; Darby, S.; McGale, P.; et al. Comparisons between different polychemotherapy regimens for early breast cancer: Meta-analyses of long-term outcome among 100,000 women in 123 randomised trials. *Lancet* **2012**, *379*, 432–444.
22. Akram, M.; Siddiqui, S.A. Breast cancer management: Past, present and evolving. *Indian J. Cancer* **2012**, *49*, 277. [CrossRef]
23. Lemieux, J.; Maunsell, E.; Provencher, L. Chemotherapy-induced alopecia and effects on quality of life among women with breast cancer: A literature review. *Psychol. Oncol.* **2008**, *17*, 317–328. [CrossRef]
24. Meganathan, P.; Fu, J.-Y. Biological Properties of Tocotrienols: Evidence in Human Studies. *Int. J. Mol. Sci.* **2016**, *17*, 1682. [CrossRef] [PubMed]
25. Wali, V.B.; Bachawal, S.V.; Sylvester, P.W. Endoplasmic reticulum stress mediates gamma-tocotrienol-induced apoptosis in mammary tumor cells. *Apoptosis* **2009**, *14*, 1366–1377. [CrossRef]
26. Samant, G.V.; Wali, V.B.; Sylvester, P.W. Anti-proliferative effects of gamma-tocotrienol on mammary tumour cells are associated with suppression of cell cycle progression. *Cell Prolif.* **2010**, *43*, 77–83. [CrossRef] [PubMed]
27. Elangovan, S.; Hsieh, T.-C.; Wu, J.M. Growth inhibition of human MDA-mB-231 breast cancer cells by delta-tocotrienol is associated with loss of cyclin D1/CDK4 expression and accompanying changes in the state of phosphorylation of the retinoblastoma tumor suppressor gene product. *Anticancer. Res.* **2008**, *28*, 2641–2647. [PubMed]
28. Constantinou, C.; Papas, A.; Constantinou, A.I. Vitamin E and cancer: An insight into the anticancer activities of vitamin E isomers and analogs. *Int. J. Cancer* **2008**, *123*, 739–752. [CrossRef] [PubMed]
29. Agarwal, M.K.; Agarwal, M.L.; Athar, M.; Gupta, S. Tocotrienol-rich fraction of palm oil activates p53, modulates Bax/Bcl2 ratio and induces apoptosis independent of cell cycle association. *Cell Cycle* **2004**, *3*, 205–211. [CrossRef]
30. Belay, A. The Potential Application of Spirulina (Arthrospira) as a Nutritional and Therapeutic supplement in Health Management. *J. Am. Nutraceutical Assoc.* **2002**, *5*, 27–48.
31. Chen, T.; Wong, Y.-S.; Zheng, W. WITHDRAWN: Induction of G1 cell cycle arrest and mitochondria-mediated apoptosis in MCF-7 human breast carcinoma cells by selenium-enriched Spirulina extract. *Biomed. Pharmacother.* **2009**. [CrossRef]
32. Hayashi, O.; Katoh, T.; Okuwaki, Y. Enhancement of Antibody Production in Mice by Dietary Spirulina platensis. *J. Nutr. Sci. Vitaminol.* **1994**, *40*, 431–441. [CrossRef]
33. Qureshi, M.A.; Garlich, J.D.; Kidd, M.T. DietarySpirulina PlatensisEnhances Humoral and Cell-Mediated Immune Functions in Chickens. *Immunopharmacol. Immunotoxicol.* **1996**, *18*, 465–476. [CrossRef]
34. Hirahashi, T.; Matsumoto, M.; Hazeki, K.; Saeki, Y.; Ui, M.; Seya, T. Activation of the human innate immune system by Spirulina: Augmentation of interferon production and NK cytotoxicity by oral administration of hot water extract of Spirulina platensis. *Int. Immunopharmacol.* **2002**, *2*, 423–434. [CrossRef]
35. Selvaduray, K.R.; Radhakrishnan, A.K.; Kutty, M.K.; Nesaretnam, K. Palm Tocotrienols Inhibit Proliferation of Murine Mammary Cancer Cells and Induce Expression of Interleukin-24 mRNA. *J. Interf. Cytokine Res.* **2010**, *30*, 909–916. [CrossRef]

36. Tomayko, M.M.; Reynolds, C.P. Determination of subcutaneous tumor size in athymic (nude) mice. *Cancer Chemother. Pharm.* **1989**, *24*, 148–154. [CrossRef]
37. Desjardins, P.; Conklin, D. NanoDrop Microvolume Quantitation of Nucleic Acids. *J. Vis. Exp.* **2010**, *45*, e2565. [CrossRef] [PubMed]
38. Hayashi, O.; Hirahashi, T.; Katoh, T.; Miyajima, H.; Hirano, T.; Okuwaki, Y. Class Specific Influence of Dietary Spirulina platensis on Antibody Production in Mice. *J. Nutr. Sci. Vitaminol.* **1998**, *44*, 841–851. [CrossRef]
39. Nesaretnam, K.; Ambra, R.; Selvaduray, K.R.; Radhakrishnan, A.; Reimann, K.; Razak, G.; Virgili, F. Tocotrienol-rich fraction from palm oil affects gene expression in tumors resulting from MCF-7 cell inoculation in athymic mice. *Lipids* **2004**, *39*, 459–467. [CrossRef]
40. Mahalingam, D.; Radhakrishnan, A.K.; Amom, Z.; Ibrahim, N.; Nesaretnam, K. Effects of supplementation with tocotrienol-rich fraction on immune response to tetanus toxoid immunization in normal healthy volunteers. *Eur. J. Clin. Nutr.* **2010**, *65*, 63–69. [CrossRef] [PubMed]
41. Lee, C.-Y.J.; Wan, J.M.-F. Vitamin E Supplementation Improves Cell-Mediated Immunity and Oxidative Stress of Asian Men and Women. *J. Nutr.* **2000**, *130*, 2932–2937. [CrossRef] [PubMed]
42. Tanaka, H.; Yoshizawa, H.; Yamaguchi, Y.; Ito, K.; Kagamu, H.; Suzuki, E.; Gejyo, F.; Hamada, H.; Arakawa, M. Successful adoptive immunotherapy of murine poorly immunogenic tumor with specific effector cells generated from gene-modified tumor-primed lymph node cells. *J. Immunol.* **1999**, *162*, 3574–3582.
43. Smyth, M.; Dunn, G.P.; Schreiber, R.D. Cancer Immunosurveillance and Immunoediting: The Roles of Immunity in Suppressing Tumor Development and Shaping Tumor Immunogenicity. *Adv. Immunol.* **2006**, *90*, 1–50. [CrossRef]
44. Duan, S.; Thomas, P.G. Balancing Immune Protection and Immune Pathology by CD8(+) T-Cell Responses to Influenza Infection. *Front. Immunol.* **2016**, *7*, 25. [CrossRef]
45. Nishikawa, H.; Sakaguchi, S. Regulatory T cells in cancer immunotherapy. *Curr. Opin. Immunol.* **2014**, *27*, 1–7. [CrossRef]
46. Curiel, T.J.; Coukos, G.; Zou, L.; Alvarez, X.; Cheng, P.; Mottram, P.; Evdemon-Hogan, M.; Conejo-Garcia, J.; Zhang, L.; Burow, M.; et al. Specific recruitment of regulatory T cells in ovarian carcinoma fosters immune privilege and predicts reduced survival. *Nat. Med.* **2004**, *10*, 942–949. [CrossRef]
47. Bates, G.J.; Fox, S.B.; Han, C.; Leek, R.D.; Garcia, J.F.; Harris, A.; Banham, A.H. Quantification of Regulatory T Cells Enables the Identification of High-Risk Breast Cancer Patients and Those at Risk of Late Relapse. *J. Clin. Oncol.* **2006**, *24*, 5373–5380. [CrossRef] [PubMed]
48. Petersen, R.P.; Campa, M.J.; Sperlazza, J.; Conlon, D.; Joshi, M.-B.; Harpole, D.H.; Patz, E.F. Tumor infiltrating Foxp3+ regulatory T-cells are associated with recurrence in pathologic stage I NSCLC patients. *Cancer* **2006**, *107*, 2866–2872. [CrossRef]
49. Surh, C.D.; Sprent, J. Homeostasis of Naive and Memory T Cells. *Immunity* **2008**, *29*, 848–862. [CrossRef]
50. Kittipatarin, C.; Khaled, A.R. Interlinking interleukin-7. *Cytokine* **2007**, *39*, 75–83. [CrossRef] [PubMed]
51. Li, B.; Chu, X.; Gao, M.; Li, W. Apoptotic mechanism of MCF-7 breast cells in vivo and in vitro induced by photodynamic therapy with C-phycocyanin. *Acta Biochim. Biophys. Sin.* **2009**, *42*, 80–89. [CrossRef]
52. Eynon, E.E.; Schlax, C.; Pieters, J. A Secreted Form of the Major Histocompatibility Complex Class II-associated Invariant Chain Inhibiting T Cell Activation. *J. Biol. Chem.* **1999**, *274*, 26266–26271. [CrossRef] [PubMed]
53. Deblandre, G.A.; Marinx, O.P.; Evans, S.S.; Majjaj, S.; Leo, O.; Caput, D.; Huez, G.A.; Wathelet, M.G. Expression Cloning of an Interferon-inducible 17-kDa Membrane Protein Implicated in the Control of Cell Growth. *J. Biol. Chem.* **1995**, *270*, 23860–23866. [CrossRef]
54. Durrant, L.G.; Spendlove, I. Immunization against tumor cell surface complement-regulatory proteins. *Curr. Opin. Investig. Drugs Lond. Engl. 2000* **2001**, *7*, 959–966.
55. Wan, L.; Pantel, K.; Kang, Y. Tumor metastasis: Moving new biological insights into the clinic. *Nat. Med.* **2013**, *19*, 1450–1464. [CrossRef] [PubMed]
56. Ravi, M.; Tentu, S.; Baskar, G.; Prasad, S.R.; Raghavan, S.; Jayaprakash, P.; Jeyakanthan, J.; Rayala, S.K.; Venkatraman, G. Molecular mechanism of anti-cancer activity of phycocyanin in triple-negative breast cancer cells. *BMC Cancer* **2015**, *15*, 1–13. [CrossRef] [PubMed]
57. Selvaduray, K.R.; Radhakrishnan, A.K.; Kutty, M.K.; Nesaretnam, K. Palm tocotrienols decrease levels of pro-angiogenic markers in human umbilical vein endothelial cells (HUVEC) and murine mammary cancer cells. *Genes Nutr.* **2011**, *7*, 53–61. [CrossRef]
58. Kunnumakkara, A.B.; Sung, B.; Ravindran, J.; Diagaradjane, P.; Deorukhkar, A.; Dey, S.; Koca, C.; Yadav, V.R.; Tong, Z.; Gelovani, J.G.; et al. γ-tocotrienol inhibits pancreatic tumors and sensitizes them to gemcitabine treatment by modulating the inflammatory microenvironment. *Cancer Res.* **2010**, *70*, 8695–8705. [CrossRef]
59. Ouhtit, A.; Gaur, R.L.; Abdraboh, M.; Ireland, S.K.; Rao, P.N.; Raj, S.G.; Al-Riyami, H.; Shanmuganathan, S.; Gupta, I.; Murthy, S.N.; et al. Simultaneous Inhibition of Cell-Cycle, Proliferation, Survival, Metastatic Pathways and Induction of Apoptosis in Breast Cancer Cells by a Phytochemical Super-Cocktail: Genes That Underpin Its Mode of Action. *J. Cancer* **2013**, *4*, 703–715. [CrossRef] [PubMed]
60. Li, F.; Ling, X. Survivin study: An update of "what is the next wave"? *J. Cell Physiol.* **2006**, *208*, 476–486. [CrossRef]
61. Nesaretnam, K.; Meganathan, P.; Veerasenan, S.D.; Selvaduray, K.R. Tocotrienols and breast cancer: The evidence to date. *Genes Nutr.* **2011**, *7*, 3–9. [CrossRef]

62. Zhang, Y.-W.; Staal, B.; Su, Y.; Swiatek, P.; Zhao, P.; Cao, B.; Resau, J.; Sigler, R.; Bronson, R.; Woude, G.F.V. Evidence that MIG-6 is a tumor-suppressor gene. *Oncogene* **2006**, *26*, 269–276. [CrossRef]
63. Lee, S.W. H–cadherin, a novel cadherin with growth inhibitory functions and diminished expression in human breast cancer. *Nat. Med.* **1996**, *2*, 776–782. [CrossRef]
64. Sohn, D.M.; Kim, S.Y.; Baek, M.J.; Lim, C.W.; Lee, M.H.; Cho, M.S.; Kim, T.Y. Expression of survivin and clinical correlation in patients with breast cancer. *Biomed. Pharmacother.* **2006**, *60*, 289–292. [CrossRef]
65. Pennati, M.; Folini, M.; Zaffaroni, N. Targeting Survivin in Cancer Therapy: Preclinical Studies. *Expert Opin. Ther. Targets* **2008**, *12*, 463–476. [CrossRef]
66. Itoh, T.; Hayashi, Y.; Kanamaru, T.; Morita, Y.; Suzuki, S.; Wang, W.; Zhou, L.; Rui, J.; Yamamoto, M.; Kuroda, Y.; et al. Clinical significance of urokinase-type plasminogen activator activity in hepatocellular carcinoma. *J. Gastroenterol. Hepatol.* **2000**, *15*, 422–430. [CrossRef]
67. Duffy, M.J.; Maguire, T.M.; McDermott, E.W.; O'Higgins, N. Urokinase plasminogen activator: A prognostic marker in multiple types of cancer. *J. Surg. Oncol.* **1999**, *71*, 130–135. [CrossRef]
68. Schmitt, M.; Harbeck, N.; Thomssen, C.; Wilhelm, O.; Magdolen, V.; Reuning, U.; Ulm, K.; Höfler, H.; Jänicke, F.; Graeff, H. Clinical Impact of the Plasminogen Activation System in Tumor Invasion and Metastasis: Prognostic Relevance and Target for Therapy. *Thromb. Haemost.* **1997**, *78*, 285–296. [CrossRef]
69. Zheng, Q.; Tang, Z.-Y.; Xue, Q.; Shi, D.-R.; Song, H.-Y.; Tang, H.-B. Invasion and metastasis of hepatocellular carcinoma in relation to urokinase-type plasminogen activator, its receptor and inhibitor. *J. Cancer Res. Clin. Oncol.* **2000**, *126*, 641–646. [CrossRef]
70. Anastasi, S.; Sala, G.; Huiping, C.; Caprini, E.; Russo, G.; Iacovelli, S.; Lucini, F.; Ingvarsson, S.; Segatto, O. Loss of RALT/MIG-6 expression in ERBB2-amplified breast carcinomas enhances ErbB-2 oncogenic potency and favors resistance to Herceptin. *Oncogene* **2005**, *24*, 4540–4548. [CrossRef]
71. Amatschek, S.; Koenig, U.; Auer, H.; Steinlein, P.; Pacher, M.; Gruenfelder, A.; Dekan, G.; Vogl, S.; Kubista, E.; Heider, K.-H.; et al. Tissue-Wide Expression Profiling Using cDNA Subtraction and Microarrays to Identify Tumor-Specific Genes. *Cancer Res.* **2004**, *64*, 844–856. [CrossRef]
72. Ferby, I.; Reschke, M.; Kudlacek, O.; Knyazev, P.; Pantè, G.; Amann, K.; Sommergruber, W.; Kraut, N.; Ullrich, A.; Fässler, R.; et al. Mig6 is a negative regulator of EGF receptor-mediated skin morphogenesis and tumor formation. *Nat. Med.* **2006**, *12*, 568–573. [CrossRef]
73. Ramdas, P.; Rajihuzzaman, M.; Veerasenan, S.D.; Selvaduray, K.R.; Nesaretnam, K.; Radhakrishnan, A.K. Tocotrienol-treated MCF-7 human breast cancer cells show down-regulation of API5 and up-regulation of MIG6 genes. *Cancer Genom.Proteom.* **2011**, *8*, 19–31.
74. Hebbard, L.W.; Garlatti, M.; Young, L.J.T.; Cardiff, R.D.; Oshima, R.G.; Ranscht, B. T-cadherin Supports Angiogenesis and Adiponectin Association with the Vasculature in a Mouse Mammary Tumor Model. *Cancer Res.* **2008**, *68*, 1407–1416. [CrossRef] [PubMed]
75. Takeuchi, T.; Misaki, A.; Chen, B.-K.; Ohtsuki, Y. H-cadherin expression in breast cancer. *Histopathology* **1999**, *35*, 87–88. [CrossRef] [PubMed]

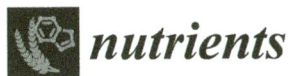

Article

YG-1 Extract Improves Acute Pulmonary Inflammation by Inducing Bronchodilation and Inhibiting Inflammatory Cytokines

Hye-Yoom Kim [1,†], Jung-Joo Yoon [1,†], Dae-Sung Kim [2], Dae-Gill Kang [1,†] and Ho-Sub Lee [1,*,†]

1. Hanbang Cardio-Renal Research Center & Professional Graduate School of Oriental Medicine, Wonkwang University, Iksan 54538, Korea; hyeyoomc@naver.com (H.-Y.K.); mora16@naver.com (J.-J.Y.); dgkang@wku.ac.kr (D.-G.K.)
2. Hanpoong Pharm and Foods Co., Ltd., Wanju 55316, Korea; kimezz@naver.com
* Correspondence: host@wku.ac.kr; Tel.: +82-63-850-6447; Fax: +82-63-850-7260
† Current address: Hanbang Cardio-Renal Syndrome Research Center, Department of Herbal Resources, Professional Graduate School of Oriental Medicine, Wonkwang University, 460 Iksan-daero, Iksan 54538, Korea.

Citation: Kim, H.-Y.; Yoon, J.-J.; Kim, D.-S.; Kang, D.-G.; Lee, H.-S. YG-1 Extract Improves Acute Pulmonary Inflammation by Inducing Bronchodilation and Inhibiting Inflammatory Cytokines. *Nutrients* **2021**, *13*, 3414. https://doi.org/10.3390/nu13103414

Academic Editor: Md Soriful Islam

Received: 1 September 2021
Accepted: 25 September 2021
Published: 28 September 2021

Publisher's Note: MDPI stays neutral with regard to jurisdictional claims in published maps and institutional affiliations.

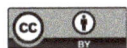

Copyright: © 2021 by the authors. Licensee MDPI, Basel, Switzerland. This article is an open access article distributed under the terms and conditions of the Creative Commons Attribution (CC BY) license (https://creativecommons.org/licenses/by/4.0/).

Abstract: YG-1 extract used in this study is a mixture of *Lonicera japonica*, *Arctic Fructus*, and *Scutellariae Radix*. The present study was designed to investigate the effect of YG-1 extract on bronchodilatation (ex vivo) and acute bronchial and pulmonary inflammation relief (in vivo). Ex vivo: The bronchodilation reaction was confirmed by treatment with YG-1 concentration-accumulation (0.01, 0.03, 0.1, 0.3, and 1 mg/mL) in the bronchial tissue ring pre-contracted by acetylcholine (10 μM). As a result, YG-1 extract is considered to affect bronchodilation by increased cyclic adenosine monophosphate, cAMP) levels through the β2-adrenergic receptor. In vivo: experiments were performed in C57BL/6 mice were divided into the following groups: control group; PM2.5 (fine particulate matter)-exposed group (PM2.5, 200 μg/kg/mL saline); and PM2.5-exposed + YG-1 extract (200 mg/kg/day) group. The PM2.5 (200 μg/kg/mL saline) was exposed for 1 h for 5 days using an ultrasonic nebulizer aerosol chamber to instill fine dust in the bronchi and lungs, thereby inducing acute lung and bronchial inflammation. From two days before PM2.5 exposure, YG-1 extract (200 mg/kg/day) was administered orally for 7 days. The PM2.5 exposure was involved in airway remodeling and inflammation, suggesting that YG-1 treatment improves acute bronchial and pulmonary inflammation by inhibiting the inflammatory cytokines (NLRP3/caspase-1 pathway). The application of YG-1 extract with broncho-dilating effect to acute bronchial and pulmonary inflammation animal models has great significance in developing therapeutic agents for respiratory diseases. Therefore, these results can provide essential data for the development of novel respiratory symptom relievers. Our study provides strong evidence that YG-1 extracts reduce the prevalence of respiratory symptoms and the incidence of non-specific lung diseases and improve bronchial and lung function.

Keywords: YG-1 extract; bronchodilation; fine particulate matter (PM2.5); acute lung injury; airway inflammation

1. Introduction

Bronchodilators are important drugs in the treatment of asthma, acute, and chronic obstructive airway disease. Beta agonists, theophylline and antimuscarinic drugs are the main drugs currently used [1]. These drugs are known to directly affect airway smooth muscle and cause bronchodilation [2]. Abnormal state of airway smooth muscle cells is involved in airway remodeling [3]. Excessive exposure to fine particulate matter (PM2.5) is gradually absorbed into the bronchi and lungs and progresses to acute respiratory distress syndrome, eventually requiring bronchodilation for respiration [4]. Therefore, it is meaningful to apply natural products with bronchodilating effect to animal models of acute bronchial and lung inflammation. Particulate matter (PM) is one of the various artificial pollutants worldwide and has recently received much attention due to its biohazard effects. PMs are classified into two groups, PM10 and PM2.5, according to their size. PM10 refers to particulate matter less than ten μm in diameter, and PM2.5 refers to particles less than 2.5 μm in diameter [4,5]. Respiratory symptoms and diseases are becoming more and more serious due to air pollution and environmental changes caused by rapid industrialization [5]. Respiratory symptoms caused by air pollution are caused by an inflammatory reaction in the bronchi with stimuli such as fine dust, which causes or worsens acute sepsis, asthma, chronic bronchitis, and airway obstruction [6,7]. Recently, exposure to PM2.5 has been identified as a major risk factor for respiratory diseases [8,9]. PM2.5 not only causes respiratory dysfunction (cough and wheezing etc.) but also worsens the condition, increasing morbidity and mortality [10,11]. Also, it was reported that PM2.5 induces airway inflammation in mice and nasal inoculation of enriched PM2.5 induces an inflammatory airway response [12]. According to various studies, short-term exposure to PM2.5 in mice is known to induce acute lung inflammation [13].

Currently, the treatment of respiratory diseases is dependent on the use of drugs such as bronchodilators and anti-inflammatory drugs, but alternative medicine using natural products with few side effects is needed [14]. Among natural products, there are many ingredients known to have antitussive expectorant effects that can treat respiratory symptoms and diseases. It has been reported that these natural products have clinical effects in relieving respiratory symptoms when administered alone or in combination [15]. Mixtures of natural products have been used for the treatment of various diseases since ancient times, and their physiologically active efficacy has been verified based on long-term experience and is widely used because there are few side effects [16]. The YG-1 extract used in this study is a mixture of *Lonicera japonica*, *Arctii Fructus*, and *Scutellariae Radix* (Table 1). *Lonicera japonica*, which accounts for a significant proportion of the YG-1 mixed extract, is known to have antipyretic, detoxifying, and sweating effects [17], and *Arctii Fructus* is used to relieve fever and sore throat [18]. In addition, *Scutellaria Radix* has anti-inflammatory, antipyretic, diuretic, and blood pressure lowering effects, and is currently used for chronic bronchitis, infectious hepatitis, and hypertension [19]. In this study, we assess the bronchodilatation (ex vivo) and acute bronchial and lung inflammation relief effects (in vivo) of YG-1 extract, a mixture of natural products (*Lonicera japonica*, *Arctii Fructus*, and *Scutellariae Radix*) widely used as antitussive expectorants in folk remedies.

Table 1. Mixing ratio of YG-1 extract.

Code	Scientific Name of Source	Ratio	Mixing Ratio
A	Lonicera japonica, Arctii Fructus	3 1	2
B	Scutellariae Radix	2.25	3

2. Materials & Methods

2.1. Preparation of YG-1 Extract

The YG-1 extract was a mixed extract containing *Lonicera japonica*, *Arctii Fructus*, and *Scutellariae Radix*, which was provided by Hanpoong (Hanpoong Pharm and Foods Co., Ltd., Wanju, Korea). Lonicera japonica, and Arctii Fructus were each added at a ratio of 3:1, and 20 times 30% alcohol was added, followed by extraction twice at 85–95 °C for 3 h each. After filtration, the extract was concentrated under reduced pressure at 60 °C or less and dried to prepare YG-A (yield 14%). *Scutellariae Radix* was extracted twice for 3 h at 85–95 °C by adding 20 times 30% alcohol, and concentrated and dried to prepare YG-B (yield 45.61%). YG-1 was prepared by mixing dried YG-A and YG-B in a ratio of 2:3 (Table 1) according to the ratio previously used in the study [20].

2.2. HPLC Analysis of YG-1

Seven reference standard components, loganin, loganic acid, sweroside, arctiin, baicalin, baicalein, and wogonin were purchased from ChemFaces (ChemFaces Biochemical, Wuhan, China), respectively. Chemical structures of these reference standard components are shown in Figure 1. HPLC analysis for the comparison of the 7 marker components in YG-1 extract was performed using HPLC instrument (I-series, LC-2030C, Shimadzu, Kyoto, Japan), PDA detector (Shimadzu, Kyoto, Japan) and LC Solution software (Version 1.24, SP1, Shimadzu, Kyoto, Japan). Analysis of loganin, loganic acid, sweroside, arctiin, baicalin, baicalein, wogonin were performed using a Capcell Pak HPLC Columns (250 × 4.6 mm I.D, C18 UG120 column, 5 µm, Osaka soda, Japan).

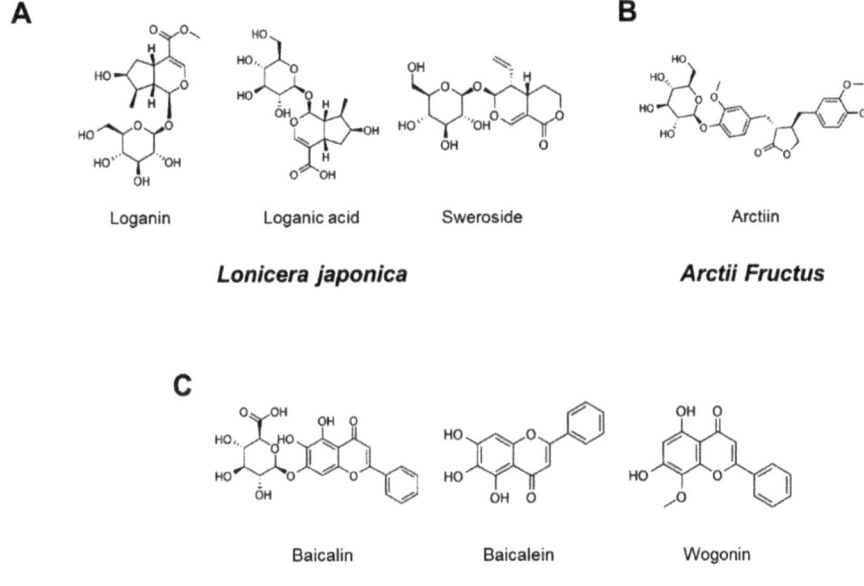

Figure 1. Chemical structures of seven marker components in YG-1 mixed extract. Loganin, logan acid, and sweroside were the main components of *Lonicera Japonica* (**A**). Aarctiin was the main components of *Arctii Fructus* (**B**). Baicalin, baicalein, and wogonin were *Scutellariae Radix* (**C**).

2.3. Isolation of Bronchial Tissue and Measurement of Bronchodilation (Ex Vivo)

After the head of a healthy male Sprague-Dawley (weighing approximately 250–300 g) was dislocated, the rib cage was excised, and the bronchi were isolated. The rapidly isolated bronchial were saturated with mixed gas (95% O_2 and 5% CO_2) in a Krebs solution (118 mM NaCl; 1.5 mM $CaCl_2$; 4.7 mM KCl; 25 mM $NaHCO_3$; 10 mM glucose; 1.1 mM $MgSO_4$; and 1.2 mM KH_2PO_4; pH 7.4 with ice-cold), remove the surrounding fat and connective bronchial tissue, and then cut into sections with a length of about 3–4 mm. At this time, be careful not to damage the bronchial smooth muscle. 5 mL of Krebs solution was placed in the chamber and maintained at 37 °C with the mixed gas. The detached bronchial ring was pulled up to a force of 1.8 g and equilibrated for 60 min. Isometric tension changes were recorded via a connected transducer (Grass FT 03, Grass Instrument Co., Quincy, MA, USA) and a Grass Polygraph recording system (Model 7E, Grass Instrument Co., West Warwick, RI, USA). The bronchodilation reaction was confirmed by treatment with YG-1 concentration-dependently (0.01, 0.03, 0.1, 0.3, and 1 mg/mL) in the bronchial tissue ring pre-contracted by acetylcholine (10 µM).

2.4. Measurement of cAMP Levels in Bronchial Tissues

After equilibrating the bronchial sections in Krebs solution for 30 min while supplying 95% O_2 and 5% CO_2 mixed gas, 3-isobutyl-1-methylxanthine (IBMX, 100 μM) and acetylcholine (100 μM) were added to equilibrate for another 5 min. Each concentration was treated with YG-1 extract (1, 2.5, and 5 mg/mL, respectively) and reacted for 10 min. In addition, KT5720 (100 uM) was pre-treated 20 min before, and YG-1 was treated with 5 mg/mL and reacted. The bronchial tissue was immediately put in liquid nitrogen to stop the reaction, and then stored at $-70\ °C$ and used to measure the cAMP concentration. After homogenizing the vascular tissue whose weight was measured in the presence of 0.1M HCl, the supernatant obtained by centrifugation at 13,000 g for 15 min was used with Dirict cAMP ELISA kit (Enzo, ADI-900-066, Biotechnologies Corp & Enzo Life Sciences, New York, NY, USA) was measured.

2.5. PM2.5-Induced Acute Lung and Bronchial Inflammation Mouse Model

After acclimatization for 7 days, all mice were randomly divided into 3 groups (*n* = 8 per group). Experiments were performed in C57BL/6 mice were divided into the following groups: control group; PM2.5-exposed group (PM2.5, 200 μg/kg/mL saline); and PM2.5-exposed + YG-1 extract (200 mg/kg/day) group. From two days before PM2.5 exposure, YG-1 extract (200 mg/kg/day) was orally administered for a total of 7 days. The YG-1 extract was exposed to PM 2.5 for 5 days from two days after the start of feeding to induce acute bronchial and lung inflammation and confirm the improvement effect of YG-1. PM2.5 purchased from Sigma Aldrich (NIST1650b, St. Louis, MO, USA) was dissolved in dimethyl sulfoxide (DMSO, 100%) and washed three times with deionized distilled water for treatment, and ultrasonic pulverization was performed for 3 min to minimize agglomeration. PM2.5 (200 μg/kg/mL saline) was exposed for 1 h for 5 days using an ultrasonic nebulizer aerosol chamber (Mass Dosing Chambers, Data Sciences International, Saint Paul, MN, USA) to instill fine dust in the bronchi and lungs, thereby inducing acute lung and bronchial inflammation. Control group received the same amount of saline used as the dosing vehicle. PM2.5 exposure procedures have been referenced based on various studies [21,22]. C57BL/6 mice were exposed to PM2.5 in the awake and uninhibited state and continuously received concentrated ambient air PM2.5 following an in vivo systemic inhalation protocol. The animals in this study were conducted after obtaining approval from the Animal Experiment Ethics Committee of Wonkwang University (ethics review number: WKU20-28).

2.6. Histological Analysis

The lung and bronchial tissues isolated from mice in each group were fixed in 10% neutral buffered formalin (10% NBF, HT501128, Merk, Darmstadt, Hessen, Germany) solution for 24 h. After perfusion fixation and paraffin embedding, paraffin blocks were cut into 6–7 μm thick tissue sections using a microtome (Thermo Electron Corporation, Pittsburg, PA, USA) and attached to slides. The lung and bronchial tissue slides were prepared using Periodic Acid Solution (PAS, VB-3005, VitroVivo Biotech, Rockville, MD, USA), Masson's trichrome (8400, BBC Biochemical, Mt Vernon, WA, USA), and orcerin (ab245881, Abcam, Cambridge, Cambs, UK) stained with a stain kit. Also, the beta-AR, TGF-beta, collagen IV proteins in lung and bronchial tissues were examined with immunohistochemical (IHC) staining. The lung and bronchial tissue slides were immune stained by mouse and rabbit specific HRP/DAB (ABC) detection IHC kit method (ab6464, Abcam, Cambridge, Cambs, UK). Tissue sections were incubated with primary antibodies of beta 2 Adrenergic Receptor (B2AR, MBS8543138, MyBioSource, San Diego, CA, USA), TGF-β, and collagen IV (Santa Cruz Biotechnology, Santa Cruz, CA, USA). Histopathological comparisons were performed with a microscope slide scanner (MoticEasyScan Pro 1, National Optical & Scientific Instruments, Inc., Schertz, TX, USA).

2.7. Western Blot Analysis and Antibodies

The lung and bronchial tissues (30–45 µg protein) were resolved on 10% SDS-PAGE (SDS-polyacrylamide gel electrophoresis) and transferred onto PVDF (polyvinylidene difluoride) western blot membranes. The membranes were washed three times with TBS-T (Tris buffered saline: 150 mM, NaCl; 10 mM, Tris-HCl; and 0.05%, Tween-20) and blocked with 5% BSA (bovine serum albumin) for 2 h. After that, it was washed again 3 times with TBS-T and reacted overnight with appropriate primary antibodies (tumor necrosis factor alpha, TNF-α; interleukin-6, IL-6; interleukin-1β, IL-1β; interleukin-18, IL-18; NOD-like receptor pyrin domain-containning protein 3, NLRP-3, apoptosis-associated speck-like protein containing a C-terminal caspase recruitment domain, ASC; caspase-1) overnight at 4 °C. TNF-α, IL-6, IL-1β, IL-18, NLRP-3, ASC, and caspase-1, and β-actin were purchased from Santa Cruz (Santa Cruz Biotechnology, Dallas, TX, USA). The next day, the membrane was washed three times with TBS-T and reacted with a secondary antibody conjugated to horseradish peroxidase (Bethyl Laboratories, Montgomery, TX, USA) for 2 hr. For the membrane reacted with the secondary antibody, the protein expression level was confirmed using an image analyzer (iBright FL100, Thermo Fisher Scientific, Waltham, MA, USA). The ImageJ program (NIH, Bethesda, MD, USA) was used to quantify protein levels by performing densitometry analysis.

2.8. Quantitative Real-Time Reverse Transcription-PCR of Lung and Bronchial Tissues

The Real-Time qRT-PCR of Lung and Bronchial Tissues

To confirm the real-time quantitative reverse transcription polymerase chain reaction (qRT-PCR) of lung and bronchial tissues, RNA was extracted from each tissue using Trizol™ Reagent (15596026, ThermoFisher Scientific, Waltham, MA, USA). The cDNAs from lung and bronchial tissues were incubated in SimpliAmp™ Thermal Cycler (A24811, ThermoFisher Scientific, Waltham, MA, USA) at 42 °C for 60 min and 94 °C for 5 min, and synthesized from mRNA through reverse transcription. The real-time qRT-PCR was performed with an initial denaturation step at 95° in a final volume of 20 µL (1 µL of cDNA sample; 1 µL of primer pair each; 8 µL, pure distilled water; 10 µL of SYBR™ Green PCR Master Mix, 4309155, ThermoFisher Scientific, Waltham, MA, USA). Reactions were performed at 95 °C for 10 min using the Step-One™ Real-Time PCR system, followed by 40 repetitions at 95 °C for 15 s and finally 60 °C for 60 s (Applied Biosystems, ThermoFisher Scientific, Waltham, MA, USA). The sequences of primers were as follows: IL-6 (forward, 5′-AACTCCATCTGCCCTTCA-3′; reverse, 5′-CTGTTGTGGGTGGTATCCTC-3′), IL-1β (forward, 5′-TTCAAATCTCACAGCAGCAT-3′; reverse, 5′-CACGGGCAAGACATAGGT AG-3′), NLRP3 (forward, 5′-CTGGAGATCCTAGGTTTCTCTG-3′; reverse, 5′-CAGGAT CTCATTCTCTTGGATC-3′), ASC (forward, 5′-CTCTGTATGGCAATGTGCTGAC-3′; reverse, 5′- GAACAAGTTCTTGCAGGTCAG-3′), Caspase 1 (forward, 5′-GAGCTGATGTTG ACCTCAGAG-3′; reverse, 5′- CTGTCAGAGAGTCTTGTGCTCTG-3′), TNF-α (forward, 5′-GCCTCTTCTCATTCCTGCTTG-3′; reverse, 5′-CTGATGAGAGGGAGGCCATT-3′), and β-actin (forward, 5-GGAGATTACTGCCCTGGCTCCTAGC-3′; reverse, 5′-GGCCGGACT CATCGTACTCCTGCTT-3′).

2.9. Statistical Analyses

All experiments were repeated at least 3 times, and statistically significant differences between group means were determined using Student's t-test. Results of experiments were expressed as mean ± standard error (S.E.). $p < 0.05$ was considered a statistically significant difference.

3. Results

3.1. HPLC Chromatograms of Compounds from YG-1 Extract

Figure 1 shows the chromatograms analyzed by high performance liquid chromatography (HPLC) for *Lonicera japonica* (loganin, loganic acid, and sweoside), *Arctii Fructus* (arctiin), and *Scutellariae Radix* (baicalin, baicaein, and wogonin) from YG-1 extract (Figure 1).

Chromatograms were detected at 254 nm for loganin, loganic acid, and sweoside, arctiin at 280 nm, and baicalin, baicalein, and wogonin at 277 nm using a photodiode array detector (Figure 2). As a result of analyzied YG-1 extract, Loganin (5.80 ± 0.16 mg/g), Loganic acid (2.38 ± 0.54 mg/g), and Sweoside (3.21 ± 0.07 mg/g) contained in *Ronica japonica*; Arctiin (42.67 ± 0.22 mg/g) contained in *Arctii Fructus*; And Baicalin, Baicaein, and Wogonin contained (sum of 3 compounds: 118.67 ± 2.34 mg/g) in *Scutellariae Radix* could be identified, respectively (Figure 2).

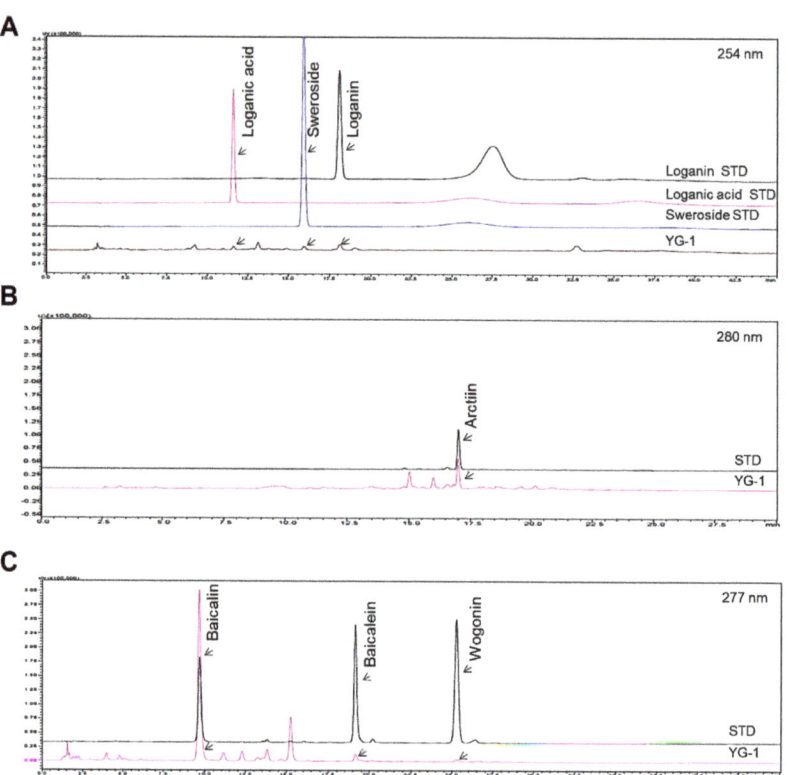

Figure 2. HPLC chromatograms showing peaks corresponding to the marker compounds, loganin, loganic acid, sweoside (**A**), arctiin (**B**), baicalin, baicaein, and wogonin (**C**) of YG-1 extract. HPLC, high performance liquid chromatography.

3.2. Concentration-Dependent Bronchodilation Effect of YG-1 Extract in Bronchial Smooth Muscle

The contraction of bronchial (tracheal) smooth muscle was induced with acetylcholine 10 μM, and the concentration-dependent bronchial relaxation effect of YG-1 extract was confirmed. As a result, bronchial smooth muscle showed a significant relaxation effect at the 5 mg/mL concentration of YG-1 extract compared to 97.58 ± 11.02% of untreated bronchial smooth muscle (Figure 3A(a). In order to examine whether YG-1 extract affects cAMP production in bronchial tissues, the amount of cAMP production was measured by treatment in a concentration-dependent manner. As a result, it was possible to confirm a significant increase in cAMP production in a concentration-dependent manner compared to the group not treated with the YG-1 extract (Figure 3A(b). In addition, the bronchial rings were pre-treated with YG-1 extract (2.5 or 5 mg/mL concentration) to determine whether contraction by acetylcholine. As a result, the YG-1 extract inhibited acetylcholine-induced contraction in a concentration-dependent manner (Figure 3B(a). Therefore, it is considered that the YG-1 extract has the effect of inhibiting bronchi contraction. Also, it is thought that the YG-1 extract has a broncho-dilating effect and is involved in cAMP production.

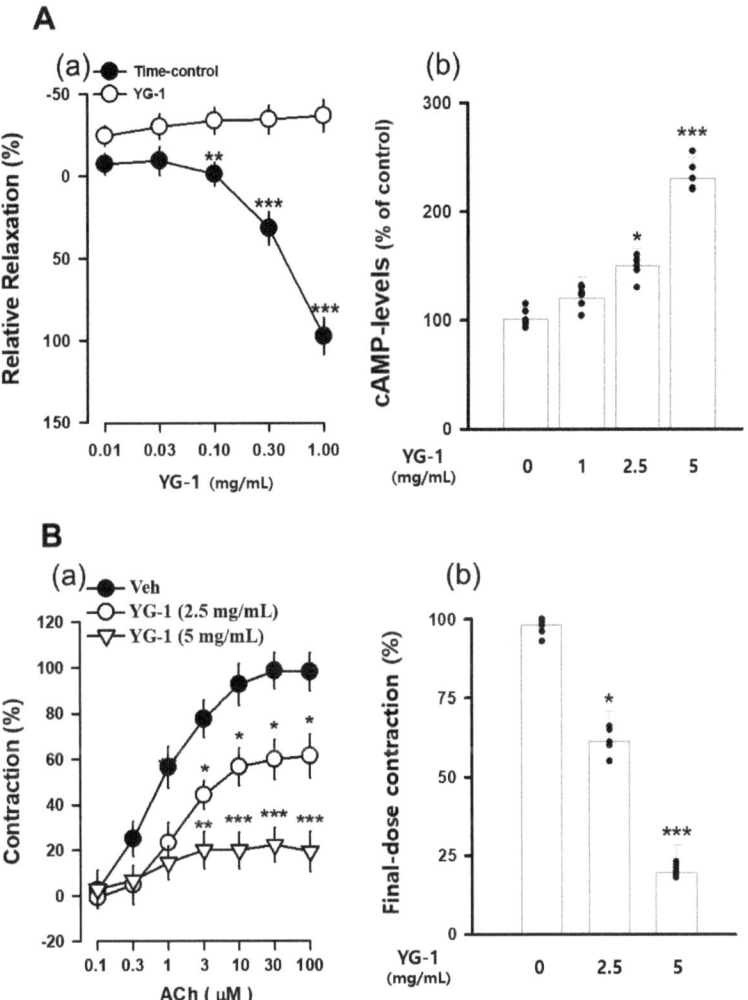

Figure 3. The concentration-accumulation treatment of YG-1 extract shows a dose-response relaxation curve (**A(a)**) in the bronchi, as shown in the bar graph (**A(b)**). Concentration-dependent bronchoconstriction response curve graph of acetylcholine with and without YG-1 treatment (**B(a)**). The bronchoconstriction effect of each group at the highest concentration of YG-1 extract was compared and graphically depicted (**B(b)**). Veh, vehicle; cAMP, cyclic adenosine monophosphate. Data are expressed as mean ± standard error. * $p < 0.05$, ** $p < 0.01$, and *** $p < 0.001$ vs. vehicle.

3.3. Effects of YG-1 Extract on Improving the β_2-Adrenergic Receptor/PKA Pathway in Bronchial Smooth Muscle

It is known that β_2-adrenergic receptors (β-AR) in the autonomic nervous system bronchodilation. To determine whether the bronchodilating effect of YG-1 extract occurs through the β-AR, the bronchodilating effect was investigated by pretreatment with propranolol (1 or 100 μM), a non-selective β_2-adrenergic antagonist. As a result, compared to the relaxation effect of the YG-1 extract, a significant blocking effect of bronchial relaxation was observed at 35.61 ± 11.01% by pretreatment with propranolol at a concentration of 100 μM (Figure 4A). In addition, it is known that smooth muscle induces relaxation by reducing Ca^{2+} levels by converting PKA to cAMP generated by the activity of adenylate cyclase (AC). As a result of confirming the bronchial relaxation effect of the YG-1 extract by pretreatment with KT5720 (10 or 100 μM), a PKA inhibitor, the relaxation effect was reduced to 35.61 ± 11.01% at the 100 M concentration (Figure 4B). As shown in Figure 3 above, YG-1 extract confirmed an increase in cAMP production in bronchial tissues. As a result of confirming whether YG-1 treatment had an effect on cAMP production when PKA blocker was treated, the amount of cAMP production increased by YG-1 treatment was significantly decreased by KT5720 (Figure 4C). Therefore, it is considered that YG-1 extract has a bronchial relaxation effect through the β2-adrenergic receptor/PKA pathway.

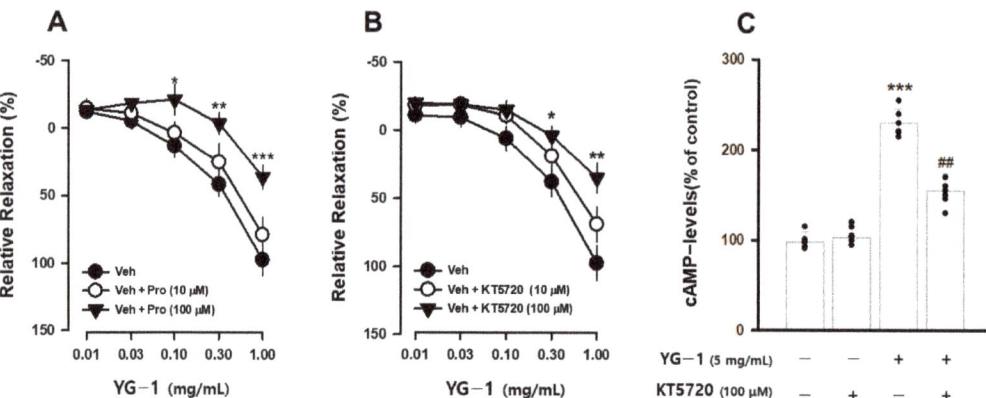

Figure 4. YG-1 extract treatment induced bronchodilation by stimulating β2 adrenergic receptor-mediated PKA activation. Bronchodilation inhibitory effect of YG-1 treatment on acetylcholine (10 μM)-induced bronchoconstriction in rats in the presence of propranolol (10 or 100 μM, **A**) and KT5720 (10 or 100 μM, **B**). The increase in cAMP production by YG-1 in the bronchi was reduced by pretreatment with KT5720 (100 μM. **C**). Veh, vehicle; Pro, propranolol, non-selective β-adrenergic receptor antagonist; KT5720, selective inhibitor of protein kinase A; cAMP, cyclic adenosine monophosphate. Data are expressed as mean ± standard error. *** $p < 0.001$, ** $p < 0.01$, * $p < 0.05$ vs. vehicle; ## $p < 0.01$ vs. YG-1.

3.4. Effect of YG-1 on Reducing Bronchial and Lung Fibrosis in PM2.5-Exposed Airway Inflammation Mice

To investigate the inflammatory effects of PM2.5 on the respiratory tract, C57Bl/6 mice were exposed to PM2.5 using a ultrasonic nebulizer aerosol chamber. After the mice were sacrificed, bronchial and lung tissues from all groups were collected and analyzed. The bronchi and lung fibrosis was confirmed using PAS (Figure 5A), masson's (Figure 5B or 6A) and orcein (Figure 6B) staining. As shown in Figures 5 and 6, significant pulmonary fibrosis was observed in the peribronchial, perivascular, and alveolar spaces of the lungs upon exposure to PM2.5. On the other hand, it was confirmed that fibrosis of the bronchi and lungs was improved by treatment with YG-1 extract.

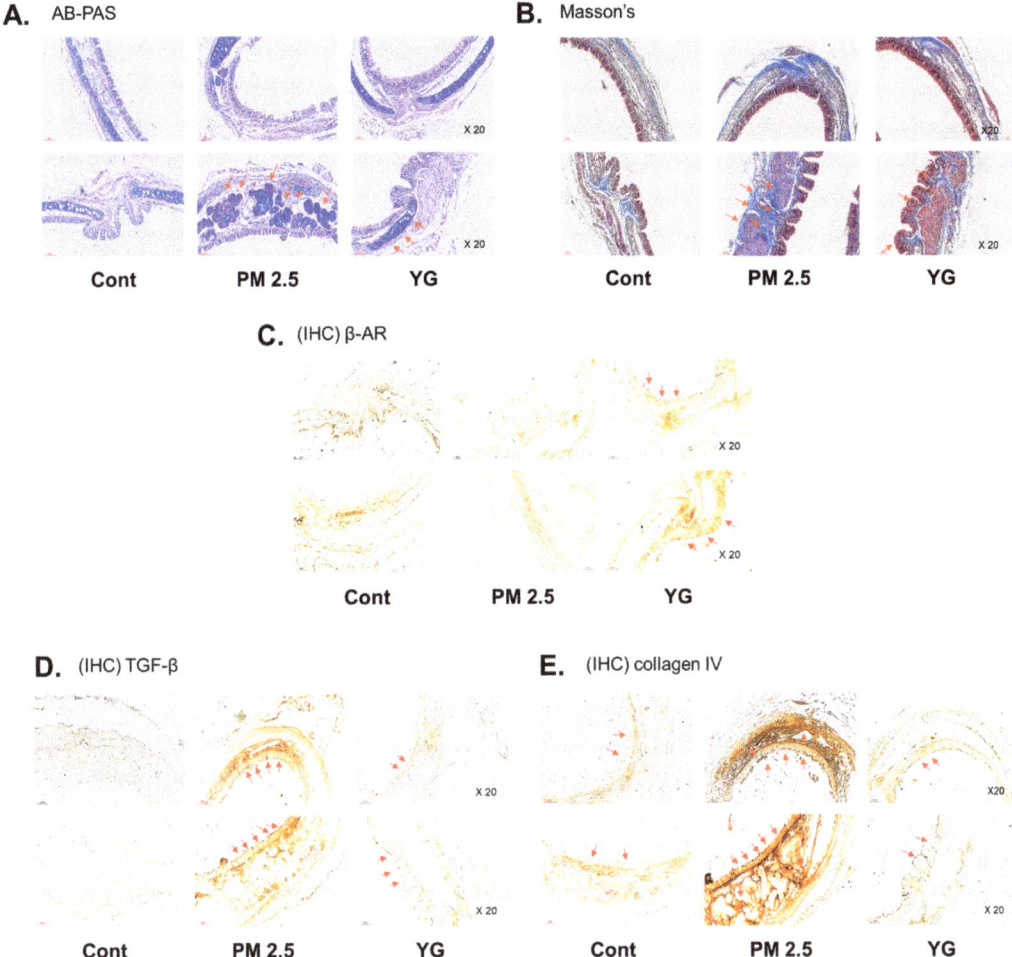

Figure 5. The effect of YG-1 extract treatment on bronchial injury in fine particulate matter (PM2.5)-stimulated mice was histologically confirmed. Representative images of AB-PAS (pseudostratified epithelium, **A**) and Masson's trichrome (collagen fibers, **B**) stained tracheal in PM2.5 stimulated mice. IHC staining was performed to examine the expression of β-AR (**C**), TGF-β (**D**), and collagen IV (**E**) in bronchial tissues. Red arrows indicate the location of pseudostratified epithelium (**A**) and collagen fibers (**B**); and β-AR, TGF-β (**C**), and collagen IV (**D**) were expressed by immunohistochemistry in tracheal. Histopathological lesions and changes were assessed by histological analyses by optical microscope (magnification ×200; n = 3~4 for each group). Cont, control; PM2.5, PM2.5 exposure mice; YG-1, PM2.5 exposure mice + YG-1 treated (200 mg/kg/daily, orally); AB-PAS, alcian blue-periodic acid-Schiff staining; Massnon's, masson's trichrome staining; IHC, Immunohistochemistry staining; β-AR, β-adrenergic receptor antagonist; TGF-β, transforming growth factor-β.

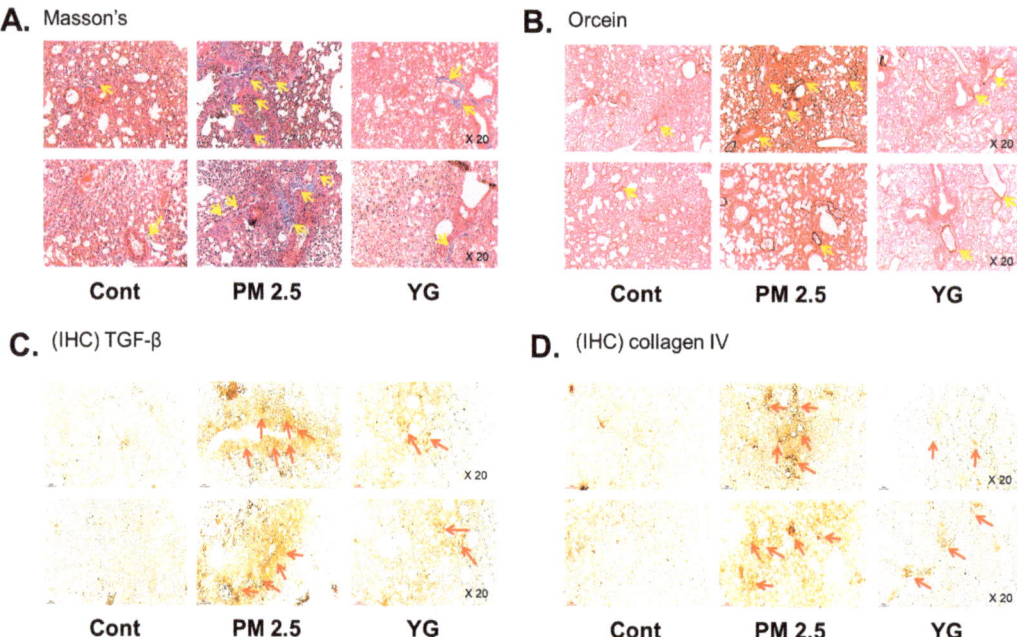

Figure 6. The effect of YG-1 extract treatment on lung injury in fine particulate matter (PM2.5)-stimulated mice was histologically confirmed. To confirm that YG extract treatment inhibited fibrosis of the PM2.5 stimulated mice, histological changes were observed by masson's trichrome (collagen fibers, **A**) and orcein (elastic fibers, **B**) staining in bronchial tissues. IHC staining was performed to examine the expression of TGF-β (**C**) and collagen IV (**D**) in lung tissues. Yellow arrows indicate the location of collagen fibers (**A**) and elastic fibers (**B**). Red arrows indicated where TGF-b (**C**) and collagen (**D**) were expressed by immunohistochemistry. Histopathological lesions and changes were assessed by histological analyses by optical microscope (magnification, ×200; (n = 3~4 for each group). Cont, control; PM2.5, PM2.5 exposure mice; YG-1, PM2.5 exposure mice + YG-1 treated (200 mg/kg/daily, orally); Massnon's, masson's trichrome staining; Orcein, orcein staining; IHC, Immunohistochemistry staining; TGF-β, transforming growth factor-β.

3.5. Effect of YG-1 on Reducing Bronchial and Lung Inflammation in PM2.5-Exposed Airway Inflammation Mice

Histopathological evaluation and pro-inflammatory cytokine levels were evaluated to confirm bronchial and lung inflammation levels. Immunohistochemistry (IHC) staining showed that YG-1 treatment significantly reduced the expression of β-AR, TGF-β, and collagen IV in PM2.5 exposure mice bronchial tissues (Figure 5C–E). As a results, the expression level of β-AR was decreased in the histological evaluation of the bronchial tissues in PM2.5 exposure mice, whereas the expression levels were increased by treatment with YG-1 (Figure 5C). In addition, IHC staining showed that YG-1 treatment significantly reduced the expression of TGF-β and collagen IV in bronchial (Figure 5D,E) and lung (Figure 6C,D) tissues of mice exposed to PM2.5. Furthermore, we investigated whether treatment of YG extract in the airways of PM2.5-exposed mice had an effect on inflammatory cytokines and NLRP3 inflammasome activation-associated protein expression and gene levels. As shown in Figures 5 and 6, PM2.5 exposure to mice increased the expression level of inflammatory cytokines in bronchia (Figure 7A(a,b) and lung tissues (Figure 8A(a,b) compared to the control group. Similarly, higher mRNA and protein levels of TNF-α, IL-1β, and IL-6 were identified in the bronchial (Figure 7B(a–c) and lung tissues (Figure 8B(a–f) of mice treated with PM2.5 (Figure 8A(a,b). Taken together, Inhibition of the NLRP3/caspase-1 pathway by YG-1 alleviated lung inflammation in PM2.5-induced mice model. It was confirmed that the treatment of YG-1 improved the activated NLRP3/caspase-1 pathway in the PM2.5-induced mice model. Thus, YG-1 treatment in mice with lung inflammation caused by PM2.5 exposure has an effect of improving inflammation.

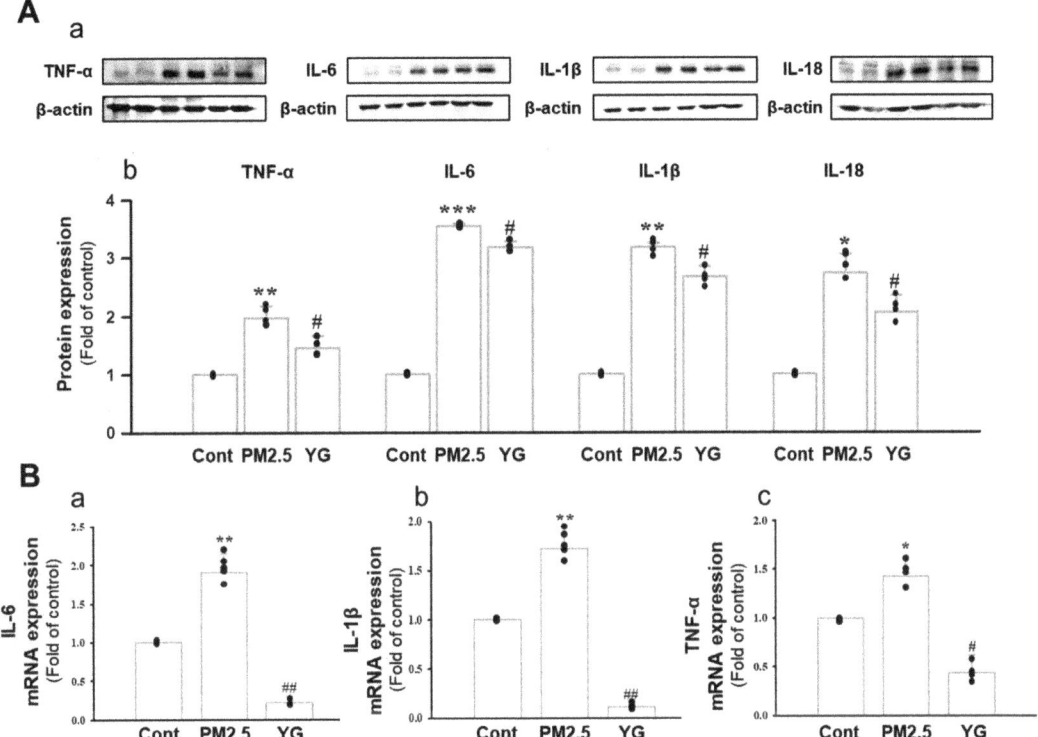

Figure 7. Treatment of YG-1 extract improved acute bronchial and lung injury in fine particulate matter (PM2.5)-stimulated mice. Increased protein expression of TNF-α, IL-6, IL-1β and IL-18 inflammatory cytokines in PM2.5-stimulated mice was improved by YG treatment (**A**). Bronchial damage in PM2.5-stimulated mice increased IL-6, IL-1β and TNF-α mRNA levels and was inhibited by YG-1 treatment (**B**). β-actin was used as loading controls for protein and mRNA expressions (n = 3~5 for each group). Cont, control; PM2.5, PM2.5 exposure mice; YG-1, PM2.5 exposure mice + YG-1 treated (200 mg/kg/daily, orally); TNF-α, tumor necrosis factor alpha; IL-6, interleukin 6; IL-1β, interleukin 1 beta; IL-18, interleukin 18. Data are expressed as mean ± standard error. * $p < 0.05$, ** $p < 0.01$, and *** $p < 0.001$ vs. control; # $p < 0.05$, ## $p < 0.01$ vs. PM2.5.

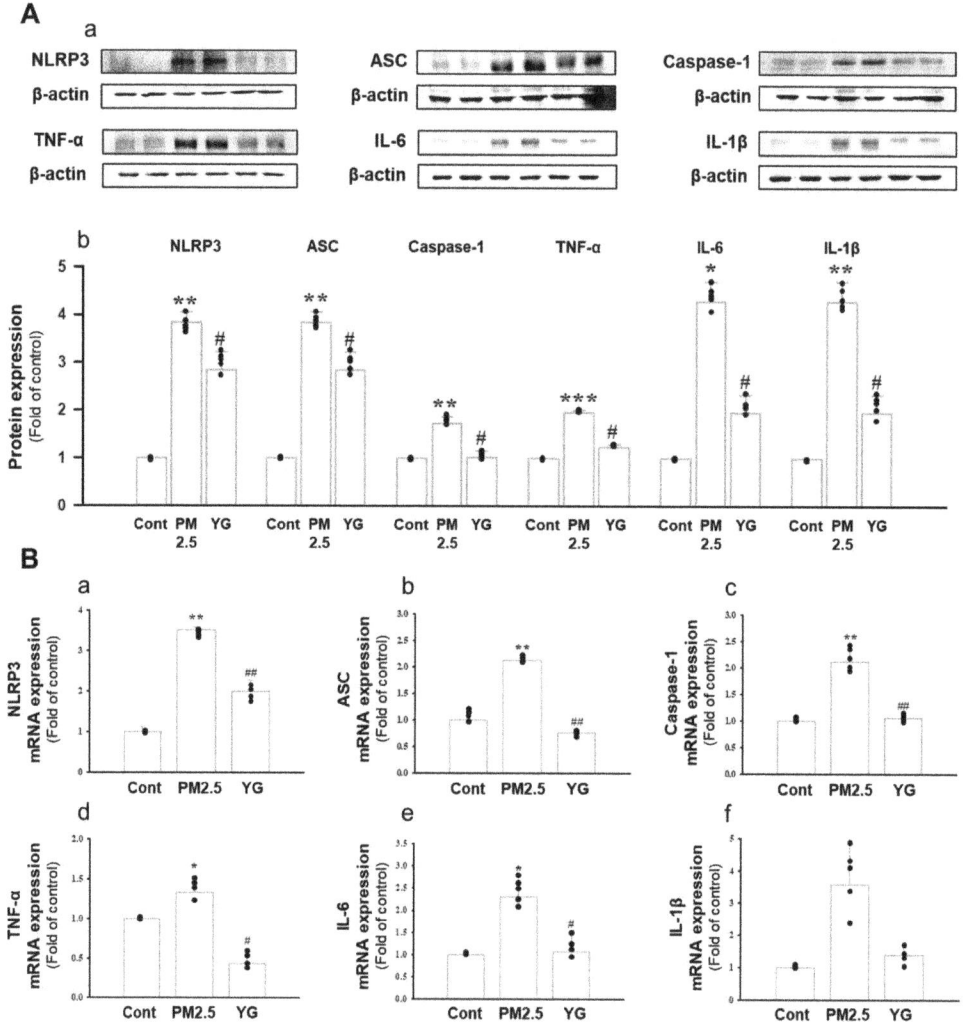

Figure 8. Treatment of YG-1 extract improved lung injury in fine particulate matter (PM2.5)-stimulated mice. Increased protein expression of NLRP-3, ASC, caspase-1, TNF-α, IL-6, and IL-1β inflammatory cytokines in PM2.5 stimulated mice was improved by YG-1 treatment (**A**). Lung injury in PM2.5 stimulated mice increased NLRP-3, caspase-1, TNF-α, IL-6, and IL-1β mRNA levels and was inhibited by YG-1 treatment (**B**). β-actin was used as loading controls for protein and mRNA expressions. Cont, control; PM2.5, PM2.5 exposure mice; YG-1, PM2.5 exposure mice + YG-1 treated (200 mg/kg/daily, orally); NLRP-3, NOD-like receptor pyrin domain-containning protein 3; ASC, apoptosis-associated speck-like protein containing a C-terminal caspase recruitment domain; TNF-α, tumor necrosis factor alpha; IL-6, interleukin 6; IL-1β, interleukin 1 beta. Data are expressed as mean ± standard error. * $p < 0.05$, ** $p < 0.01$, *** $p < 0.001$ vs. control; # $p < 0.05$, ## $p < 0.01$ vs. PM2.5.

4. Discussion

This study was conducted using YG-1 extract mixed with *Lonicera japonica, Arctii Fructus,* and *Scutellariae Radix*, which are natural products used for respiratory diseases in actual clinical practice. The YG-1 mixed extract was prepared so that natural products could create synergy, and the bronchodilation effect of the YG-1 extract was confirmed. We also evaluated the anti-inflammatory effects of YG-1 in a mouse model of acute bronchial and lung inflammation exposed in PM2.5 exposure mice.

The two most common bronchodilators used to reverse airway constriction act through stimulation of β_2-adrenergic receptors (such as salmeterol) or antagonism of muscarinic receptors (such as ipratropium) [23]. In our study, the relaxation effect of YG-1 is mediated through β2-adrenergic receptor stimulation. When β-adrenergic receptor (β_2-AR) and protein kinase A were blocked by propranolol and KT5720, the bronchodilation effect induced by YG-1 was specifically inhibited. When β_2-AR and protein kinase A were blocked by propranolol and KT5720 [24], YG-1 induced bronchodilatation was inhibited.

It is generally accepted that stimulation of β_2-adrenergic receptors increases cyclic adenosine monophosphate (cAMP) levels to mediate airway smooth muscle cell relaxation by activating adenylyl cyclase via the receptor-associated G protein. Respiratory disorders, such as asthma and sore throat, induce contraction of airway smooth muscle cells and airway hyperresponsiveness [25]. To alleviate these acute and chronic airway constrictions, β-adrenergic agonists that relax airway smooth muscle cells are usually administered [24]. The mechanism of action of cAMP is to induce airway smooth muscle cell expansion through stimulation of protein kinase A (PKA) [26,27]. Acts via the cAMP-linked intracellular pathway in airway smooth muscle relaxation, suggesting that it may be an important secondary messenger in bronchodilation [28]. Our study found that increased cAMP production due to YG-1 treatment was significantly reduced by PKA blockers, which resulted in bronchial dilation through beta-AR/PKA pathways. Therefore, YG-1 extract is considered to be of sufficient value as a bronchodilator.

Excessive exposure to PM2.5 gradually adsorbs to the bronchi and lungs and progresses to acute respiratory distress syndrome, eventually requiring bronchodilation for breathing [29,30]. Therefore, YG-1 extract with bronchodilating effect was applied to animal models of acute bronchial and pulmonary inflammation. PM2.5 is a very tiny particle size that can reach almost any organ in the body through blood flow [30]. In particular, the respiratory airway is a tissue that PM2.5 directly affects through respiration. High PM2.5 concentrations in the atmosphere have been reported to increase heart and respiratory diseases [31].

Inflammation is a complex pathophysiological process, and it is the expression of a biological defense mechanism against various types of infection or irritants among in vivo metabolites [32]. The main symptoms of the inflammatory reaction are fever, redness, pain, and edema. Nonsteroidal anti-inflammatory drugs are mainly used for the treatment of symptoms, but they are accompanied by various side effects such as gastrointestinal disorders and renal toxicity [33]. Inflammation releases mediators that can induce organ contraction, mucus secretion, and structural changes. TGF-β has been shown to affect many structural cells in vitro and in vivo and implicated in asthma and other inflammatory and immune-mediated lung and bronchial remodeling processes. [34]. We confirmed the increase in airway smooth muscle expression of TGF-1 through the dyeing of bronchial tubes and lung tissue, and confirmed that it was improved by YG-1 extract. TGF-b1 is widely known in many institutions. When structural immune cells and asthma deteriorate, TGF-β1 expression increases in the airway epithelial, which is the main expression area [35,36] Because, PM2.5 has a wide impact on human health [37], it is very important of research to evaluate the improvement effectiveness of YG-1 extracts in PM2.5 inhalation acute lung inflammation-causing mice. Our study used C57BL/6 mice to evaluate the potential mechanism of acute lung inflammation induced by PM2.5 and to confirm the efficacy of YG-1. Additionally, actors involved in the regulation of the proinflammatory cytokines, and IL-1β were also investigated in this model. Exposure to PM2.5 is characterized by the appearance of emphysema and inflammation [38]. In our study, lung histopathology and proinflammatory cytokine levels were detected to assess lung inflammation. As shown in Figures 5 and 6, PM2.5 exposure revealed marked pulmonary inflammation in the peribronchial, perivascular and alveolar spaces of the lung. Previous studies have confirmed that the inflammasome promotes inflammation in a mouse model of PM2.5-induced lung inflammation and that the chronic inflammatory response triggered by various immune cells is important [39,40]. The NOD-like receptor protein 3 (NLRP3) inflammasome is an intracellular multiprotein complex that includes NLRP3, apoptotic speck protein (ASC) and pro-caspase-1 [41]. Pro-interleukin-1β (IL-1β) and pro-IL-18 are converted to mature bioactive forms and released into the extracellular space [36]. IL-1β is a pro-inflammatory cytokine involved as an effector of the NLRP3 inflammasome and is known to increase the incidence of respiratory diseases induced by PM2.5 [42]. As reported in several studies, PM2.5 exposure is known to induce pulmonary inflammation by inducing IL-1β signaling activation [43], and YG-1 extract was found to reduce this in our study. In addition, activation of the NLRP3 inflammasome is known to accelerate pulmonary fibrosis caused by airborne particulate matter [44]. Also, Airway remodeling, one of the main characteristics, shows an increase in airway smooth muscle mass [45]. By contrast, YG extract was confirmed to reduce fibrosis. Various studies have shown that activation of the NLRP3/caspase-1 pathway contributes to the inflammatory response through the onset of diseases such as airway inflammation and chronic obstructive pulmonary disease including pulmonary fibrosis [44]. In addition, it has been reported that TLR4 mainly contributes to the cytokine production induced by PM2.5 [45]. It is known that NLRP3 activates caspase-1 to cleavage pro-IL-1β into mature IL-1β, thereby increasing the expression of inflammatory cytokines to induce inflammation [46,47]. Therefore, in our study, profibrotic pro-inflammatory cytokines such as IL-1β, IL-6, IL-8, and TNF-a [48] were increased in mice exposed to PM2.5. On the other hand, treatment with YG-1 extract decreased the expression of profibrotic cytokines induced by PM2.5 stimulation. Our results suggest that YG-1 extract targeting β-AR signaling in PM2.5-induced airway formation and lung inflammation reduces the production of inflammatory cytokines (IL-6, IL-8, and IL-1β) (Figure 9). Therefore, YG-1 extract is an effective therapeutic strategy for PM2.5-related airway and lung inflammation.

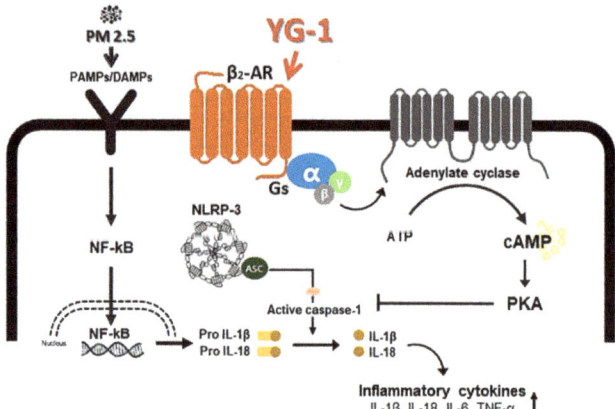

Figure 9. A schematic diagram of the effect of YG-1 extract on airway remodeling in fine particulate matter (PM2.5)-stimulated mice. YG-1 extract improved bronchial and lung inflammation by inhibiting NLRP3/caspase-1 signaling through $β_2$-adrenergic receptor stimulation in PM2.5 stimulated mice. Cont, control; PM2.5, fine particulate matter; Gs, G protein; α, G protein alpha subunit; β, G protein beta subunit; γ, G protein gamma subunit; $β_2$-AR, $β_2$ adrenergic receptor; ATP, adenosine triphosphate; cAMP, cyclic adenosine monophosphate; PKA, protein kinase A; NF-κB, nuclear factor kappa-light-chain-enhancer of activated B cells; Gs, G-protein subtype; NLRP-3, NOD-like receptor pyrin domain-containning protein 3; IL-. 1β, Interleukin 1 beta; IL-18, Interleukin 18; TNF-α, tumor necrosis factor alpha.

However, two major limitations of this study currently need to be acknowledged and addressed. First, unfortunately, chemical compounds were analyzed for YG-1 extract, but related studies were not performed. Second, since our results were conducted only on acute lung and bronchial inflammation caused by PM2.5, including the bronchodilatation effect of YG-1, additional studies on chronic diseases are needed.

5. Conclusions

In summary, YG-1 extract is considered to have an effect of bronchodilation by increased cAMP levels through the β2-adrenergic receptor/PKA pathway. In addition, PM2.5 exposure was involved in airway remodeling and inflammation, suggesting that YG-1 treatment improves acute bronchial and pulmonary inflammation by inhibited the inflammatory cytokines. Therefore, these results can provide basic data for the development of novel respiratory symptom relievers.

Author Contributions: H.-S.L. important comments and discussions; D.-S.K. performed extraction and compositional analysis of YG-1 extract; H.-Y.K. and J.-J.Y. designed and conducted experiments and analyzed the data. H.-Y.K. wrote the original text. H.-S.L. and D.-G.K. edited the manuscript. All authors have read and agreed to the published version of the manuscript.

Funding: Our research was supported by the National Research Foundation of Korea (NRF-2017R1A5 A2015805 to H.S.L.; NRF-2019R1I1A3A01062432 to H.Y.K.).

Institutional Review Board Statement: The study was conducted according to the guidelines of the Declaration of Helsinki, and approved by the Animal Experiment Ethics Committee of Wonkwang University (protocol code, WKU20-28; and date of approval, 30 March 2021)

Informed Consent Statement: Informed consent was obtained from all subjects involved in the study.

Data Availability Statement: Not applicable.

Acknowledgments: The authors would like to thank D.S. Kim of Hanpoong Pharm and Foods Co. (Wanju, Korea) for providing the YG-1 extract.

Conflicts of Interest: The authors declare they have no conflict of interest.

References

1. Matera, M.G.; Page, L.; Calzetta, P.; Cazzola, M. Pharmacology and therapeutics of bronchodilators revisited. *Pharmacol. Rev.* **2020**, *72*, 218–252. [CrossRef] [PubMed]
2. Cazzola, M.; Page, C.P.; Calzetta, L.; Matera, M.G. Pharmacology and therapeutics of bronchodilators. *Pharmacol. Rev.* **2012**, *64*, 450–504. [CrossRef] [PubMed]
3. An, S.S.; Fredberg, J.J. Biophysical basis for airway hyperresponsiveness. *Can. J. Physiol. Pharmacol.* **2007**, *85*, 700–714. [CrossRef] [PubMed]
4. Xing, Y.F.; Xu, Y.H.; Shi, M.H.; Lian, Y.X. The impact of PM2.5 on the human respiratory system. *J. Thorac. Dis.* **2016**, *8*, E69–E74. [PubMed]
5. Kim, H.H. Allergic rhinitis, sinusitis and asthma—Evidence for respiratory system integration. *Korean J. Pediatr.* **2007**, *50*, 335–339. [CrossRef]
6. Shin, D.C. Health effects of ambient particulate matter. *J. Korean Med. Assoc.* **2007**, *50*, 175–182. [CrossRef]
7. Kim, D.S.; Bae, G.; Kim, S.K.; LEE, H.S.; Kim, Y.J.; Lee, S.H. Retrospective drug utilization review of antibiotics for respiratory tract infection(RTI) in ambulatory outpatient care. *Korean J. Clin. Pharm.* **2012**, *22*, 291–303.
8. Atkinson, R.W.; Carey, I.M.; Kent, A.J.; Van Staa, T.P.; Anderson, H.R.; Cook, D.G. Long-term exposure to outdoor air pollution and the incidence of chronic obstructive pulmonary disease in a national English cohort. *Occup. Environ. Med.* **2015**, *72*, 42–48. [CrossRef]
9. Zhao, B.; Zheng, H.; Wang, S. Change in household fuels dominates the decrease in PM2.5 exposure and premature mortality in China in 2005. *Proc. Natl. Acad. Sci. USA* **2018**, *115*, 12401–12406. [CrossRef]
10. Schultz, E.S.; Litonjua, A.A.; Melen, E. Effects of long-term exposure to traffic-related air pollution on lung function in children. *Curr. Allergy Asthma Rep.* **2017**, *17*, 41. [CrossRef]
11. Huang, W.; Wang, G.; Lu, S.E. Inflammatory and oxidative stress responses of healthy young adults to changes in air quality during the Beijing olympics. *Am. J. Respir. Crit. Care Med.* **2012**, *186*, 1150–1159. [CrossRef]
12. Ogino, K. Allergic airway infammation by nasal inoculation of particulate matter (PM2.5) in nc/nga mice. *PLoS ONE* **2014**, *9*, e92710. [CrossRef]

13. Wang, H. The acute airway infammation induced bypm2.5 exposure and the treatment of essential oils in balb/c mice. *Sci. Rep.* **2017**, *7*, 44256. [CrossRef]
14. Mahemuti, G.; Zhang, H.; Li, J.; Tieliwaerdi, N.; Ren, L. Efficacy and side effects of intravenous theophylline in acute asthma: A systematic review and meta-analysis. *Drug Des. Devel. Ther.* **2018**, *12*, 99–120. [CrossRef]
15. Huang, J.; Pansare, M. New treatments for asthma. *Pediatr. Clin. N. Am.* **2019**, *66*, 925–939. [CrossRef]
16. Mushtaq, S.; Abbasi, B.H.; Uzair, B.; Abbasi, R. Natural products as reservoirs of novel therapeutic agents. *EXCLI J* **2018**, *4*, 420–451.
17. Lee, Y.C.; Kwon, T.H.; Ok, I.S.; Seo, C.W.; Kim, Y.J.; Roh, S.S.; Seo, Y.B. The experimental studies on the immunomodulational effects of Lonicerae Caulis et Folium: The effects of Lonicerae Caulis et Folium on cytokines production in mice splenocytes. *Korea J. Herbol.* **2005**, *20*, 141–149.
18. Nam, J.Y.; Kim, D.G.; Lee, J.Y. Effects of Woobangja on anti-allergic inflammation. *J. Pediatrics Korean Med.* **2006**, *20*, 241–255.
19. Cho, S.H.; Kim, Y.R. Antimicrobial characteristics of Scutellariae Radix extract. *J. Korean Soc. Food Sci. Nutr.* **2001**, *30*, 964–968.
20. Song, I.B.; Na, J.Y.; Song, K.B.; Kim, S.H.; Lee, J.H.; Kwon, Y.B.; Kim, D.K.; Kim, D.S.; Jo, H.K.; Kwon, J.K. Effects of extract mixture (Yg-1) of anti-inflammatory herbs on LPS-induced acute inflammation in macrophages and rats. *J. Korean Soc. Food Sci. Nutr.* **2015**, *44*, 49–505. [CrossRef]
21. Wu, H.; Yang, S.; Wu, X.; Zhao, J.; Zhao, J.; Ning, Q.; Xu, Y.; Xie, J. Interleukin-33/ST2 signaling promotes production of interleukin-6 and interleukin-8 in systemic inflammation in cigarette smoke-induced chronic obstructive pulmonary disease mice. *Biochem. Biophys. Res. Commun.* **2014**, *450*, 110–116. [CrossRef]
22. Sun, Q.; Yue, P.; Deiuliis, J.A.; Lumeng, C.N.; Kampfrath, T.; Mikolaj, M.B.; Cai, Y.; Ostrowski, M.C.; Lu, B.; Parthasarathy, S. Ambient air pollution exaggerates adipose inflammation and insulin resistance in a mouse model of diet-induced obesity. *Circulation* **2009**, *119*, 538–546. [CrossRef] [PubMed]
23. Lee, M.K.; Lim, K.H.; Millns, P.; Mohankumar, S.K.; Ng, S.T.; Tan, C.S. Bronchodilator effects of Lignosus rhinocerotis extract on rat isolated airways is linked to the blockage of calcium entry. *Phytomedicine* **2018**, *42*, 172–179. [CrossRef] [PubMed]
24. Sozzani, S.; Agwu, D.E.; McCall, C.E.; O'Flaherty, J.T.; Schmitt, J.D.; Kent, J.D.; McPhail, L.C. Propranolol, a phosphatidate phosphohydrolase inhibitor, also inhibits protein kinase C. *J. Biol. Chem.* **1992**, *267*, 20481–20488. [CrossRef]
25. Global Initiative for Asthma. *Global Strategy for Asthma Management and Prevention National Institute of Health 2002*; NIH: Bethesda, MD, USA, 2002; No. 02-3659.
26. Yang, C.M.; Hsu, M.C.; Tsao, H.L.; Chiu, C.T.; Ong, R.; Hsieh, J.T.; Fan, L.W. Effect of cAMP elevating agents on carbachol-induced phosphoinositide hydrolysis and calcium mobilization in cultured canine tracheal smooth muscle cells. *Cell Calcium.* **1996**, *19*, 243–254. [CrossRef]
27. Hoiting, B.H.; Meurs, H.; Schuiling, M.; Kuipers, R.; Elzinga, C.R.; Zaagsma, J. Modulation of agonist-induced phosphoinositide metabolism, Ca^{2+} signalling and contraction of airway smooth muscle by cyclic AMP-dependent mechanisms. *Br. J. Pharmacol.* **1996**, *117*, 419–426. [CrossRef]
28. McGrogan, I.; Lu, S.; Hipworth, S.; Sormaz, L.; Eng, R.; Preocanin, D.; Daniel, E.E. Mechanisms of cyclic nucleotide-induced relaxation in canine tracheal smooth muscle. *Am. J. Physiol.* **1995**, *268*, L407–L413. [CrossRef]
29. Gao, Y.; Lv, J.; Lin, Y.; Li, X.; Wang, L.; Yin, Y.; Liu, Y. Effects of beta-adrenoceptor subtypes on cardiac function in myocardial infarction rats exposed to fine particulate matter (PM 2.5). *Biomed. Res. Int.* **2014**, *2014*, 308295. [CrossRef]
30. Nel, A. Air pollution-related illness: Effects of particles. *Science* **2005**, *308*, 804–806. [CrossRef]
31. Kyung, S.Y.; Jeong, S.H. Particulate-matter related respiratory diseases. *Tuberc. Respir. Dis.* **2020**, *83*, 116–121. [CrossRef]
32. Aghasafari, P.; George, U.; Pidaparti, R. A review of inflammatory mechanism in airway diseases. *Inflamm. Res.* **2019**, *68*, 59–74. [CrossRef]
33. Bonini, M.; Usmani, O.S. The role of the small airways in the pathophysiology of asthma and chronic obstructive pulmonary disease. *Ther. Adv. Respir. Dis.* **2015**, *9*, 281–293. [CrossRef]
34. Coker, R.K.; Laurent, G.J.; Shahzeidi, S.; Hernandez-Rodriguez, N.A.; Pantelidis, P.; Du Bois, R.M.; Jeffery, P.K.; McAnulty, R.J. Diverse cellular TGF-beta 1and TGF-beta 3 gene expression in normal human and murine lung. *Eur. Respir. J.* **1996**, *9*, 2501–2507. [CrossRef]
35. Fukatsu, H.; Koide, N.; Tada-Oikawa, S. NF-κB inhibitor DHMEQ inhibits titanium dioxide nanoparticle-induced interleukin-1β production: Inhibition of the PM2.5-induced inflammation model. *Mol. Med. Rep.* **2018**, *18*, 5279–5285. [CrossRef]
36. Xu, F.; Qiu, X.; Hu, X. Effects on IL-1β signaling activation induced by water and organic extracts of fine particulate matter (PM(2.5)) in vitro. *Environ. Pollut.* **2018**, *237*, 592–600. [CrossRef]
37. Feng, S.; Gao, D.; Liao, F.; Zhou, F.; Wang, X. The health effects of ambient PM2.5 and potential mechanisms. *Ecotoxicol. Environ. Saf.* **2016**, *128*, 67–74. [CrossRef]
38. Zheng, X.Y.; Tong, L.; Shen, D. Airborne bacteria enriched PM2.5 enhances the inflammation in an allergic adolescent mouse model induced by ovalbumin. *Inflammation* **2020**, *43*, 32–43. [CrossRef]
39. Li, C.; Chen, J.; Yuan, W.; Zhang, W.; Chen, H.; Tan, H. Preventive effect of ursolic acid derivative on particulate matter 2.5-induced chronic obstructive pulmonary disease involves suppression of lung inflammation. *IUBMB Life* **2020**, *72*, 632–640. [CrossRef]
40. Zhu, Y.; Zhu, C.; Yang, H.; Deng, J.; Fan, D. Protective effect of ginsenoside Rg5 against kidney injury via inhibition of NLRP3 inflammasome activation and the MAPK signaling pathway in high-fat diet/streptozotocin-induced diabetic mice. *Pharmacol. Res.* **2020**, *155*, 104746. [CrossRef]

41. Zhou, Y.; Zhang, C.Y.; Duan, J.X. Vasoactive intestinal peptide suppresses the NLRP3 inflammasome activation in lipopolysaccharideinduced acute lung injury mice and macrophages. *Biomed. Pharmacother.* **2020**, *121*, 109596. [CrossRef]
42. Provoost, S.; Maes, T.; Pauwels, N.S. NLRP3/caspase-1-independent IL-1beta production mediates diesel exhaust particle-induced pulmonary inflammation. *J. Immunol.* **2011**, *187*, 3331–3337. [CrossRef] [PubMed]
43. Chen, H.; Ding, Y.; Chen, W.; Feng, Y.; Shi, G. Glibenclamide alleviates inflammation in oleic acid model of acute lung injury through NLRP3 inflammasome signaling pathway. *Drug Des. Devel. Ther.* **2019**, *13*, 1545–1554. [CrossRef] [PubMed]
44. Zheng, R.; Tao, L.; Jian, H. NLRP3 inflammasome activation and lung fibrosis caused by airborne fine particulate matter. *Ecotoxicol. Environ. Saf.* **2018**, *163*, 612–619. [CrossRef] [PubMed]
45. Postma, D.S.; Timens, W. Remodeling in asthma and chronic obstructive pulmonary disease. *Proc. Am. Thorac. Soc.* **2006**, *3*, 434–439. [CrossRef]
46. Lucas, K.; Maes, M. Role of the toll like receptor (TLR) radical cycle in chronic inflammation: Possible treatments targeting the TLR4 pathway. *Mol. Neurobiol.* **2013**, *48*, 190–204. [CrossRef]
47. Kingston, H.G.; Dungan, M.L.; Sarah, A.; Jones, A.; Harris, J. The role of inflammasome-derived IL-1 in driving IL-17 responses. *J. Leukoc. Biol.* **2013**, *93*, 489–497.
48. Kong, F. Curcumin represses NLRP3 inflammasome activation via TLR4/MyD88/NF-κB and P2X7R Signaling in PMA induced macrophages. *Front. Pharmacol.* **2016**, *7*, 00369. [CrossRef]

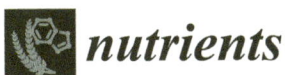

Review

Natural Products for Pancreatic Cancer Treatment: From Traditional Medicine to Modern Drug Discovery

Ahyeon Kim [1,†], Jiwon Ha [1,†], Jeongeun Kim [1], Yongmin Cho [2,3], Jimyung Ahn [2], Chunhoo Cheon [3], Sung-Hoon Kim [2], Seong-Gyu Ko [3] and Bonglee Kim [1,2,3,*]

[1] College of Korean Medicine, Kyung Hee University, Seoul 02447, Korea; ahyeon8022@khu.ac.kr (A.K.); jiwooonha@khu.ac.kr (J.H.); kje654@khu.ac.kr (J.K.)
[2] Department of Pathology, College of Korean Medicine, Kyung Hee University, Seoul 02447, Korea; ymcho@khu.ac.kr (Y.C.); skyajm911@khu.ac.kr (J.A.); sungkim7@khu.ac.kr (S.-H.K.)
[3] Korean Medicine-Based Drug Repositioning Cancer Research Center, College of Korean Medicine, Kyung Hee University, Seoul 02447, Korea; hreedom@khu.ac.kr (C.C.); epiko@khu.ac.kr (S.-G.K.)
* Correspondence: bongleekim@khu.ac.kr; Tel.: +82-2-961-9217
† These authors contributed equally to this work.

Abstract: Pancreatic cancer, the seventh most lethal cancer around the world, is considered complicated cancer due to poor prognosis and difficulty in treatment. Despite all the conventional treatments, including surgical therapy and chemotherapy, the mortality rate is still high. Therefore, the possibility of using natural products for pancreatic cancer is increasing. In this study, 68 natural products that have anti-pancreatic cancer effects reported within five years were reviewed. The mechanisms of anti-cancer effects were divided into four types: apoptosis, anti-metastasis, anti-angiogenesis, and anti-resistance. Most of the studies were conducted for natural products that induce apoptosis in pancreatic cancer. Among them, plant extracts such as *Eucalyptus microcorys* account for the major portion. Some natural products, including *Moringa*, Coix seed, etc., showed multi-functional properties. Natural products could be beneficial candidates for treating pancreatic cancer.

Keywords: pancreatic cancer; natural product; traditional medicine; apoptosis; angiogenesis; metastasis; drug resistance

Citation: Kim, A.; Ha, J.; Kim, J.; Cho, Y.; Ahn, J.; Cheon, C.; Kim, S.-H.; Ko, S.-G.; Kim, B. Natural Products for Pancreatic Cancer Treatment: From Traditional Medicine to Modern Drug Discovery. *Nutrients* **2021**, *13*, 3801. https://doi.org/10.3390/nu13113801

Academic Editor: Md Soriful Islam

Received: 22 September 2021
Accepted: 21 October 2021
Published: 26 October 2021

Publisher's Note: MDPI stays neutral with regard to jurisdictional claims in published maps and institutional affiliations.

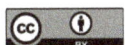

Copyright: © 2021 by the authors. Licensee MDPI, Basel, Switzerland. This article is an open access article distributed under the terms and conditions of the Creative Commons Attribution (CC BY) license (https:// creativecommons.org/licenses/by/ 4.0/).

1. Introduction

Pancreatic cancer is a disease in which malignant cancer cells develop in the tissue of the pancreas. Due to concealed clinical manifestation, limited treatment options, and side effects, pancreatic cancer is considered one of the most difficult cancers to treat. Jaundice, belly or back pain, poor appetite, and weight loss are typical signs and symptoms of pancreatic cancer [1]. The cure rate for this disease is only 9%, and if not treated, the median survival of patients with metastatic disease is only about three months worldwide [2]. According to GLOBOCAN 2018, 458,918 cases were newly diagnosed, and 432,242 deaths were reported worldwide in 2018. These rates account for 2.5% and 4.5% of all cancer cases globally in 2018. Pancreatic cancer was estimated to be the seventh most common cancer in both men and women. Meanwhile, pancreatic cancer was more common in developed countries, including Europe, North America, East Asia, and Australia [3].

Surgical resection is well known as the most effective treatment for pancreatic cancer. Because there are many cases in which surgical resection is not available due to late presentation, chemotherapy is often used as adjuvant treatment [4]. FOLFIRINOX and gemcitabine/albumin-bound nab-paclitaxel are considered the first-line treatment against pancreatic cancer. For patients with BRCA1/2 and PALB2 mutations, gemcitabine/cisplatin is a suitable treatment. Because the selection of an available treatment depends on a number of factors, including patient preference, comorbidities, goals of treatment, and predictive biomarkers, treatment is not quite so simple in fact [2]. In addition, the risk of recurrence and the possibility of side effects remain. Therefore, using only existing drugs is not enough for covering pancreatic cancer, and it is essential to develop some new drugs.

Traditional medicine around the world, including China, Japan, Thailand, India, and Korea, is drawing attention these days. Traditional Chinese medicine (TCM) has been widely used in China using treatments accumulated over thousands of years. Thus, TCM occupies an important position throughout traditional medicine. Traditional Thai medicine (TTM) is a Buddhism-based health care system in Thailand that includes herbal medicine, massage, midwifery, etc. [5]. Ayurveda medicine in India, which emphasizes 'balance', has been with Indians in their daily lives for more than 5000 years [6]. Traditional Korean medicine (TKM) is a unique medicine that has developed independently for 5000 years [7]. TKM has established its own medical identity, through *Euibangyoochui*, *Donguibogam* compiled by Jun Heo and Sasang constitutional medicine established by Je-ma Lee [8]. Treatments of TKM such as acupuncture, moxibustion, and herbal medicine are still widely used today. TKM attracted worldwide attention with the growth of complementary and alternative medicine (CAM). In particular, natural product-based herbal medicine is currently expected to be a novel treatment of several diseases including cancer, due to its effectiveness and lack of serious side effects [9].

Anticancer effects of natural products are being proved through experimental studies in various types of cancers, such as lung, breast, colon, and prostate cancer. Several natural compounds, including curcumin, resveratrol, berberine, baicalein, dioscin, wogonin, piperine, etc., were reported to have an anti-cancer effect [10–16]. In addition, natural product-derived compounds are known to induce apoptosis in cancer cells rather than in normal cells [17]. Thus, natural products will play a key role as a novel cancer treatment for the next decade.

Most representative anti-cancer mechanisms include: apoptosis, anti-metastasis, anti-angiogenesis, resistance, etc. Apoptosis or programmed cell death (PCD) is a prime cellular mechanism to control cell proliferation and remove harmful or unnecessary cells from an organism [18]. Apoptosis can be regulated by targeting Bcl-2 family members and caspases. Meanwhile, some defects in the process of apoptosis can lead to tumor metastasis and resistance [19]. Metastasis means that malignant cancer cells spread from primary tumors to other sites, thereby resisting treatment and causing organ dysfunction [20]. Anti-angiogenesis is a process that inhibits novel blood vessels formed in pre-existing ones. Resistance is a mechanism that decreases the effect of anticancer drugs, typically driven by irreversible genetic mutations [21].

Therefore, we aim to review the experimental studies about natural products against pancreatic cancer, analyzing original research in terms of apoptosis, anti-metastasis, anti-angiogenesis, and resistance. Only studies published in the last five years were included in this paper. Several natural compounds which were combined with radiotherapy or enhanced the anticancer activity of gemcitabine are also reviewed. Furthermore, our present study included clinical trials which were conducted to evaluate the efficacy and safety of natural products when treating pancreatic cancer.

2. Apoptosis Inducing Natural Products

Apoptosis, known as programmed cell death is regarded as a significant component of numerous processes including defense mechanisms like immune responses, when cells are damaged by disease or toxic agents [22]. Inadequate apoptosis, too much or too little, can lead to a variety of diseases, including many types of cancer such as pancreatic cancer. Apoptosis is one of the major target mechanisms when treating cancer. It has been observed that a wide variety of natural products trigger apoptosis, but they do not affect the cell lines to die in the same mechanism.

2.1. Apoptosis Inducing Fungi

Five natural products from fungi were reported to have an apoptotic effect on pancreatic cancer cells (Table 1).

Table 1. Apoptosis inducing fungi.

Classification	Compound/Extract	Source	Cell Line/Animal Model	Dose; Duration	Efficacy	Mechanism	Reference
Fungus	Agaricus blazei Murrill water extract	Agaricus blazei Murrill	MIA PaCa-2, PCI-35, PK-8	0.005, 0.015, 0.045%(w/v); 48 h	Induction of apoptosis	↑c-caspase-3, -9, c-PARP	[23]
Fungus	Chaetospirolactone	Chaetomium sp. NF00754	HPDE6c-7, AsPC-1, PANC-1	100 nM; 18 h	Induction of apoptosis	↑c-caspase-3, -8, -9 ↓EZH2	[24]
			AsPC-1-bearing BALB/c mice	0.075 mg/kg; 28 days		↑c-caspase-3	
Fungus	Dicatenarin	Penicillium pinophilum	MIA PaCa-2	20 µg/mL; 48 h	Induction of apoptosis	↑cytochrome c, caspase-3	[25]
Fungus	Skyrin	Penicillium pinophilum	MIA PaCa-2	50 µg/mL; 48 h	Induction of apoptosis	↑cytochrome c, caspase-3	
Fungus	Xylarione A (-) 5-methylmellein	Xylaria psidii	MIA PaCa-2	10, 30, 50 µm; 24 h	Induction of apoptosis	↓MMP	[26]

c-caspase, cleaved caspase; PARP, poly adenosine diphosphate ribose polymerase; MMP (ΔΨm), Mitochondrial membrane potential; ↑—up-regulation; ↓—down-regulation.

Agaricus blazei Murrill is the most frequently used medicinal mushroom in Japan. Matsushita et al. showed that its water extract (AbE) induced cell cycle arrest and increased nuclear fragmentation [22]. Cleavages of caspase-3, -9, and PARP1 indicate that AbE induces apoptosis via caspase-dependent pathway. In addition, overexpression of the genes which encode proapoptotic proteins, such as DEDD2, DAPK3, and NLRP1, was observed after AbE treatment.

Chaetospirolactone is a natural product that is isolated from the endophytic fun-gus *Chaetomium* sp. NF00754 [23]. Both in vitro and in vivo, chaetospirolactone induced apoptosis without interrupting the normal pancreatic cells of HPDE6c-7 cell line. Chaetospirolactone treatment sensitized AsPC-1 and PANC-1 cells, which are TRAIL (Tumor necrosis factor-related apoptosis inducing ligand)-resistant cells. As a result, TRAIL-mediated apoptosis occurred in a dose-dependent manner, and cleaved bands of caspase-8, -9, and -3 were detected.

Dicatenarin and Skyrin, secondary metabolites from fungus *Penicillium pinophilum*, induced apoptosis via reactive oxygen species (ROS)-mediated mitochondrial pathway in MIA PaCa-2 cells [24]. The activation of cytochrome c and caspase-3 and the loss of MTP were observed. Because of an additional phenolic hydroxyl group at C-4, dicatenarin could generate more ROS. Thus, dicatenarin is slightly more effective than skyrin as a pancreatic cancer treatment.

Both Xylarione A and (-) 5-methylmellein, which were isolated from fungus *Xylaria psidii*, induced cell cycle arrest and led to apoptosis [25]. Hence, 10, 30, and 50 µm of these compounds were treated for 24 h in MIA PaCa-2 cells. As a result, the MMP (mitochondrial membrane potential, ΔΨM) loss was observed, indicating that these compounds triggered apoptosis through mitochondrial damage.

2.2. Apoptosis Inducing Marine Sponge

One compound from the marine sponge was reported to have an apoptotic effect on pancreatic cancer cells (Table 2). Leiodermatolide, isolated from a marine sponge *Leiodermatium*, was treated to identify apoptosis in AsPC-1, BxPC-3, MIA PaCa-2, and PANC-1 cells [27]. In this study, cleavage of caspase-3 was most remarkable after 24 h of Leiodermatolide treatment in BxPC-3 and MIA PaCa-2 cells. In an orthotopic xenograft mouse model of pancreatic cancer, reduction of tumor weight was successful. However, the survival rate was not significantly increased.

Table 2. Apoptosis inducing marine sponge.

Classification	Compound/ Extract	Source	Cell Line/ Animal Model	Dose; Duration	Efficacy	Mechanism	Reference
Marine sponge	Leiodermatolide	*Leiodermatium*	AsPC-1, BxPC-3, MIA PaCa-2, PANC-1	10 nM; 24 h	Induction of apoptosis	↑c-caspase-3	[27]
			L3.6pl cells bearing mice	10 mg/kg; 3 weeks	Reduction of tumor weight		

↑—up-regulation.

2.3. Apoptosis Inducing Plants

Forty-three plant extracts and their compounds were reported to have apoptotic effects on pancreatic cancer cells (Table 3).

2.3.1. Natural Compounds from Plants

In a study, *Andrographis paniculata* 70% EtOH extracts showed 21 known compounds [28]. Lee et al. demonstrated that 14-deoxy-11,12-didehydroandrographolide (compound 17) had the strongest preferential toxicity against PANC-1 and PSN-1 cell lines. When the cell lines were treated with compound 17, apoptosis-like cell death appeared in a time- and dose-dependent manner.

The compound 2′,4′-Dihydroxy-6′-methoxy-3′,5′-dimethylchalcone (DMC) originated from *Cleistocalyx operculatus* [29]. When PANC-1 cells were exposed to 3, 10, and 30 μM of DMC for 48 h, activation of Bax, cytochrome c, c-caspase-3, -9, and c-PARP, and reduction of Bcl-2 were observed.

In addition, 5,7-dihydroxy-3,6,8-trimethoxyflavone (flavone A), extracted from *Gnaphalium elegans*, triggered apoptosis through the mitochondrial intrinsic pathway in PANC-28 cells which are relatively differentiated pancreatic cancer cells [30]. Meanwhile, 3,5-dihydroxy-6,7,8-trimethoxyflavone (flavone B), extracted from *Achyrocline bogotensis*, induced apoptosis through the extrinsic pathway in Mia-PaCa-2 cells which are relatively poorly differentiated pancreatic cancer cells.

Zhang et al. demonstrated that 8-Chrysoeriol mainly targets and inhibits Bcl-2, showing cytotoxicity against SW1990 cells overexpressed with Bcl-2 [31]. After SW1990 cells were exposed to 50 and 100 μM of 8-Chrysoeriol for 24 h, the rate of apoptotic cell death increased. Notably, at 100 μM, the rate surged to 79.8%.

Tian et al. reported that various cardiac glycosides, derived from seeds of *Thevetia peruviana*, had inhibitory effects on three cancer cell lines, namely P15, MGC-803, and SW1990, and one normal hepatocyte cell, LO2 [32]. Cardiac glycosides also turned out to have a selective inhibitory effect on three tumor cells.

Crocetinic acid, extracted from *Crocus sativus*, inhibited the proliferation of pancreatic cancer cells [33]. Fraction 5 had the strongest anti-cancer effect both in vitro and in vivo among five fractions isolated from commercial crocetin. In vitro, five fractions were treated to MiaPaCa-2 cells. In vivo, 6–8-weeks old athymic female mice bearing MiaPaCa-2 cells were treated with 0.5 mg/kg crocetinic acid for 21 days. Crocetinic acid up-regulated c-caspase 3 and Bax, and down-regulated PCNA, p-EGFR, p-AKT, and Bcl2, leading to apoptosis.

As a kind of steroid sapogenin, diosgenin is derived from *Solanum, Dioscorea,* and *Costus* species [34]. Diosgenin induced apoptotic cell death and cell cycle arrest in Patu8988 and PANC-1 cells. EZH2, which is known to be an oncogenic protein of several cancers, and its target vimentin was down-regulated in pancreatic cancer cells after diosgenin treatment.

Echinacoside (ECH), which is isolated from stems of *Cistanchessalsa*, induced apoptosis by elevating ROS and reducing MMP in SW1990 cells [35]. ROS elevation and MMP decrease have been reported to be necessary for the induction of apoptosis. Moreover, Wang et al. investigated that ECH upregulated the expression of Bax, which is triggered by the tumor suppressor p53. Further, ECH triggers apoptosis via mitogen-activated protein kinase (MAPK) pathway, suppressing JNK and ERK1/2 activity, while enhancing p38 activity. However, ECH did not affect AKT activity, which is also an important mechanism in cell proliferation.

Elemene, extracted from *Zingiberaceae* plants, inhibited cell proliferation and induced cell cycle arrest in a dose-dependent manner in BxPC-3 and PANC-1 cells [36]. Elemene treatment also had an apoptotic effect on in vivo model. In this study, up-regulation of p53 (tumor suppressor gene) and down-regulation of Bcl-2 (apoptosis-related gene) in BxPC-3 bearing BALB/c nude mice model were observed by Western blot method.

MicroRNAs (miRNA) are small non-coding RNA molecules which function in the post-transcriptional regulation of gene expression, and their functions are related to mRNA molecules [37]. Wang et al. demonstrated that grape seed proanthocyanidins (GSPs), an active component of *Vitis vinifera* (grape) seed, inhibited the growth in PANC-1 by modulating miRNA expression. GSPs down-regulated miRNA-SS3, SS12, and SS24, and also down-regulated CDK6, EGFR, MSH6, and DNMT1. This indicated that the negative co-expression correlations between DE miRNAs and target genes showed that GSPs may play an anti-cancer role by regulating miRNAs' expression.

Guha et al. demonstrated that hydroxychavicol induces apoptosis through JNK-dependent and caspase-mediated pathway [38]. The expression of c-caspase-3, -8, -9, c-Bid, c-PARP, and Bax increased, while the expression of Bcl-2 was suppressed in MIA PaCa-2 and PANC-1 cells after hydroxychavicol treatment. Notably, the activation of caspase-8 and -9 indicates that both extrinsic and intrinsic apoptotic pathways were induced in the hydroxychavicol-treated model.

Hyperoside and hypoxoside, which are natural prodrugs, induced caspase-dependent apoptosis against MIA PaCa-2 and INS-1 pancreatic cancer cells [39]. Activation of cleaved capase-3, a key factor of apoptosis, was remarkable in this study. These compounds also caused G2/M cell cycle arrest and a hydrolyzed form of hyperoside and hypoxoside showed selective cytotoxicity.

Icariin, purified from traditional chinese medicine *Herba Epimedii*, induced apoptosis and inhibited migration and proliferation in PANC-2 cells [40]. This study also included an in vivo experiment, treating 120 mg/kg of icariin in C57BL/6 mice for 11 days. The result showed that icariin affects the tumor immune microenvironment, thus inhibiting pancreatic cancer growth.

Isothiocyanates, major compounds of cruciferous vegetables, have been widely known to have cancer prevention effects [41]. Luo et al. showed that Methyl4-(2-isothiocyanatoethyl) benzoate (compound 6) and N-Ethyl-4-(2-isothiocyanatoethyl) benzamide (compound 7) especially had a more apoptotic effect in PANC-1 but were less noxious to non-cancer cells. Compound 7 up-regulated ROS, and down-regulated GSH, resulting in apoptosis of pancreatic cancer cells.

Mastic gum resin (MGR), isolated from *Pistacia atlantica* subspecies kurdica, at concentrations from 0.01 to 100 μM for 72 h enhanced apoptosis in PANC-1 [42]. Rahman demonstrated that the resin had the anti-proliferative effect not only in pancreatic cancer cells, but also in bile duct cancer, gastric adenocarcinoma, and colonic cancer.

Monogalactosyl diacylglycerol (MGDG), extracted from a spinach, induced apoptosis in cancer cells when it is used alone or with radiation [43]. The combination of MGDG and radiation resulted in a higher percentage of apoptosis than each single treatment, and also inhibited tumor growth in a mouse xenograft model. Meanwhile, up-regulated gene expression of cytochrome c, c-PARP, c-caspase-3, and Bax and down-regulation of Bcl-2 were observed in MIA PaCa-2 cells when treated with MGDG.

Wang et al. reported that piperlongumine, originated from the fruit of the pepper *Piper longum*, up-regulated the level of procaspase-3 and c-PARP in BxPC-3, PANC-1, and AsPC-1 cells [44]. In addition to in vitro experiments, in vivo model also showed anticancer activity against pancreatic cancer. In BxPC-3 bearing BALB/c mice treated with 10 mg/kg of piperlongumine for 21 days, tumor growth was significantly inhibited. When piperlongumine is combined with gemcitabine in vitro and In vivo, an apoptotic effect was enhanced. The expression of Bcl-2, Bcl-xL, survivin, XIAP, c-Myc, cyclin D1, COX-2, VEGF, and matrix metalloproteinase-9 (MMP-9), all of which are regulated by NF-κB, was decreased after combination treatment.

Karki et al. demonstrated that piperlongumine, an anti-cancer natural compound found in *Piper longum*, induced apoptosis and inhibited cell growth by inducing ROS in PANC-1 with 5 to 15 μmol/mL treatment [45]. In PANC-1 cells, a piperlongumine-induced ROS decrease triggered a down-regulation of miR-27a, miR-20a, and miR-17, which are miRNAs regulated by cMyc. Moreover, this results in the downregulation of Sp1, Sp3, and Sp4. These mechanisms are critically related to the action of piperlongumine against pancreatic cancer cells. L3.6pL bearing athymic nu/nu mice were treated with piperlongumine in the amount of 30 mg/kg for 21 days. Accompanying down-regulation of Sp1, Sp3, and Sp4, piperlongumin induced inhibition of tumor weight, without affecting body weight. Cotreatment with glutathione was effective both in vitro and in vivo.

Zhang et al. demonstrated that RN1, a polysaccharide from the flower of *Panax notoginseng*, inhibited PDAC cell growth both in vitro and In vivo, which is highly related to Gal-3 [46]. RN1 had a dose-dependent apoptotic effect on AsPC-1 and BxPC-3 cells, while having no effect on other cancer cells such as L-02 (normal liver cell line) and HPDE6-C7 (normal pancreatic cell line). RN1 specifically inhibited Gal-3 expression by binding to Gal-3, which inhibited the activation of the EGFR/ERK signaling pathway as well. Gal-3 expression was also inhibited by Runx1 In vitro. RN1 inhibited Gal-3 expression and down-regulated EGFR/ERK/Runx1 signaling In vivo. Thus, RN1 works as a novel Gal-3 inhibitor and is expected to be a potent anti-pancreatic cancer cell treatment via multiple mechanisms and pathways.

Rottlerin, which is isolated from *Mallotus philippinensis*, triggered cellular apoptosis in Patu8988 and PANC-1 cells [47]. An increase of cytochrome c release was observed. This compound also induced cell cycle arrest, inhibited cell proliferation, and delayed cell migration and invasion. When Skp2 (S-phase kinase associated protein 2) is overexpressed, cancer growth could not be suppressed effectively. In this study, the inactivation of Skp2 was significant after rottlerin treatment, indicating that rottlerin could be a potential agent for pancreatic cancer therapy.

Sugiol, a kind of diterpene, showed antiproliferative activity and induced apoptosis in Mia-PaCa2 cells [48]. Bax elevation and Bcl-2 depression suggest that sugiol triggered apoptosis through mitochondrial pathway. When the concentration of sugiol increased, intracellular ROS was up-regulated, whereas MMP level was down-regulated.

Several anticancer activities of Withaferin A (WA, a steroidal lactone isolated from *Withania somnifera*) and Carnosol (CA; an ortho-diphenolic diterpene included in rosemary, sage, and oregano) were demonstrated in this study [49]. WA and CA induced early apoptosis in AsPC-1 cells. However, late apoptosis and necrosis were insignificant. In terms of the HGF-mediated c-Met signaling pathway, phosphorylation of c-Met and Akt was attenuated. WA and CA also had an inhibitory effect on cell proliferation, cell migration, and cell cycle arrest.

Li et al. investigated whether WA suppresses proteasome activity and induces ER stress [50]. This WA-induced ER stress resulted in cellular apoptosis, and up-regulation of c-caspase-3, -8, -9, c-PARP1 was observed in PANC-1 and MIA PaCa-2 cells. Meanwhile, when WA is combined with a series of ER stress aggravators, c-PARP level elevates, and cell viability decreases, suggesting that the treatment enhanced apoptotic effect.

2.3.2. Plants Extracts

Bitter apricot ethanolic extract (BAEE) originated from *Prunus armeniaca* L. led to apoptosis through a mitochondrial-dependent pathway [51]. Therefore, the Bax/Bcl-2 ratio and level of caspase-3 were both increased in PANC-1 cells. To determine cell cytotoxicity, apoptosis, and necrosis, PANC-1 (human pancreatic cancer cells) and 293/KDR (normal epithelial cells) were used in this study. All cellular apoptosis occurred without affecting normal epithelial cells.

Non-polar stem extracts (SN) of *Clinacanthus nutans* were effective for inducing apoptosis in AsPC-1, BxPC-3, and SW1990 cells [52]. This compound up-regulated the level of Bax and down-regulated the level of Bcl-2, cIAP-2, and XIAP. The synergistic effect occurred when SN extracts were combined with gemcitabine, thereby improving anti-pancreatic cancer activity compared to those treated respectively.

Qian et al. showed that In vitro, pre-treatment with coix seed emulsion (CSE) significantly up-regulated caspase-3, c-PARP, and Bax, leading to the synergetic effect of gemcitabine in three types of pancreatic cancer cell lines: BxPC-3, PANC-1, and AsPC-1 [53]. Moreover, the pre-treatment down-regulated anti-apoptotic substances like Bcl-2, survivin, and COX-2. In vivo, co-treatment of coix seed emulsion and gemcitabine had a more potent apoptotic effect than using them separately. Six-week old male nude BALB/c mice bearing human BxPC-3 cells were treated with 12.5 mL/kg CSE for 24 days. This resulted in a decrease in p65. Conclusively, despite the CSE dose-dependently induced apoptotic effect in pancreatic cancer cell lines, the combination of CSE and gemcitabine turned out to be potent in pancreatic cancer than using them separately.

Cordifoliketones A is a compound extracted from Tsoong, the roots of *Codonopsis cordifolioidea* [54]. Luan et al. showed that treatment with cordifoliketones A inhibited growth and induced apoptosis of AsPC-1, BxPC-3, and PANC-1 both in vitro and in vivo. In vitro, treatment of 2, 4, and 6 µg/mL cordifoliketones A to three types of PDAC cells for 24 and 48 h turned out to have an apoptotic effect. Moreover, 6 µg/mL cordifoliketones A-treated groups showed stronger apoptosis compared to the other groups which were treated with different doses. Additionally, cordifoliketones A did not affect normal human cells. In vivo, BALB/c nude mice bearing human AsPC-1, BxPC-3, and PANC-1 cells alone (placebo) and mice bearing the same PDAC cells with the treatment with cordifoliketones A (control) were compared. It was proven that the control had a slower PDAC proliferation rate than the placebo.

Bhuyan et al. reported that *Eucalyptus microcorys* leaf aqueous extract had an antiproliferative effect against pancreatic cancer cells [55]. F1, which is one of the five major fractions of the extract, had an especially prominent apoptotic effect against MIA PaCa-2. F1 up-regulated Bak, Bax, c-PARP, and c-caspase-3, and down-regulated Bcl-2, procaspase-3, which led to apoptosis. Moreover, gemcitabine and F1 showed a synergistic apoptotic effect when combined.

Another study by Bhuyan et al. demonstrated that selected Eucalyptus species inhibited the growth of various cancer cells including lung and pancreatic cancer cells by more than 80% [56]. Aqueous and ethanolic *Eucalyptus microcorys* leaf extract, ethanolic *Eucalyptus microcorys* fruit extract, and *Eucalyptus saligna* ethanolic extract had an apoptotic effect in MIA PaCa-2. MIA PaCa-2, treated with 100 µg/mL aqueous *Eucalyptus microcorys* leaf and fruit extract for 24 h, showed significant apoptosis compared to other extracts. Growth inhibition was much stronger when MIA PaCa-2 was treated with 100 µg/mL than 50 µg/mL. The selected Eucalyptus species had a great apoptotic effect in MIA PaCa-2 compared to BxPC-3 and CFPAC-1.

Pak et al. showed that the herbal mixture ethanol extract (H3) from *Meliae Fructus*, the bark of *Cinnamomum cassia*, and *Sparganium rhizome* had an antitumor effect in vitro and in vivo in PANC-1 cells [57]. H3 inhibited proliferation of PANC-1, induced apoptosis, induced G0/G1 cell cycle arrest, and down-regulated apoptosis-related mRNAs like CXCR4, JAK2, and XIAP. Moreover, the anticancer activity of H3 was confirmed by up-regulation of cytochrome c and down-regulation of COX-2. In vivo, five-week old BALB/c nude mice bearing human PANC-1 cells were divided into four groups: control, treated with H3, gemcitabine, and H3+gemcitabine. The group treated with only H3 showed significant necrotic cell death and RBC-containing cavities in tumor tissue. H3 up-regulated cytochrome c and down-regulated COX-2 In vivo.

Ethyl acetate extract of *Inula helenium* L. (EEIHL) inhibited the proliferation of pancreatic cancer cells and activated apoptosis in CFPAC-1 cells [58]. EEIHL treatment up-regulated mRNA level of E-cadherin, and down-regulated mRNA level of Snail, which leads to cell adhesion. Additionally, EEIHL down-regulated the phosphorylation of STAT3 and AKT. A low concentration of EEIHL induced cell arrest and high concentration of EEIHL enhanced apoptosis by the phosphorylation mechanism.

Aqueous leaf extract of *Moringa oleifera* has been reported to exhibit anticancer activity [59]. When this compound is combined with radiation, the expression of PARP-1, Bcl-2, COX-2, and p65 protein is down-regulated, increasing the inhibitory effect on tumor growth. In vivo, PANC-1 bearing mice treated with 1.5 mg/g *moringa* showed the smallest tumor volume compared with control, 0.5 mg/g, and 1.0 mg/g groups, suggesting that *moringa* suppressed tumor growth in a dose-dependent manner.

The root bark of *Paeonia suffruticosa* is known to inhibit the growth of cancer and metastasis [60]. Liu et al. reported that treatment of *P. suffruticosa* aqueous extracts (PS), aqueous extract from *Paeonia suffruticosa*, augmented caspase-3, -8, and -9, showing the activation of apoptosis. PS-elevated ROS and accumulated ER stress lead to inhibition of autophagy and proteasomes, which triggers apoptosis of PANC1, AsPC-1, and BxPC-3 cells.

Pterospermum acerifolium ethanolic bark extract induced apoptosis and cytotoxic effect in PANC-1 cells by up-regulating mitochondrial-mediated ROS production [61]. *P. acerifolium* bark extract also showed apoptosis against lung cancer cells (A549). The extract up-regulated ROS generation and arrested both types of cancer cells by inducing early apoptosis of cells before the G1 phase. Additionally, PANC-1 cells were more sensitive to *P. acerifolium* bark extract than A549.

Polyphenol-rich extract of *Salvia chinensis* is reported to exhibit an inhibitory effect on breast, lung, and colon cancer cells [62]. This compound also induced cell cycle arrest and apoptosis in MIA PaCa-2 cells. The increase of cytochrome c release and the loss of MMP suggest that this compound leads to a mitochondrial apoptotic pathway.

The extract of *Sedum sarmentosum Bunge* (SSBE), originated from traditional Chinese herbal medicine, is known to have antiviral, anticancer, and anti-inflammatory properties [63]. This compound activated the expression of caspase-3, -8, Bax, and Bad, and suppressed the level of Bcl-2 in PANC-1 cells at a dose of 100 μg/mL. SSBE-treated PANC-1 cells also showed a p53 increase and a c-Myc decrease. In animal xenograft models of pancreatic cancer, tumor weight was reduced by inhibition of Hedgehog signaling after SSBE treatment.

Total flavonoid aglycones extract (TFAE), derived from *Radix Scutellariae*, has been previously reported to suppress lung cancer [64]. Liu et al. showed that TFAE also had anticancer activity against pancreatic cancer [65]. After TFAE treatment, cleavages of caspase-3, -9, PARP, and Bid increased whereas Bax and Bcl-2 were unchanged in BxPC-3 cells. Inhibition of TFAE-induced autophagy increases apoptosis, suggesting that autophagy and apoptosis are in a cross-regulatory relationship. Meanwhile, the mice with 150 mg/kg TFAE had the strongest inhibitory effect against tumor growth, compared with the mice which were treated with lower doses.

2.3.3. Formulations

F35, isolated from *Inula helenium* L., is a mixture of alloalantolactone, alantolacton, isoalantolactone in a ratio of 1:5:4 [66]. Its anti-cancer activity was investigated in two types of pancreatic cancer cells: PANC-1, SW1990, and was compared with isoalantolactone's anti-tumor activity. Even though isoalantolactone is the main component from *Inula helenium* L., it is hard to gain pure isoalantolactone by current methods. Fortunately, F35, which is relatively easy to extract, strongly inhibited the growth of PANC-1 and SW1990 with a treatment of 8 μg/mL of F35 at 48 h. In addition, when treated with 6 μg/mL of F35 for 24 h, both groups of cells showed mitochondrial-dependent apoptotic activity, just as they were treated with isoalantolactone. Treating PANC-1 and SW1990 with 2 μg/mL of F35 for 24 h eliminated colony formation and with 2 or 4 μg/mL of F35 for 24 h inhibited migration.

Apoptosis, also called programmed cell death, is a well-known mechanism for treating various cancers, including pancreatic cancer. Forty-nine substances were reported to induce apoptosis in pancreatic cancer. The apoptotic mechanisms of natural products were illustrated in Figure 1. Most of the substances belonged to the plant, except for five fungus and one marine sponge. The pancreatic cancer cell lines commonly used for apoptosis were MIA PaCa-2, PANC-1, AsPC-1, and BxPC-3. In vivo, BALB/c mice were mainly used as an animal model. As a result, the rate of apoptotic cell death increased after treatment, mostly in a dose- and time-dependent manner.

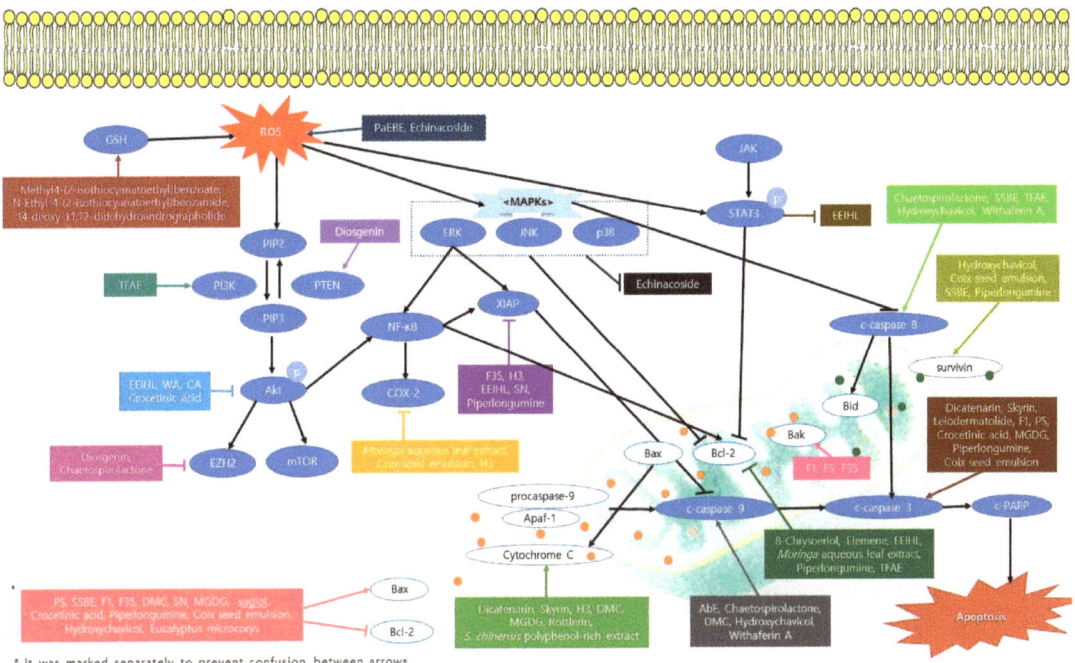

* It was marked separately to prevent confusion between arrows.
The drugs in the pink box act on the case-dependent pathway by regulating Bax and Bcl-2.

Figure 1. Schematic diagram of apoptotic mechanisms of various natural products against pancreatic cancer. The intrinsic apoptotic pathway is regulated primarily by anti-apoptotic Bcl-2 family of proteins. Bcl-2 inhibits release of mitochondrial cytochrome c. Cytochrome c which is released from the mitochondrial intermembrane forms the apoptosome complex in the cytosol with Apaf-1 and procaspase-9, leading to caspase-9 activation. Caspase-9 then activates effector caspases, resulting in some cleavages of cellular proteins and finally cell death by apoptosis. Several natural products such as 8-Chrysoeriol, Elemene, EEIHL, *Moringa* aqueous leaf extract, Piperlongumine, TFAE, PS, SSBE, F1, F35, DMC, SN, MGDG, sugiol, Crocetinic acid, Coix seed emulsion, Hydroxychavicol, and *Eucalyptus microcorys* down-regulated Bcl-2. Dicatenarin, Skyrin, H3, DMC, MGDG, Rottlerin, S. chinensis polyphenol-rich extract induced cytochrome c release to the cytosol. Some drugs affected on caspase-3, 8, and 9 straight without going through the process. Meanwhile, MAPKs signaling pathway, stimulated by ROS, could also inhibit anti-apoptotic Bcl-2 proteins. In addition to MAPKs, several processes triggered by ROS act directly or indirectly on apoptosis.

Chaetospirolactone, xylarione A, (-) 5-methylmellein, 2′,4′-Dihydroxy-6′-methoxy-3′,5′-dimethylchalcone (DMC), 3,5-dihydroxy-6,7,8-trimethoxyflavone (flavone B), 5,7-dihydroxy-3,6,8-trimethoxyflavone (Flavone A), cardiac glycosides, elemene, hydroxychavicol, hypoxoside, mastic gum resin (MGR), Methyl4-(2-isothiocyanatoethyl)benzoate (compound 6), monogalactosyl diacylglycerol, N-Ethyl-4-(2-isothiocyanatoethyl)benzamide (compound 7), piperlongumin, RN1, withaferin A, bitter apricot ethanolic extract, *Eucalyptus microcorys* aqueous extract (F1), and *Salvia chinensis* polyphenol-rich extrac, showed almost no cytotoxicity in normal cells while having an apoptotic effect on pancreatic cancer cells [24,26,29,30,32,36,38,39,41–44,46,49,51,55,62]. The rest of the studies on the apoptosis of pancreatic cells did not handle experiments on normal cells, so additional tests are required. However, the researchers pointed out that additional in vivo experiment is necessary to ensure the safety and effectiveness of these substances.

Seventeen substances, namely Chaetospirolactone, leiodermatolide, cordifoliketones A, diosgenin, elemene, icariin, monogalactosyl diacylglycerol, piperlongumin, RN1, withaferin A, coix seed emulsion, herbal mixture extract (H3), *Moringa* aqueous leaf extract, *Paeonia suffruticosa* aqueous extracts (PS), *Sedum sarmentosum Bunge* extract, and total flavonoid aglycones extract, were investigated for their anti-cancer effects in mice models [24,27,34,36,40,43–46,50,51,53,54,57,59,60,63,65]. The rest of the studies had only in vitro experiments. Some studies suggested that clinical trials with natural compounds are needed. Meanwhile, because leiodermatolide and monogalactosyl diacylglycerol showed toxicity when treated with high doses, a further investigation with low doses experiment was suggested [27,43].

In in vitro experiments, fifteen substances, 8-Chrysoeriol, elemene, mastic gum resin, RN1, bitter apricot ethanolic extract (BAEE), coix seed emulsion, *Eucalyptus microcorys* aqueous extract, *Eucalyptus microcorys* leaf ethanolic extract, *Eucalyptus microcorys* fruit aqueous extract, *Eucalyptus saligna* ethanolic extract, *Moringa* aqueous leaf extract, *Paeonia suffruticosa* aqueous extracts (PS), *Salvia chinensis* polyphenol-rich extract, *Pterospermum acerifolium* ethanolic bark extract (PaEBE), and *Sedum sarmentosum Bunge*, extract were conducted at a high concentration of 60 µg/mL or higher [31,36,42,46,53,56,59–63]. In such cases, when applied to humans, the amount of medicine could be far abundant, which requires attention.

Besides inducing apoptosis, most of the substances had an inhibitory effect on tumor growth such as suppressing cell proliferation or inducing cell cycle arrest. Some substances were also effective in preventing metastasis, angiogenesis, and chemoresistance. Moreover, several natural products potentiated the anticancer activity of gemcitabine with a synergistic effect.

Table 3. Apoptosis inducing plants.

Classification	Compound/Extract	Source	Cell Line/Animal Model	Dose; Duration	Efficacy	Mechanism	Reference
Plant	14-deoxy-11,12-didehydroandrographolide	*Andrographis paniculata*	PANC-1, PSN-1	6.25, 12.5, 25, 50, 100 µM; 12, 16, 20, 24 h	Induction of apoptosis	↓GSH	[28]
Plant	2′,4′-Dihydroxy-6′-methoxy-3′,5′-dimethylchalcone (DMC)	*Cleistocalyx operculatus* buds	PANC-1	3, 10, 30 µM; 48 h	Induction of apoptosis	↑Bax, cytochrome c, c-caspase-3, -9, c-PARP ↓Bcl-2	[29]
Plant	3,5-dihydroxy-6,7,8-trimethoxyflavone (flavone B)	*Achyrocline bogotensis*	Mia PaCa-2	40 µM; 6 h	Induction of apoptosis and cell cycle arrest	↑p-ERK, p-c-JUN ↓pS6	[30]
Plant	5,7-dihydroxy-3,6,8-trimethoxyflavone (flavone A)	*Gnaphalium elegans*	PANC-28	40 µM; 6 h		↓p-ERK, pS6, p-Bad, Bcl-xL, Bcl-2	
Plant	8-Chrysoeriol		SW1990	50, 100 µM; 24 h	Induction of apoptosis	↓Bcl-2	[31]
Plant	Cardiac glycosides	seed of *Thevetia peruviana*	SW1990		Inhibition of proliferation of tumor cell lines		[32]
Plant	Carnosol	*Rosmarinus officinali*, *Salvia carnosa*, *Origanum vulgare*	AsPC-1	1 µM; 48 h	Induction of apoptosis		[49]
Plant	Crocetinic acid	*Crocus sativus*	MIA PaCa-2	1, 10, 25, 50 µM; 72 h	Induction of apoptosis Inhibition of proliferation	↑c-caspase 3, Bax ↓CD133, DCLK-1, Shh, PCNA, p-EGFR, p-AKTa, Bcl-2	[33]
Plant			MIA PaCa-2 bearing athymic nude-mice	0.5 mg/kg; 30 days	Inhibition of pancreatic cancer growth	↑c-caspase 3 ↓PCNA, p-EGFR, p-AKT, Bcl-2	
Plant	Diosgenin	*Solanum, Dioscorea, Costus* species	Patu8988, PANC-1	50, 75 µM; 48 h	Induction of apoptosis	↓EZH2, vimentin ↑PTEN	[34]
Plant			PANC-1 bearing mice	20 mg/kg; 4 weeks	Inhibition of tumor growth	↑PTEN ↓EZH2, vimentin	
Plant	Echinacoside	Stems of *Cistanchessalsa*	SW1990	20, 50, 100 µM; 5 days	Induction of apoptosis	↑ROS, Bax, p38 ↓MMP, JNK, ERK1/2	[35]

Table 3. Cont.

Classification	Compound/Extract	Source	Cell Line/Animal Model	Dose; Duration	Efficacy	Mechanism	Reference
Plant	Elemene	Zingiberaceae	BxPC-3, PANC-1	15, 30, 60 μg/mL; 12 h	Inhibition of cell proliferation, Induction of cell cycle arrest		[36]
			BxPC-3 bearing BALB/c mice	20, 40, 60 mg/kg; 18 days	Inhibition of cell proliferation, Induction of cell cycle arrest	↑p53 ↓Bcl-2	
Plant	Grape seed proanthocyanidins (GSPs)	Vitis vinifera	PANC-1	20 μg/mL; 3, 12, 24 h	Induction of apoptosis	↓miRNA-SS3, SS12, SS24 ↓CDK6, EGFR, MSH6, DNMT1	[37]
Plant	Hydroxychavicol	Piper betle	MIA PaCa-2	100 μM; 48 h	Induction of apoptosis	↑c-caspase -8, -9, c-Bid	[38]
			MIA PaCa-2, PANC-1	50, 100 μM; 48 h	Induction of apoptosis	↑c-caspase-3, -8, -9, c-Bid, c-PARP, Bax ↓Bcl-2, survivin	
Plant	Hyperoside		MIA PaCa-2	50 μM; 48 h	Induction of caspase-dependent apoptosis	↑c-caspase-3	[39]
Plant	Hypoxoside		INS-1	25 μM; 48 h		↑c-caspase-3	
Plant	Icariin	Herba Epimedii	PANC-2	100, 150, 200 μM; 48 h	Induction of apoptosis		[40]
			PANC-2 bearing C57BL/6 mice	120 mg/kg; 11 days	Inhibition of pancreatic tumor progression		
Plant	Methyl4-(2-isothiocyanatoethyl)benzoate	Cruciferous vegetables	PANC-1	10 μM; 72 h	Induction of apoptosis	↑ROS ↓GSH	[41]
	N-Ethyl-4-(2-isothiocyanatoethyl)benzamide						
Plant	Mastic gum resin	Pistacia atlantica	PANC-1	20, 40, 60, 80, 100 μg/mL; 72 h	Induction of cytotoxicity		[42]

Table 3. *Cont.*

Classification	Compound/Extract	Source	Cell Line/Animal Model	Dose; Duration	Efficacy	Mechanism	Reference
Plant	Monogalactosyl diacylglycerol	Spinach	MIA PaCa-2	25, 50, 75 μM; 24 h	Induction of apoptosis	↑cytochrome c, c-PARP, Bax, c-caspase-3 ↓Bcl-2	[43]
Plant	Piperlongumine	*Piper longum*	MIA PaCa-2 bearing BALB/cAJcl-nu/nu mice	2 mg; 23 days	Inhibition of tumor growth		[44]
			BxPC-3, PANC-1, AsPC-1	5, 10, 20, 30, 40 μmol/L; 24, 48, 72 h	Induction of apoptosis Enhancement of gemcitabine-induced apoptosis	↑procaspase-3, c-PARP ↓Bcl-2, Bcl-xL, survivin, XIAP	
			BxPC-3 bearing BALB/c mice	10 mg/kg; 21 days	Inhibition of tumor growth Enhancement of gemcitabine-induced apoptosis		
Plant	Piperlongumine	*Piper longum*	PANC-1	5, 10, 15 μmol/mL; 24, 48 h	Induction of apoptosis, Inhibition of cell proliferation	↓miR-27a, miR-17/miR-20a ↑c-PARP, ROS	[45]
			L3.6pL bearing athymic nu/nu mice	30 mg/kg; 21 days	Inhibition of tumor growth	↓miR-27a, miR-17/miR-20a ↓Sp1, Sp3, Sp4	
Plant	RN1	Flower of *Panax notoginseng*	AsPC-1, BxPC-3	62.5, 125, 250, 500, 1000 μg/mL; 48 h	Inhibition of PDAC cell growth	↓Galectin-3, EGFR, ERK, Runx1	[46]
			BxPC-3 bearing BALB/c nude mice	0.5, 20 mg/kg; 46 days		↓Galectin-3, Ki-67, EGFR, ERK, Runx1	
Plant	Rottlerin	*Mallotus phillippinensis*	Patu8988	4 μM; 48 h	Induction of apoptosis	↑cytochrome c ↓Skp2	[47]
			PANC-1	3 μM; 48 h			

Table 3. Cont.

Classification	Compound/Extract	Source	Cell Line/Animal Model	Dose; Duration	Efficacy	Mechanism	Reference
Plant	Sugiol		MIA PaCa-2	7.5, 15, 30 μM; 48 h	Induction of apoptosis and cell cycle arrest Increase of ROS production	↑Bax ↓Bcl-2, MMP	[48]
Plant	Withaferin A	Withania somnifera	AsPC-1	1 μM; 48 h	Induction of apoptosis	↑c-caspase-3, -8, -9, c-PARP1	[49]
Plant	Withaferin A	Withania somnifera	PANC-1, MIA PaCa-2	0.5, 1, 2.5, 5 μM; 24 h	Induction of apoptosis		[50]
Plant			PANC-1 bearing BALB/c mice	4 mg/kg; 24 days	Enhancement of the therapeutic efficacy of ER stress aggravators		
Plant	Bitter apricot ethanolic extract	Prunus armeniaca L.	PANC-1	704 μg/mL; 72 h	Induction of apoptosis	↑Bax, caspase-3 ↓Bcl-2	[51]
Plant	Clinacanthus nutans non-polar stem extracts (SN) and gemcitabine combination	Clinacanthus nutans	BxPC-3, SW1990	5 μg/mL (and/or 5 μg/mL of gemcitabine); 48 h	Induction of apoptosis Enhancement of gemcitabine-induced apoptosis	↑Bax ↓Bcl-2, cIAP-2, XIAP	[52]
Plant	Coix seed emulsion	Coix lacryma-jobi	BxPC-3	1.50–10 mg/mL; 48 h	Induction of apoptosis	↑caspase-3, c-PARP, Bax ↓Bcl-2, survivin, COX-2	[53]
Plant			PANC-1	1.75–10 mg/mL; 48 h			
Plant			AsPC-1	1.80–10 mg/mL; 48 h			
Plant			BxPC-3 bearing nude BALB/c mice	12.5 mL/kg; 24 days		↓p65, Ki-67	
Plant	Cordifoliketones A	Codonopsis cordifolvidea	AsPC-1, BxPC-3, PANC-1	2, 4, 6 μg/mL; 24, 48 h	Induction of apoptosis	↑Bax, Bad, caspase-3, -8, -9 ↓Bcl-2, Bcl-xL	[54]
Plant			AsPC-1, BxPC-3, PANC-1 bearing BALB/c nude mice	20, 80, 120, 240 M/kg; 27 days			

Table 3. Cont.

Classification	Compound/Extract	Source	Cell Line/Animal Model	Dose; Duration	Efficacy	Mechanism	Reference
Plant	Eucalyptus microcorys aqueous extract (F1)	Leaf of Eucalyptus microcorys	MIA PaCa-2	100, 150 µg/mL; 48 h	Induction of cell cycle arrest and apoptosis	↑Bak, Bax, c-PARP, c-caspase-3 ↓Bcl-2, procaspase-3	[55]
Plant	Eucalyptus microcorys leaf aqueous extract	Leaf of Eucalyptus microcorys	MIA PaCa-2, BxPC-3, CFPAC-1	50, 100 µg/mL; 24 h	Induction of apoptosis		[56]
	Eucalyptus microcorys leaf ethanolic extract						
	Eucalyptus microcorys fruit aqueous extract	Fruit of Eucalyptus microcorys					
	Eucalyptus saligna ethanolic extract	Eucalyptus saligna					
Plant	Herbal mixture ethanol extract (H3)	Meliae Fructus, bark of Cinnamomum cassia, Sparganium rhizome	PANC-1	0.05 mg/mL; 72 h	Induction of apoptosis Induction of cell cycle arrest	↑cytochrome c ↓COX-2, CXCR4, JAK2, XIAP	[57]
			PANC-1 bearing BALB/c nude mice	200 mg/kg; 31 days	Inhibition of tumor growth	↑cytochrome c ↓COX-2	
Plant	Inula helenium L. ethyl acetate extract (EEIHL)	Inula helenium L.	CFPAC-1	2, 4, 6 µg/mL; 24 h	Inhibition of proliferation Inhibition of cell migration	↑p-AKT, p-STAT3 ↑E-cadherin, c-PARP ↓Snail, XIAP,	[58]
					Mitochondrial-dependent apoptosis	↑Bim ↓Bcl-2, Mcl-1	
Plant	Moringa aqueous leaf extract	Moringa oleifera (Moringa)	PANC-1	1.8 mg/mL; 24 h	Induction of apoptosis	↓Bcl-2, COX-2	[59]
			PANC-1 bearing CD-1 mice	0.5, 1.0, 1.5 mg/g; 6 weeks	Inhibition of tumor growth		
Plant	Paeonia suffruticosa aqueous extracts (PS)	Paeonia suffruticosa	PANC-1, AsPC-1, BxPC-3	750 µg/mL; 72 h	Induction of autophagy	↑caspase-3, -8, -9, c-caspase-3, DAPK3	[60]
			AsPC-1 bearing mice	0.9, 1.8 g/kg; 21 days	Inhibition of cell cycle progression and cell migration	↓Cyclin, CDK	

Table 3. Cont.

Classification	Compound/Extract	Source	Cell Line/Animal Model	Dose; Duration	Efficacy	Mechanism	Reference
Plant	*Pterospermum acerifolium* ethanolic bark extract (PaEBE)	Bark of *Pterospermum acerifolium*	PANC-1	50, 75 µg/mL; 24 h	Induction of apoptosis	↑ROS	[61]
					Induction of mitochondrial-mediated cell death	↓MMP	
				50 µg/mL; 24 h	Induction of cell cycle arrest		
Plant	*Salvia chinensis* polyphenol-rich extract	*Salvia chinensis*	MIA PaCa-2	20, 40, 60, 80 µg/mL; 48 h	Induction of apoptosis	↑cytochrome c ↓MMP	[62]
Plant	*Sedum sarmentosum* Bunge extract (SSBE)	*Sedum sarmentosum* Bunge	PANC-1	100 µg/mL; 24 h	Induction of apoptosis	↑Bax, Bad, caspase-3, -8, p53 ↓Bcl-2, c-Myc, survivin	[63]
			PANC-1 bearing BALB/c mice	10, 100 mg/kg; 30 days	Inhibition of tumor growth		
Plant	Total flavonoid aglycones extract	*Radix Scutellariae*	BxPC-3	3.2, 6.4, 12.8 µg/mL; 24 h	Induction of apoptosis	↑c-caspase-3, -8, c-PARP, c-Bid	[65]
			BxPC-3-bearing BALB/c nu/nu mice	50, 100, 150 mg/kg; 56 days	Induction of apoptosis and autophagy	↑c-caspase-3, c-PARP, LC3-II ↓p62	
				8 µg/mL; 48 h	Inhibition of proliferation		
Plant	F35 (alloalantolactone, alantolacton, isoalantolactone [1:5:4])	*Inula helenium* L.	PANC-1, SW1990	6 µg/mL; 24 h	Induction of mitochondrion-related apoptosis	↑Bak ↓Bcl-2, Mcl-1, XIAP	[66]
				2, 4 µg/mL; 24 h	Inhibition of colony-formation and migration		

GSH, Glutathione; c-caspase, cleaved caspase; Bax, Bcl-2-associated X protein; Bcl-2, B-cell lymphoma 2; PARP, Poly Adenosine diphosphate Ribose Polymerase; p-ERK, phospho-Extracellular-related kinase; p-c-JUN, phospho-c-Jun; pS6, phospho-S6; p-Bad, phosphor-Bad; COX-2, Cyclooxygenase-2; cIAP-2, Cellular inhibitor of apoptosis 2; XIAP, X-Linked Inhibitor of Apoptosis; DCLK-1, Doublecortin-like kinase 1; Shh, Sonic hedgehog signaling molecule; PCNA, Proliferating Cell Nuclear Antigen; EGFR, Epidermal Growth Factor Receptor; AKT, Protein kinase B(PKB); EZH2, Enhancer of Zeste Homolog 2; PTEN, Phosphatase and tensin homolog; ROS, Reactive Oxygen Species; MMP (∆Ψm), Mitochondrial membrane potential; E-cadherin, Epithelial cadherin; Mcl-1, Myeloid cell leukemia 1; CDK6, Cell division protein kinase 6; MSH6, MutS Homolog 6; DNMT1, DNA Methyltransferase 1; CXCR4, C-X-C Motif Chemokine Receptor 4; JAK2, Janus Kinase 2; c-Bid, cleaved-Bcl-2 homology 3 interacting domain death agonist; DAPK3, Death-Associated Protein Kinase 3, ↑—up-regulation; ↓—down-regulation.

3. Metastasis Inhibiting Natural Products

To acquire metastatic features, cancer cells change their characteristics, leading to epithelial mesenchymal transition (EMT). EMT makes cancer cells to be founded in other tissues. Metastasis can be responsible for cancer-related death [67]. Thus, it is important to regulate this process, and we focused on both natural products and their compounds that contribute to anti-metastasis (Table 4).

Cheng et al. reported that *Poria cocos*-derived compound polyporenic acid and its extract have inhibitory effect of metastasis in PANC-1 cells [68]. A decrease in cell division cycle protein 20 homolog (CDC20) that has been unveiled to associate with invasion was observed by both treatments.

Zhang et al. reported that a novel natural compound terphenyllin has an anti-metastatic effect in both in vitro and in vivo [69]. A transwell assay and PANC-1 orthotopic model were used to measure the anti-cancer efficacies of terphenyllin. As a result, it was observed that treatment of terphenyllin reduced invasion as well as migration in HPAC and PANC-1. In vivo and histological data also showed the reduction of metastasis.

Novel compound cordifoliketones A, isolated from roots of *Codonopsis cordifolioidea*, showed an anti-cancer effect via the regulation of migration and invasion as well as apoptosis [54]. In the results of the invasion and migration assay, the reduction of invasion and migration in pancreatic ductal adenocarcinoma cells by cordifoliketones A was observed.

The expressions of C-X-C chemokine receptor type 4 (CXCR4) and cyclooxygenase-2 (COX-2) are increased after radiation therapy and facilitate metastasis of pancreatic cancer cells [70]. Aravindan et al. demonstrated that *Hormophysa triquertra* polyphenol (HT-EA) treatment represses irradiation-induced translation of CXCR4, COX-2, β-catenin, and matrix metalloproteinase-9 (MMP-9), Ki-67. Especially, repressions of CXCR4 and COX-2 lead to down-regulations of cancer cell migration and invasion. These results suggest that HT-EA would alleviate the dissemination of pancreatic cancer cells resistant to radiation-therapy.

Radiation has been commonly used for cancer therapy in decades. Hagoel et al. reported that combined with radiation and *moringa* aqueous leaf extract showed synergistic inhibitory activity in metastasis of PANC-1 cells [59]. As for migration and invasion, *moringa* treatment inhibited by 61.6% and 63.7% compared to control, respectively. Moreover, reductions in migration (56.4%) and invasion (39.8%) were observed by *moringa* combined with 4 Gy in comparison to control.

Dephosphorylation of cofilin by slingshot homologs (SSH) associates with actin depolymerization [71]. This change in actin dynamics can be responsible for invadopodia, protrusions observed invasive cancer cell. Lee et al. reported that a novel compound, sennoside A, contributes to a reduction in metastasis by acting as a slingshot inhibitor. After treatment, up-regulation of p-cofilin was confirmed in MIA PaCa-2 and PANC-1 cells. Furthermore, an in vivo study trans-planting PANC-1 cell into the spleens showed that sennoside A induced a prominent reduction of liver metastasis compared to control.

Pei et al. investigated whether a natural product toosendanin has anti-cancer activity on pancreatic cancer and reported that inhibition of migration and invasion was observed by this natural product both in vitro and in vivo [72]. The levels of E-cadherin, known as epithelial marker, increased, whereas those of mesenchymal markers, including vimentin, Snail, and ZEB, decreased. In addition, it was found that toosendanin attenuated the phosphorylation of AKT and mTOR as well as PRAS40 and p70S6K.

Table 4. Metastasis inhibiting natural products.

Classification	Compound/Extract	Source	Cell Line/Animal Model	Dose; Duration	Efficacy	Mechanism	Reference
Fungus	Polyporenic acid	*Poria cocos*	PANC-1	30, 60 μM; 24 h	Inhibition of metastasis	↓CDC20	[68]
Fungus	*Poria cocos* EtOH extract			30, 60 μg/mL; 24 h			
Fungus	Terphenyllin		PANC-1, HPAC	25 μM; 24 h	Inhibition of invasion and migration		[69]
			SCID mice bearing PANC1 orthotopic tumors	20 mg/kg/day; 5 weeks	Inhibition of metastasis		
Plant	Cordifoliketones A	*Codonopsis cordifolioidea*	AsPC-1, BxPC-3, PANC-1	2, 4, 6 μg/mL; 12 h	Inhibition of invasion and migration		[54]
Plant	*Hornophysa triquetra* polyphenol	*Hornophysa triquetra*	PANC-1, PANC-3.27, BxPC-3, MIA PaCa-2	100 μg/mL; 24 h	Inhibition of	↓CXCR4, COX-2, β-catenin, MMP-9, Ki-67, BAPX, PhPT-1, MEGF10	[70]
			MIA PaCa-2 bearing NCr-nu/nu nude mice	10 mg/kg; 3 weeks	resistant cell migration/invasion		
Plant	*Moringa oleifera* leaves water extract	Leaves of *Moringa oleifera*	PANC-1	0.4, 0.8, 1.8 mg/mL; 24 h, 2, 4 Gy radiation	Inhibition of metastasis		[59]
			MIA PaCa-2, PANC-1	10 μmol/L; 24 h	Inhibition of invadopodia formation	↑p-cofilin	
Plant	Sennoside A	*Rheum rhabarbarum*	PANC-1	10 μM; 20 m	Inhibition of invasion and migration		[71]
			PANC-1-Luc bearing BALB/c nu/nu mice	10 mg/kg; 10 days	Inhibition of metastasis		
Plant	Toosendanin		AsPC-1, PANC-1	50, 100, 200 nM; 24 h	Inhibition of invasion and migration	↑E-cadherin ↓Vimentin, ZEB1, Snail, p-AKT, p-PRAS40, p-mTOR, p-p70S6K	[72]
			PANC-1 bearing BALB/c mice	0.2 mg/kg; 28 days	Inhibition of EMT	↑E-cadherin ↓Vimentin, ZEB1, Snail	

CDC20, cell division cycle protein 20; CXCR-4, C-X-C chemokine receptor type 4; COX-2, cyclooxygenase-2; MMP-9, matrix metalloproteinase-9; BAPX, bagpipe homeobox homolog; PhPT-1, phosphohistidine phosphatase-1; MEGF10, multiple EGF-like domains 10; EMT, epithelial mesenchymal transition; ZEB1, zinc finger E-box-binding homeobox 1; PRAS, proline rich protein; mTOR, mammalian target of rapamycin; ↑, up-regulation; ↓, down-regulation.

To sum up, eight substances derived from plants and fungi showed anti-metastatic activities against pancreatic cancer. The anti-metastatic mechanisms of natural products were illustrated in Figure 2. When compared to studies on apoptotic effect of natural substances, studies on metastasis are scarce. Among them, Poria co-cos showed that its extract and their compound polyporenic acid exert anti-metastatic potency. Moreover, CDC20, commonly known as cell division cycle associated factor, has been shown to participate in invasion. However, data concerning whether the empirical doses are toxic against normal cell lines remain necessary. The study of *Hormophysa triquetra* polyphenol elucidated that the polyphenol inhibited cell migration of pancreatic cancer cells In vitro. However, when 100 μg/mL of polyphenol was applied on PANC-1, PANC-3.27, BxPC-3, and MIA PaCa-2, a somewhat high concentration of over 60 μg/mL was observed. Treatment of *moringa* leaf extract with PANC-1 inhibited metastasis, but a synergistic effect was observed when combined with radiation. This suggests that natural products and their compounds combined with radiation could be effectively used for cancer therapy. Reflecting a partial interaction, the in vitro study has a limitation in that it does not represent whole sophisticated interactions. Thus, subsequent studies comprising an in vivo model appear to be needed. Of the studies mentioned above table, Pei et al. presented evidence supporting the anti-cancer activity of toosendanin from a molecular perspective both in vitro and in vivo. Notably, this study showed hallmarks of EMT, including Snail, vimentin, and E-cadherin.

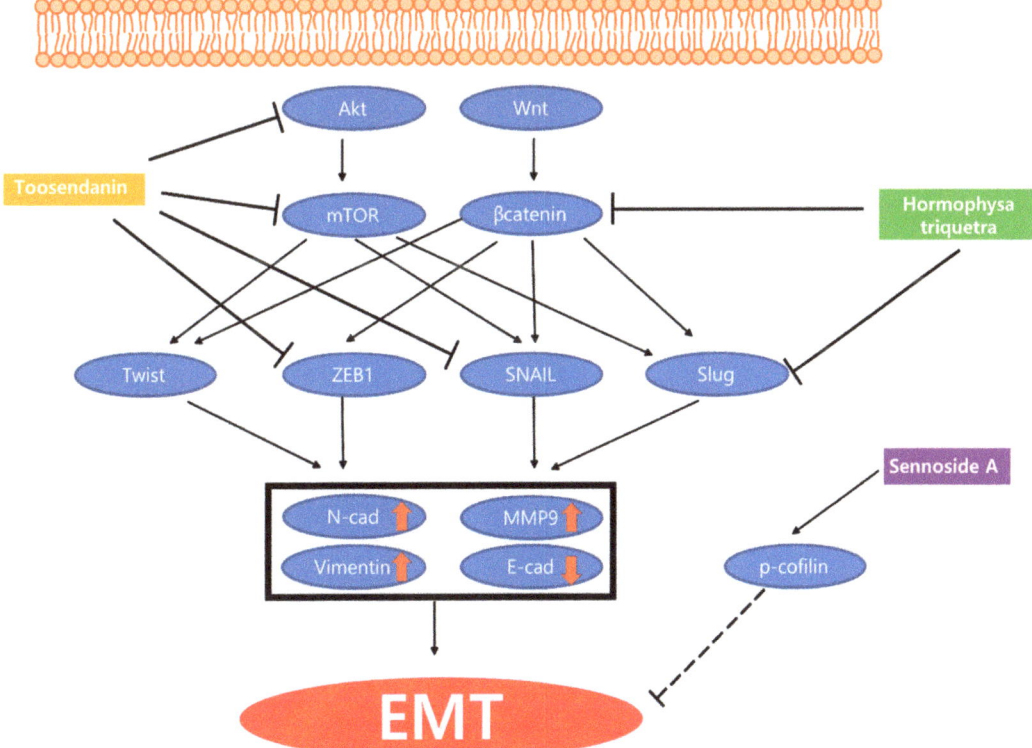

Figure 2. Schematic diagram of anti-metastasis mechanisms of various natural products against pancreatic cancer.

4. Angiogenesis Inhibiting Natural Products

Angiogenesis is the formation of new blood vessels, and the tumor is provided with oxygen and nutrition by newly formed vessels. This is attributed to the growth of cancer cells and metastasis to other organs [73]. Thus, it is essential to down-regulate angiogenesis in cancer therapy. Various natural products have been demonstrated to regulate angiogenesis (Table 5).

Danggui-Sayuk-Ga-Osuyu-Saenggang-Tang (DSGOST) is a mixture of herbal extract used in Traditional Korean medicine [73]. Human umbilical vascular endothelial cells and human dermal microvascular endothelial cells were treated with DSGOST 100 μg/mL for 72 h with/without 50 ng/mL of vascular endothelial growth factor (VEGF). The treatment inhibited VEGF-dependent tube formation in both cases. In PANC-28 xenograft BALB/c nude mice model, injection of DSGOST at a dose of 100 μg with 100 ng/μL of VEGF down-regulated newly formed vessel number in the tumor, as measured by vascular permeability assays. For bioluminescence imaging analyses, DSGOST was orally administered at a dose of 20 mg/kg and repressed tumor growth. These results indicate that DSGOST mitigates vascular leakages caused by VEGF and thereby inhibits tumor growth.

SH003 is a mixture that contains *Astragalus membranaceus*, *Angelica gigas*, and *Trichosanthes Kirilowii* Maximowicz [74]. Choi et al. investigated whether the SH003 inhibits VEGF-induced tumor angiogenesis. Human umbilical vein endothelial cells were treated with SH003 at doses of 10, 20, and 50 μg/mL for 24 h, and VEGF was prevented from binding to VEGFR2. As a result, cell migration, invasion, and tube formation were suppressed through this mechanism. As assessed by vascular leakage assays in vivo PANC-28 bearing nude mice model, VEGF-induced vessel permeability was inhibited after an injection of SH003 at 20 μg. When SH003 was orally administered at a dose of 2 mg/kg, a reduction of tumor growth was detected in bioluminescence imaging analyses, while the bodyweight of the mice was not affected.

There were two types of research associated with anti-angiogenesis effect. DSGOST and SH003 were mixtures of various kinds of natural products and all of their contents were derived from plants [73,74]. Both materials were investigated by the same researchers who mainly investigated VEGF-related mechanisms. DSGOST and SH003 were treated to HUVECs in vitro and to PANC-28 bearing BALB/c nude mice in vivo. Both were demonstrated to down-regulate the metastasis by inhibition of angiogenesis without any effect on pancreatic tumor cell viability. In the case of DSGOST, inhibition of angiogenesis was observed at an extremely high concentration 100 μg/mL, higher than 60 μg/mL. Moreover, studies to investigate cytotoxicity to normal cells are required for DSGOST and SH003.

Table 5. Angiogenesis inhibiting natural products.

Classification	Compound/Extract	Source	Cell Line/Animal Model	Dose; Duration	Efficacy	Mechanism	Reference
Plant	Danggui-Sayuk-Ga-Osuyu-Saenggang-Tang (DSGOST)	Angelica gigas, Cinnamomum cassia Blume, Paeonia lactiflora Pallas, Akebia quinata var. polyphylla Nak., Asarum sieboldii var. seoulense Nakai, Glycyrrhiza uralensis Fischer, Zizyphus jujuba var. inermis Rehder, Evodia rutaecarpa var. bodinieri Huang, Zingiber officinale Rosc.	HUVECs, HDMECs	100 µg/mL; 72 h	Inhibition of migration Inhibition of tube formation	↓p-VEGFR2, p-FAK, p-SRC, p-AKT, p-IKKα/β, p-IκBα, p-NF-κB, MMP-9	[73]
			PANC-28 bearing BALB/c nude mice	20 mg/kg; 49 days 100 µg; 0.5 h	Inhibition of angiogenesis	↑c-caspase-3 ↓Ki-67, p-VEGFR2, MMP-9	
Plant	SH003	Astragalus membranaceus, Angelica gigas, Trichosanthes Kirilowii Maximowicz	HUVECs	10, 20, 50 µg/mL; 24 h	Inhibition of angiogenesis	↑c-caspase-3 ↓p-VEGFR2, MMP-9, p-FAK, p-SRC, p-ERK, p-AKT, p-STAT3	[74]
			PANC-28 bearing BALB/c nude mice	2 mg/kg; 49 days 20 µg; 0.5 h		↑c-caspase-3 ↓Ki-67, p-VEGFR2, MMP-9	

HUVECs, human umbilical vascular endothelial cells; HDMECs, human dermal microvascular endothelial cells; p-VEGFR2, phosphorylated vascular endothelial growth factor 2; p-FAK, phosphorylated focal adhesion kinase; p-AKT, phosphorylated protein kinase B; p-IKKα/β, phosphorylated inhibitor of nuclear factor kappa-B kinaseα/β; p-NF-κB, phosphorylated nuclear factor kappa B; MMP-9, matrix metallopeptidase 9; p-ERK, phosphorylated extracellular signal-regulated kinase; p-STAT3, phosphorylated signal transducers and activators of transcription 3; ↑—up-regulation; ↓—down-regulation.

5. Resistance Inhibiting Natural Products

Although various therapies have been developed against cancer, including chemotherapy, radiation therapy, and so forth, pancreatic cancer is still deadly and represents 10% of the five-year survival rate [75]. Resistance is known to occur in gemcitabine treatment, which is the most common anti-cancer drug [76,77]. The drug resistance makes gemcitabine ineffective, and it consequently leads to difficulties in the successful treatment of cancer. For this reason, only 12% of patients treated with gemcitabine showed anti-cancer efficacy [78]. Therefore, new substances which enhance the efficacy of the anti-cancer drug and suppress drug resistance are needed [79]. There were 10 natural products demonstrated to regulate factors inducing resistance and promote the efficacy of anti-cancer therapy (Table 6). The anti-resistance mechanisms of natural products were illustrated in Figure 3.

Terpinen-4-ol is a kind of monoterpene derived from mainly tee-tree oil [80]. Shapira et al. investigated the anti-cancer effect of terpinen-4-ol on pancreatic cancer in vitro and in vivo. A synergistic tumor growth inhibition effect was observed when the compound was combined with oxaliplatin, fluorouracil, or gemcitabine, which are the general anti-cancer medicines. Especially, when gemcitabine was combined with terpinen-4-oil at a concentration of 0.01%, the tumor growth inhibition effect was increased to 60–85%. In vivo, this substance reduced the tumor volume and weight in the colorectal DLD1 cancer cell xenograft model. Moreover, it was demonstrated that terpinen-4-ol inhibited colorectal, gastric, even prostate cancer growth as well as the growth of pancreatic cancer.

Scalarin, derived from *Euryspongia* cf. *rosea*, showed a reduction of receptor for advanced glycation end products (RAGE) [81]. RAGE level was down-regulated when PANC-1 and MIA PaCa-2 were exposed to 10 µg/mL of scalarin for 24 h. This result suggests that scalarin diminishes the drug resistance and proliferation of pancreatic cancer cells. However, RAGE-associated factors, such as Bcl-xL, p-ERK 1/2, p-NFκB, and p-STAT3, were not modified by scalarin, so researchers suggested that it may be because of other mechanisms associated with RAGE.

Somasagara et al. demonstrated that an increase of phosphorylated AKT and ERK1 is associated with gemcitabine resistance [82]. Bitter melon juice inhibited the phosphorylation of AKT and ERK1/2. When gemcitabine-resistant AsPC-1 cells were treated with bitter melon juice, cell viability was diminished through targeting AKT mediated pathway.

Activation of NF-κB induced by gemcitabine was abolished by pretreatment of coix seed emulsion (CSE) [53]. CSE pretreatment, as agents which down-regulate NF-κB, reduced resistance to gemcitabine and increased sensitivity to gemcitabine in pancreatic cancer cells. Such pretreatment also activated proteins which induce apoptosis, such as caspase-3, c-PARP, and Bax, and reduced counteracting factors, such as Bcl-2, survivin, and COX-2. Consistent with in vitro study, CSE administration combined with gemcitabine treatment indicated a 68% decrease of tumor weight on BxPC-3 xenograft models at a dose of 12.5 mg/kg, which is superior to each treatment alone.

Gemcitabine-induced ABC transporters were previously reported to cause drug resistance [76]. Qian et al. demonstrated that coix seed extract downregulated the expression of ABCB1 and ABCG2 and induced sensitivity to gemcitabine. The coix seed extract treatment elevated gemcitabine accumulation in BxPC-3 cells, while down-regulating drug efflux and elimination. In BxPC-3 and PANC-1 at a dose of coix seed extract 10 mg/mL for 24 and 48 h combined with gemcitabine 3 µg/mL, the level of IC50 of gemcitabine was significantly decreased. This result suggests that the compound induces a synergistic anti-cancer effect with gemcitabine.

Table 6. Resistance inhibiting natural products.

Classification	Compound/Extract	Source	Cell Line/Animal Model	Dose; Duration	Efficacy	Mechanism	Reference
Plant	Terpinen-4-ol		COLO357, PANC-1, MIA-PaCa	0.005, 0.01, 0.05, 0.1%; 72 h	Inhibition of tumor growth Sensitization of gemcitabine	↓RAGE	[80]
Animal	Scalarin	Euryspongia cf. rosea	PANC-1, MIA PaCa-2	10 µg/mL; 24 h	Inhibition of autophagy		[81]
Plant	Bitter melon juice	Momordica charantia	AsPC-1	1–4%; 24, 48 h	Inhibition of viability	↓p-AKT, p-ERK1/2, p-PI3K, p-PTEN	[82]
Plant	Coix seed emulsion	Coix lachryma-jobi	PANC-1	4.0 mg/mL; 72 h	Sensitization of gemcitabine	↑caspase-3, c-PARP, Bax ↓NF-κB, Bcl-2, survivin, COX-2	[53]
			BxPC-3 bearing BALB/c nude mice	12.5 mL/kg; 24 days			
Plant	Coix seed extract	Coix lachryma-jobi	BxPC-3, PANC-1	10 mg/mL; 24, 48 h	Sensitization of gemcitabine	↓ABCB1, ABCC2	[76]
			BxPC-3 bearing BALB/c nude mice	12.5 mL/kg; 3 weeks			
Plant	Enzyme-treated asparagus extract		KLM1-R	2 mg/mL; 120 h	Sensitization of gemcitabine	↓HSP27, p-HSP27	[77]
Plant	EriB/ethanol extract	Isodon eriocalyx	SW1990	2.5 µM; 24 h	Sensitization of gemcitabine	↑c-caspase 3, c-PARP, p-JNK ↓p-PDK1, p-AKT1	[79]
Plant	Oat bran ethanol extract	Avena sativa L.	PANC-1, MIA PaCa-2	40 µg/mL; 72 h	Sensitization of gemcitabine	↑p-AMPK, p21, p27 ↓p-JNK, cyclin D1, CDk4, RRM1, RRM2	[78]
Plant	Pao Pereira extract	Geissospermum vellosii	PANC-1, MIA PaCa-2	50, 100 µg/mL; 48 h	Inhibition of tumor spheroid formation Reduction of pancreatic CSCs	↓ CD44, CD24, EpCam, Nanog, β-catenin, BCL2L2, COX-2	[83]
			PANC-1 bearing nude mice.	20 mg/kg; 3 weeks	Reduction of pancreatic CSCs		
Plant	Qingyihuaji	Herba Scutellariae barbatae, Herba Hedyotidis, Rhizoma Arisaematis erubescentis, Herba seu Radix Gynostemmatis pentaphylli, Fructus Amomi Rotundus	CFPAC-1	40 µg/L; 24, 48, 72h	Sensitization of gemcitabine Inhibition of proliferation Decrease of migration	↑lncRNA AB209630 ↓miR-373, EphB2, Nanog	[84]
			CFPAC-1 bearing nude mice	40 g/kg; 28 days	Sensitization of gemcitabine Inhibition of proliferation		
Plant	Rauwolfia vomitoria root extract	Rauwolfia vomitoria	PANC-1, MIA PaCa-2	50, 100, 200 µg/mL; 48 h	Inhibition of tumor spheroid formation Reduction of pancreatic CSCs	↓CD24, EpCam, Nanog, β-catenin	[85]
			PANC-1 bearing athymic NCr-nu/numice	20 mg/kg; 5 week	Reduction of tumorigenicity		

CSCs, pancreatic cancer stem-like cells; RAGE, receptor for advanced glycation end products; c-PARP, cleaved-poly ADP ribose polymerase; Bax, Bcl-2-associated X protein; NF-κB, nuclear factor kappa B; Bcl-2, B-cell lymphoma-2; COX-2, cyclooxygenase-2; ABCB1, ATP-binding cassette B1; ABCC2, ATP-binding cassette G2; HSP27, heat-shock protein 27; p-JNK, phosphorylated c-Jun N-terminal kinase; PDK1, pyruvate dehydrogenase kinase 1; AKT1, protein kinase B1; CDk4, cyclin-dependent kinase 4; RRM1, ribonucleotide reductase subunit M1; RRM2, ribonucleotide reductase subunit M2; EpCam+, epithelial cell adhesion molecule+; ↑—up-regulation; ↓—down-regulation.

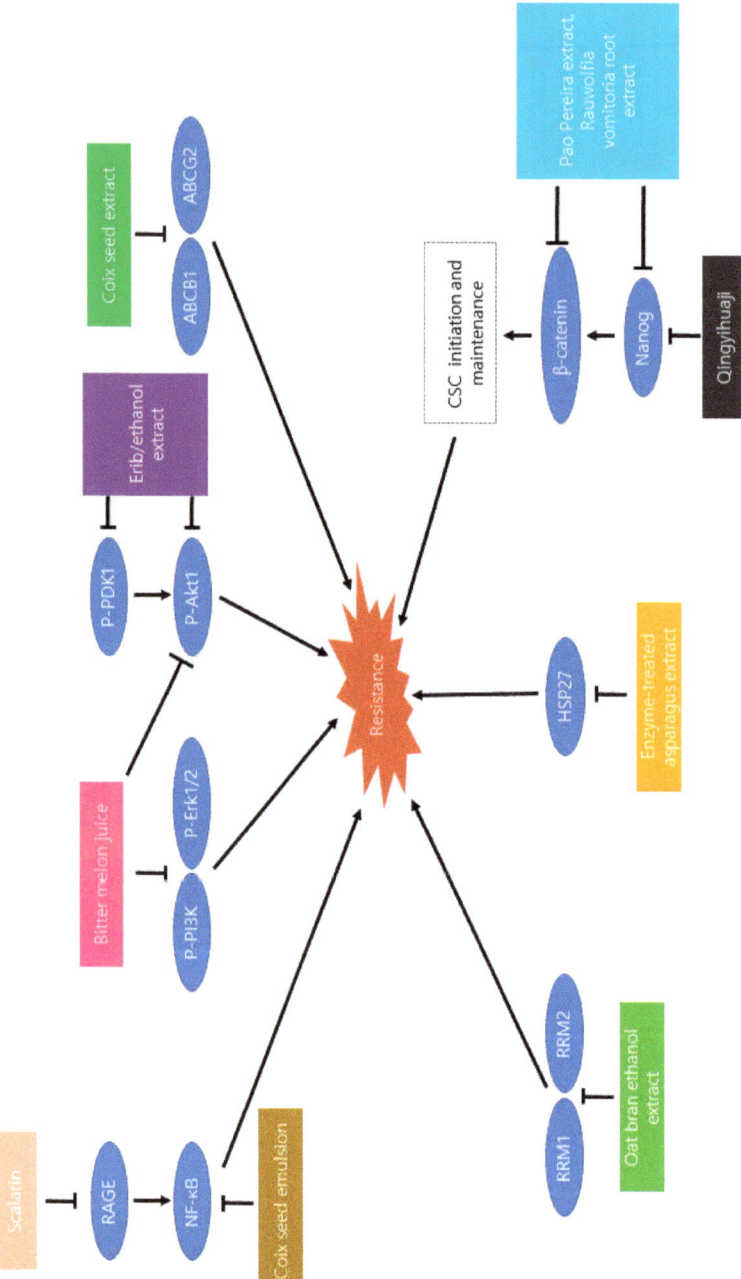

Figure 3. Schematic diagram of anti-resistance mechanisms of various natural products against pancreatic cancer.

Enzyme-treated asparagus extract (ETAS) is known to induce heat-shock protein (HSP) 70 [77]. Shimada et al. investigated the regulation effect of ETAS on HSP27, which was previously demonstrated to causes gemcitabine resistance. When ETAS was treated to gemcitabine-resistant KLM1-R cell line at 2 mg/mL for 120 h, the expression of HSP27 and p-HSP27 (serine 78) were mitigated. This result suggests that ETAS would show a synergistic effect with gemcitabine and would be used to induce the sensitivity of gemcitabine on drug-resistant cancer cells.

Based on previous studies of the effectiveness of Eriocalyxin B (EriB) in treating pancreatic cancer, Li et al. studied whether EriB could assist the function of gemcitabine against SW1990 cells [79]. EriB, the ethanol extract of *Isodon eriocalyx*, stimulated gemcitabine-induced apoptosis and anti-proliferative effect. Among the mixtures of gemcitabine and EriB in various concentrations, 25 μM gemcitabine/1.25 μM EriB combination exhibited a remarkably synergistic effect on SW1990 cells. Especially when 2.5 μM of EriB was treated alone, phosphorylation of AKT was diminished, whereas AKT and PDK1 were both inhibited from phosphorylation when EriB was combined with 25 μM of gemcitabine.

Oat bran ethanol extract (OBE) was elucidated to overcome drug resistance by reduction of RRM1 and RRM2 levels, which was expressed higher in MIA PaCa-2 cells treated with gemcitabine than those were not [78]. The viability and proliferation of gemcitabine-resistant pancreatic cancer cells were selectively disrupted, as compared with normal pancreatic cells. Additionally, OBE induced the apoptosis of pancreatic cancer cells by the activation of AMPK and inactivation of JNK. Consistent with this, OBE increased the cell accumulation in the G0/G1 phase and death of pancreatic cancer cells in flow cytometry analysis and a TUNEL assay of MIA PaCa-2 and PANC-1 cells.

Another study of Pao Pereira extract derived from *Geissospermum vellosii*, was conducted to investigate the inhibitory effect on tumor spheroid formation by Dong et al. [83]. The anti-resistance effect of the Pao Pereira extract was proved by examining pancreatic cancer stem-like cells (CSCs) surface markers and tumor spheroid assay. As a result, surface markers such as CD44+ CD24+ EpCam+ were diminished, and IC50 of Pao was 27 μg/mL in spheroids inhibition. At a higher concentration of 100 μg/mL, it completely inhibited spheroid formation on PANC-1 and MIA PaCa-2. Pao reduced β-catenin and Nanog by down-regulation of BCL2L2, COX-2, and several kinds of mRNA levels related to CSCs, such as Dppa4, Esrrb, and Tcl1. In vivo, the expression of CSCs and tumorigenicity were reduced in the PANC-1 xenograft nude mice model. However, the CSCs inhibitory mechanism of Pao was also not clearly identified in the present study.

Qingyihuaji is an extract of five herbs; *Scutellariae barbatae, Hedyotdis, Arisaematis erubescentis, Gynostemmatis pentaphylli*, Amomi Rotundus [84]. Chen et al. reported that Qingyihuaji elevated the expression of lncRNA AB209630 while inhibited that of miR-373, EphB2, Nanog. Gemcitabine-resistant CFPAC-1 treated with Qingyihuaji combined 30 ng/L of gemcitabine showed synergistic effects on cell proliferation and migration. In vivo, the combination of Qingyihuaji and gemcitabine showed a greater antitumor effect than separately treating them.

CSCs are related to cause drug resistance and metastasis in pancreatic cancer [85]. Dong et al. reported that *Rauwolfia vomitoria* root extract treatment reduced β-catenin and Nanog which initiate and maintain CSCs. The reduction of β-catenin and Nanog indicates that the compound inhibits tumor spheroid formation of CSCs. The extract exerted complete inhibition of the tumor spheroid in PANC-1 at a dose of 200 μg/mL, and in MIA PaCa-2 at a higher concentration of 100 μg/mL. At lower than each concentration, a reduction of tumor spheroid was shown in both PANC-1 and MIA PaCa-2. It also was demonstrated to suppress tumor formation in a NCr-nu/nu mice model at a dose of 20 mg/kg.

Scalarin was originated from a marine sponge whereas the remaining ten were from the plant [81]. Terpinen-4-ol was the only one effective at resistance to anti-EGFR therapy [80]. Coix seed emulsion and coix seed extract were extracted from the same natural product [53,76]. Moreover, there was no statement about sources of ETAS [77]. When

OBE was treated on hTERT-immortalized human pancreatic epithelial nestin-expressing (HPNE) cells obtained from a normal pancreatic duct, cytotoxicity was not found at less than 40 µg/mL [78]. Both *Rauwolfia vomitoria* root extract and Pao Pereira extract had less impact on MRC-5 epithelial cells that are not cancer cells than pancreatic cancer cells at concentrations of 567 µg/mL and 547 µg/mL [83,85]. Terpinen-4-ol, scalarin, bitter melon juice, coix seed emulsion, coix seed extract, ETAS, EriB/ethanol extract, and Qingyihuaji were not tested for confirmation of cytotoxicity in normal cells [53,76,77,79–82,84]. There was a lack of in vivo tests regarding scalarin, bitter melon juice, OBE, ETAS, and EriB/ethanol extract [77–79,81,82]. Additional studies about these need to be carried out in order to be used for an adjuvant to clinical chemotherapy.

6. Clinical Trials

There were seven clinical trials of natural products against pancreatic cancer from 2009 to 2020, and five types of natural products were tested (Table 7). Phase 1–3 pancreatic cancer clinical trials were targeted, and a majority of the clinical trials of phase 2 were conducted. Most of them were completed, while one was yet recruiting participants.

In a study, 15 patients with gemcitabine-refractory advanced pancreatic cancer were the subjects of UMIN000005787, a clinical trial that took place in Japan [86]. GBS-01, extracted from the fruit of *Arctium lappa* L., was administered orally once a day until the disease progresses or unacceptable toxicity occurs. None of the patients treated with GBS-01 showed any signs of dose-limiting toxicities (DLTs). The main adverse effects were the increase of γ-glutamyl transpeptidase and hyperglycemia. The trial was a non-randomized, unblinded, and uncontrolled study, executed from 16 June 2011 to 5 May 2014. According to the clinical trial results, the recommended dose of GBS-01 was 12.0 g q.d, and the clinical safety of GBS-01 monotherapy was confirmed in pancreatic cancer patients who were difficult to treat with gemcitabine therapy [87]. The co-treatment of gemcitabine and GBS-01 can also be a promising therapy for pancreatic cancer patients, as gemcitabine has anti-tumor effects on cancer cells under oxygen and glucose-rich conditions, while GBS-01 has the ability to remove the resistance of cancer cells.

Non-randomized, open-label study NCT00192842 expected that curcumin, extracted from *Curcuma longa Linn*, could aid the efficacy of gemcitabine [88]. The patients were administered gemcitabine once a week and had 8 g of curcumin orally every day. The study started in July 2004 and was primarily completed in November 2007. The result of this trial was not posted.

The phase 2 clinical trial NCT00094445 started on November 2004 and results were updated on 28 August 2020 [89]. A total of 50 patients suffering from pancreatic cancer were administered 8 g of oral curcumin every day for eight weeks. In total, 44 patients completed the study. About 20% of the patients had severe adverse events including cardiac disorders (chest pain, multiple pulmonary emboli, atrial fibrillation etc.), gastrointestinal disorders (GI hemorrhage, abdomen pain etc.), dehydration, or pain. About 13% of the patients had no serious adverse events like gastrointestinal disorders (vomiting, nausea) or edema.

The aim of the phase 2 clinical trial NCT00837239 was to compare the effect of two types of treatment against pancreatic cancer: the combination of HuaChanSu plus gemcitabine, and gemcitabine plus placebo [90]. Both groups were administered 1000 mg/m^2 gemcitabine once a week and then skipping a week, for a cycle of 28 days. One group was additionally treated with HuaChanSu, 20 mL/m2 for a total 500 mL, given 2 h infusion, 5 days a week (3 weeks), and skipping a week. The other group was the placebo group, additionally treated with saline. It was a randomized, placebo-controlled, and blinded study, started in June 2007 and primarily completed in July 2012. According to the results of randomized clinical trials, locally advanced pancreatic or metastatic pancreatic cancer patients' outcomes were not improved when treated with the combination of huachansu and gemcitabine [91]. So, the co-treatment of hwachansu and gemcitabine against advanced pancreatic cancer is not recommended. Kanglaite, an oil extract from *Coicis Semen*, was used in phase 2 NCT00733850 clinical trial [92]. It was targeted to 85 adults suffering from pancreatic cancer. The experimental group was administered kanglaite injection plus gemcitabine, and the compared group was administered only gemcitabine. This was a randomized, open-label, interventional study, that occurred from August 2008 to June 2014. The clinical trial report was sent to the FDA, and the phase 3 clinical trial is expected. According to the results, the combination of 30 g kanglaite injection per day and a standard therapy of gemcitabine has been demonstrated to encourage clinical evidence of proliferation effects and a well-controlled safety profile [93].

The phase 3 clinical trial ISRCTN70760582 targeted 434 adults suffering from four pancreatic cancers [94]. Mistletoe therapy was predicted to enhance the survival rate and improve the life quality of the patients. Iscador Qu Spezial (IQuS), subcutaneous injection of an extract of *Viscum album* L., was given to the patients three times a week for 12 months, and all patients were followed up for 12 months. This trial started on 1 January 2009 and ended on 31 December 2014. According to the result, mistletoe is an effective supplementary treatment for locally advanced or metastatic pancreatic cancer in that mistletoe treatment noticeably improved the quality of life in patients suffering from the disease [95].

Iscador Qu, extracted from *Viscum album* L., is planned to be used to pancreatic cancer patients in phase 3 clinical trial NCT02948309 [96]. This study is present recruiting patients and is estimated to be completed in June 2021. Half of the patients will be administered Iscador Qu by subcutaneous injections and the other half will be the placebo group. The result of the trial was not posted.

There are seven clinical trials for treating pancreatic cancer using natural products. Those conducted in the US were five: two of them published in the last 10 years, three of them in the last five years. One was conducted in the UK, 11 years ago, the other one in Japan, six years ago. Curcumin and Iscador Qu (Mistletoe extract) were tested twice each. One of the studies was phase 1, four were phase 2, and two were phase 3. Six out of seven trials were completed, and four of them posted results. There were evident gaps in the number of participants among the clinical trials. Four clinical trials had recruited more than 80 people, while two trials had about 15 participants. In three out of seven trials, Curcumin and GBS-01 were administered orally, and the rest were administered by subcutaneous injections.

Table 7. Clinical trials of natural products against pancreatic cancer.

Compound/Extract	Source	Phase	Patients	Status	Results	Registry Number	Reference
GBS-01	Fruit of *Arctium lappa*	Phase 1	Pancreatic Cancer (≥20 yrs) 15 participants	Completed	Safe up to 12 g per day Favorable response	UMIN000005787	[86]
Curcumin	*Curcuma longa* Linn	Phase 2	Pancreatic Cancer (≥18 yrs) 17 participants	Completed	Partial response 1 Stable disease 4 Tumor progression 6 Discontinued 5 Dose reduced 2	NCT00192842	[88]
Curcumin	*Curcuma longa* Linn	Phase 2	Pancreatic Cancer (≥18 yrs) 50 participants	Completed	The six-month survival rate was 15.9% (7/44)	NCT00094445	[89]
Huachansu/Bufo toad skin water extract	*Bufo gargarizans*	Phase 2	Pancreatic Cancer (≥18 yrs) 80 participants	Completed	Median overall survival Experimental: 160 days Control: 156 days Not statistically significant ($p = 0.339$)	NCT00837239	[90]
Kanglaite/oil extract	*Coicis Semen*	Phase 2	Pancreatic Cancer (≥18 yrs) 85 participants	Completed	Progression-free survival Experimental: 112 days Control: 58 days	NCT00733850	[92]
Iscador Qu Spzial	*Viscum album*	Phase 3	Pancreatic Cancer (≥18 yrs) 434 patients	Completed	Mistletoe treatment improve the global health status significantly	ISRCTN70760582	[94]
Iscador Qu/Mistletoe extract	*Viscum album* L.	Phase 3	Pancreatic Cancer (≥18 yrs) 290 participants	Recruiting	N/A	NCT02948309	[96]

N/A, not available.

7. Discussion

Despite continuous research on the treatment of pancreatic cancer, the proportion of patients overcoming pancreatic cancer has not improved noticeably. Therefore, recognizing a novel treatment is needed, and we found that the therapy of pancreatic cancer using the natural products has been meaningful. We analyzed original research in terms of apoptosis, anti-metastasis, anti-angiogenesis, and anti-resistance. Additionally, we reviewed the clinical trials practiced in various countries.

7.1. Anti-Cancer Mechanisms of Natural Products

In total, 68 drugs were reviewed for their anti-cancer effects against pancreatic cancer. The mechanisms of anticancer were divided into four categories, namely apoptosis, anti-metastasis, anti-angiogenesis, and anti-resistance, with a significant proportion of drugs related to apoptosis. MIA PaCa-2, PANC-1, AsPC-1, or BxPC-3 pancreatic cancer cell lines were usually used in in vitro studies, with several studies including in vivo experiments, usually using BALB/c mice as an animal model.

Apoptosis, known as programmed cell death, plays a significant role in health and disease [22]. Inappropriate apoptosis may occur in various diseases, including many types of cancer like pancreatic cancer. However, not all researches had in vivo studies, but 17 were effective in a mice model [24,27,33,34,36,40,43–46,50,53,54,57,59,60,63,65]. Fifteen substances were administered at a high concentration of 60 μg/mL or higher, which demands attention when applied to humans [31,36,42,46,51,53,55,56,59–63]. Twenty substances conducted cytotoxicity experiments [24,26,29,30,36,38,41–44,46,49–51,53,55,62]. The rest of the studies require additional toxicity tests to normal pancreatic cancer cells. In the case of leiodermatolide, it showed low efficacy on cell survival [27]. Even though the administration of leiodermatolide exhibited potent cytotoxicity compared to control groups or gemcitabine groups, it was not completely preventable due to the possibility of toxicity. If administered less, it will be possible to increase the survival rate and get accurate results for efficacy. Notably, 8-Chrysoeriol as a natural dietary product potentially targeting BCL-2 could serve as a lead compound for SW1990 pancreatic cancer therapy [31]. In addition, echinacoside (ECH) induced apoptosis by elevating ROS and reducing MMP in SW1990 cells [35]. However, since SW1990 cell lines do not have the mutation of p53, which triggers the upregulation of Bax, additional investigation is needed to determine whether ECH is available for suppressing tumors.

Metastasis, the tendency of cancer cells to spread to different organs, is a sign of cancer that is distinguished from benign tumors [97]. Seven natural products that originated from plants and fungi were observed to have anti-metastasis-related mechanisms in pancreatic cancer. Six compounds had one or no mechanism, which encourages additional studies about specific mechanisms. Still, it is widely known that the downregulation of CDC20 plays an important role in the cell cycle. Several reports described inhibition of metastasis in both cell lines and in vivo [69,71,72]. However, the remaining studies require in vivo experiments. Moreover, *Poria cocos* extract and its compound polyporenic acid seem to require data indicating whether the empirical doses are noxious to normal cell lines. About half of the products were administered to the cancer cell line at an abnormally large amount, treated with a dose of 60 μg/mL or more [59,68].

Angiogenesis, which supports the growth of cancer cells and metastasis to other organs, should be down-regulated when treating cancer [73]. Two compounds included successful in vivo experiments, but there was no cytotoxicity test [73,74]. One out of two compounds was tested with a concentration of 100 μg/mL [73].

Since pancreatic cancer is highly resistant to chemotherapy and radiation therapy, anti-resistance is one of the decisive factors in cancer treatment [70]. Ten natural products that are related to anti-resistance were reviewed. Half of the studies not only included in vitro experiments, but also in vivo experiments [53,70,76,85]. Moreover 60% of the compounds were administered in high doses on cancer cell lines, which demands attention when applied to humans [53,70,76,77,83,85]. Notably, coix seed extract (10 mg/mL), coix seed emulsion (4.0 mg/mL), and enzyme-treated asparagus extract (2 mg/mL) were way beyond the standard, 60 µg/mL. Pao Pereira extract and *Rauwolfia vomitoria* root extract were assessed in highly reliable studies conducted in vitro, in vivo, and even with normal cytotoxicity tests.

7.2. Clinical Trials of Natural Products against Pancreatic Cancer

Although there is original research about 68 products in this review, seven clinical trials have been given a registry number and internationally recognized. Even if the substances used in clinical trials were not included in this review, they have been experimentally studied for their anti-cancer effects for a long time or have been used in clinical trials for cancers other than pancreatic cancer [98–101]. Therefore, among the studies in this review, particularly highly reliable substances are worth testing in clinical trials.

Since Pao Pereira extract has various anti-cancer effects, such as inducing apoptosis, increasing sensitivity to gemcitabine, and suppressing tumor growth in vivo, a clinical trial dealing with the administration of Pao Pereira extract plus gemcitabine is recommended. *Isodon eriocalyx* ethanol extract showed good effects in induction of apoptosis and anti-resistance, and also was effective in suppressing proliferation. Thus, clinical trials can be conducted if successful results are achieved in in vivo studies.

7.3. Multi-Functional Natural Products

Among the natural products, several products were multi-functional natural products, which have treated pancreatic cancer through two or more mechanisms. Emulsion and extract from *Coix lacryma-jobi* showed an outstanding effect in the treatment of pancreatic cancer in apoptosis and anti-resistance. In particular, the reliability of both studies was raised by including in vivo experiments as well as in vitro experiments. Although abnormally high doses were administered in vitro, emulsion or extract from *Coix lacryma-jobi* have been the subject of completed clinical trials as kanglaite and proven to be acceptable to humans. Natural products that treat pancreatic cancer through apoptosis and anti-metastasis are Cordifoliketones A and *Moringa* aqueous leaf extract. In anti-metastasis, both extracts require additional experiments due to the lack of in vivo experiments. *Moringa* aqueous leaf extract showed great anti-cancer effects, especially when combined with radiation therapy. In addition, many of the natural substances in anti-resistance had other effects, such as the induction of apoptosis or inhibition of tumor growth as well as the effect on resistance. Oat bran ethanol extract (OBE), *Isodon eriocalyx*, Coix seed emulsion, *Rauwolfia*, and Terpinen-4-ol were demonstrated to induce the apoptosis of pancreatic cancer cells. *Isodon eriocalyx* was especially also effective in suppressing proliferation. Furthermore, *Pao Pereira* extract was demonstrated to induce apoptosis in a previous study. According to the experimental study reviewed in this paper, *Pao Pereira* extract was proven to increase sensitivity to gemcitabine apart from the induction of apoptosis, suppressing tumor growth.

7.4. Anti-Inflammatory and Anti-Tumor Effects of Natural Products

The mechanisms of the reviewed natural products suggest that they are somewhat related to anti-inflammatory activity. Resveratrol acts to activate anti-inflammatory reactions through modulation of enzymes and pathways that produce mediators of inflammatory reactions, and also induces programmed cell death in activated immune cells. Resveratrol, which has no side effects even at high concentrations, has significant potential to be used as an alternative therapy against cancer and inflammatory diseases [14,15,102]. Curcumin is known to have a significant anti-inflammatory effect by blocking NF-κB signals at several stages, and shows great potential in the anti-tumor effect by inhibiting I-κB kinase [16,103]. It can be seen shown that anti-inflammatory mechanisms, including the NF-κB mechanism of natural products and natural products with anti-inflammatory effects, are strongly related.

7.5. miRNA Regulating Natural Products

The manipulation of miRNAs is known to be useful in the treatment of diseases, especially cancer [16,37]. Therefore, in the present review, we noted the papers related to miRNAs, but this had drawbacks in that only two out of the 68 natural products considered involved mechanisms of miRNAs, which were concentrated on apoptosis [37,45]. Additionally, poorly regulated miRNAs have the potential to cause pancreatic cancer, the dysregulated miR-646 and MIIP expression being associated with the exacerbation of pancreatic cancer [104].

7.6. Strengths and Limitations

In this review article, various anti-cancer mechanisms of pancreatic cancer were systematically analyzed and the source, cell line, animal model, dose, duration, efficacy, and mechanism of the natural compound in each paper were arranged clearly. Notably, the tables were divided into seven sections based on the anti-cancer mechanism and the sources of natural products. Anti-tumor activity by modulating miRNAs was separated from other mechanisms. Most of the reviews in the last 10 years were based on immunotherapy. Yue et al. reported a similar review about treating pancreatic cancer with the combination of natural products and chemotherapeutic agents like gemcitabine [105]. They only reviewed the studies that had the anti-cancer mechanism of apoptosis, but we analyzed the studies of the four different anti-cancer mechanisms and the clinical trials additionally. In particular, we not only dealt with the study of synergetic effect with anti-cancer drugs, but also focused on the inherent anti-cancer efficacy of natural products. In addition, pancreatic cancer treatment using natural products has a great advantage of being effective in various mechanisms and producing synergistic effects. Fortunately, there were no papers on natural products that cause pancreatic cancer.

Limitations exist in this review, which does not include papers older than five years after publication, and only studies written in English have been reviewed. In addition, the research on compounds and extracts was mostly reviewed. Moreover, among the reviewed papers, in vitro experiments were performed in all the cited studies, but not all of the papers conducted in vivo experiments, so further investigation is suggested. The possibility that the concentrations of natural substances that were effective in in vitro experiments may not be effective in actual clinical practice cannot be excluded. Since natural products have multi-compound and multi-target characteristics, additional mechanistic studies are needed, and further studies on bioavailability and drug delivery systems are also needed.

7.7. Future Research Directions for Natural Product Treatment against Pancreatic Cancer

In future studies on pancreatic cancer treatment, studies on synergistic effects related to existing anti-cancer drugs or studies on natural products that suppress side effects of anti-cancer drugs are needed. Natural products that can treat various symptoms, such as loss of appetite and weight loss related to cachexia due to pancreatic cancer, should be studied. When the natural products of the studies and clinical trials were searched at nifds.go.kr, several drugs were found to have been used as traditional medicines in China, Japan, and Korea. These drugs suggest that modern cancer treatment ideas can be obtained from traditional medicine [34,44,45,57,58,60,66,68,73,74,86,88,89,94,96]. Additionally, since there have been many studies on the effects of natural products inhibiting resistance, this field is promising and noteworthy.

8. Methods

Original research regarding the effects of TKM or natural products on pancreatic cancer were collected from PubMed and Google scholar. When searching for relevant original research, we included "natural product", "pancreatic cancer", "apoptosis", "metastasis", "angiogenesis", and "cancer drug resistance" as keywords. After the initial search, we only included studies between July 2015 and April 2020. We selected studies that fit into the following criteria: (1) research based on in vitro or in vivo to demonstrate anti-cancer effects of natural products; (2) research containing experiments using natural products derived from fungi, marine sponges, or plants; (3) statically significant researches whose p values were less than 0.05; (4) researches written in English.

Clinical trials about natural products against pancreatic cancer were collected from clinicaltrials.gov, isrctn.com, and umin.ac.jp/ctr/. Clinical trials conducted in other countries rather than the USA were additionally searched in PubMed. When searching for clinical trials, "pancreatic cancer" and "natural product" were used as keywords. We only included studies between February 2009 and April 2020. Subsequently, we collected clinical trials suitable to the following criterion: (1) clinical trials that include administration of natural-derived treatment.

9. Conclusions

In this study, 68 natural products that treated pancreatic cancer were classified and organized by their various anti-cancer mechanisms. The anti-cancer effects of natural products and regulations in related factors for each anti-cancer mechanism were easily summarized. Therefore, the recent research trend in pancreatic cancer treatment using natural products can be easily recognized. Natural products have high potential in treating pancreatic cancer by having a synergetic effect with conventional anti-cancer drugs and inherent anti-cancer efficacy themselves. Nevertheless, many cases are limited to in vitro studies, and for natural products to make a greater contribution to the treatment of pancreatic cancer, further in vivo studies and clinical trials are needed.

Author Contributions: Conceptualization, A.K., J.H., J.K., Y.C. and B.K.; methodology, A.K.; investigation, A.K., J.H., J.K. and Y.C.; writing—original draft preparation, A.K., J.H., J.K. and Y.C.; writing—review and editing, C.C. and B.K.; visualization, A.K., J.H., J.K. and Y.C.; supervision, J.A., S.-H.K., S.-G.K. and B.K.; project administration, B.K.; funding acquisition, S.-G.K. and B.K. All authors have read and agreed to the published version of the manuscript.

Funding: This research was supported by Basic Science Research Program through the National Research Foundation of Korea (NRF) funded by the Ministry of Education (NRF-2020R1I1A2066868), the National Research Foundation of Korea (NRF) grant funded by the Korea government (MSIT) (No. 2020R1A5A2019413), a grant of the Korea Health Technology R&D Project through the Korea Health Industry Development Institute (KHIDI), funded by the Ministry of Health & Welfare, Republic of Korea (grant number: HF20C0116), and a grant of the Korea Health Technology R&D Project through the Korea Health Industry Development Institute (KHIDI), funded by the Ministry of Health & Welfare, Republic of Korea (grant number: HF20C0038).

Institutional Review Board Statement: Not applicable.

Informed Consent Statement: Not applicable.

Data Availability Statement: Not applicable.

Conflicts of Interest: The authors declare no conflict of interest.

Abbreviations

c-caspase	cleaved caspase
c-PARP	cleaved poly adenosine diphosphate ribose polymerase
Bax	Bcl-2-associated X protein
Bcl-family	B cell lymphoma-family
miRNA	microRNA
BRCA1/2	breast cancer susceptibility gene 1/2
PALB2	partner and localizer of BRCA2

TCM	Traditional Chinese Medicine
TTM	Traditional Thai Medicine
TKM	Tracitional Korean Medicine
CAM	Complementary and Alternative Medicine
PCD	programmed cell death
AbE	*Agaricus blazei* Murrill water extract
DAPK3	death-associated protein kinase 3
NLRP1	NACHT, LRR, and PYD domains-containing protein 1
TRAIL	tumor necrosis factor-related apoptosis inducing ligand
ROS	reactive oxygen species
MMP	mitochondrial membrane potential
compound 17	14-deoxy-11,12-didehydroandrographolide
DMC	$2',4'$-Dihydroxy-$6'$-methoxy-$3',5'$-dimethylchalcone
flavone A	5,7-dihydroxy-3,6,8-trimethoxyflavone
flavone B	3,5-dihydroxy-6,7,8-trimethoxyflavone
PCNA	proliferating cell nuclear antigen
EGFR	epidermal growth factor receptor
AKT	protein kinase B (PKB)
EZH2	enhancer of Zeste homolog 2
ECH	Echinacoside
MAPK	mitogen-activated protein kinase
GSPs	grape seed proanthocyanidins
CDK6	cell division protein kinase 6
MSH6	MutS homolog 6
DNMT1	DNA methyltransferase 1
JNK	c-Jun N-terminal kinase
c-Bid	cleaved-Bcl-2 homology 3 interacting domain death agonist
GSH	Glutathione
MGR	mastic gum resin
MGDG	monogalactosyl diacylglycerol
XIAP	X-linked inhibitor of apoptosis
COX-2	cyclooxygenase 2
VEGF	vascular endothelial growth factor
MMP-9	matrix metalloproteinase 9
NF-κB	nuclear factor kappa B
RN1	a polysaccharide from the flower of *Panax notoginseng*
Gal-3	Galectin-3
ERK	extracellular signal-regulated kinase
Runx1	Runt-related transcription factor 1
Skp2	S-phase kinase associated protein 2
WA	Withaferin A
CA	Carnosol
HGF	hepatocyte growth factor
c-Met	mesenchymal-epithelial transition factor
BAEE	Bitter apricot ethanolic extract
SN	non-polar stem extracts
cIAP-2	cellular inhibitor of apoptosis 2
CSE	coix seed emulsion
F1	*Eucalyptus microcorys* aqueous extract
H3	herbal mixture ethanol extract
CXCR-4	C-X-C motif chemokine receptor 4
JAK2	Janus kinase 2
RBC	red blood cell
EEIHL	ethyl acetate extract of *Inula helenium* L.
STAT3	signal transducers and activators of transcription 3
PS	*Paeonia suffruticosa* aqueous extracts

SSBE	the extract of *Sedum sarmentosum* Bunge	
TFAE	total flavonoid aglycones extract	
F35	alloalantolactone, alantolacton, isoalantolactone [1:5:4]	
PaEBE	*Pterospermum acerifolium* ethanolic bark extract	
p-c-JUN	phospho-c-Jun	
pS6	phospho-S6	
DCLK-1	doublecortin-like kinase 1	
Shh	sonic hedgehog signaling molecule	
PTEN	phosphatase and tensin homolog	
E-cadherin	epithelial cadherin	
Mcl-1	myeloid cell leukemia 1	
EMT	epithelial mesenchymal transition	
CDC20	cell division cycle protein 20	
CXCR-4	C-X-C chemokine receptor type 4	
HT-EA	*Hormophysa triquertra* polyphenol	
SSH	slingshot homologs	
ZEB	zinc finger E-box-binding homeobox	
mTOR	mammalian target of rapamycin	
PRAS	proline rich protein	
BAPX	bagpipe homeobox homolog	
PhPT-1	phosphohistidine phosphatase 1	
MEGF10	multiple EGF-like domains 10	
DSGOST	Danggui-Sayuk-Ga-Osuyu-Saenggang-Tang	
HUVECs	human umbilical vascular endothelial cells	
HDMECs	human dermal microvascular endothelial cells	
VEGFR2	vascular endothelial growth factor 2	
p-FAK	phosphorylated focal adhesion kinase	
p-IKKα/β	phosphorylated inhibitor of nuclear factor kappa-B kinaseα/β	
RAGE	receptor for advanced glycation end products	
ABC	ATP-binding cassette	
ABCB1	ATP-binding cassette B1	
ABCG2	ATP-binding cassette G2	
ETAS	enzyme-treated asparagus extract	
HSP	heat-shock protein	
EriB	Eriocalyxin B	
PDK1	pyruvate dehydrogenase kinase 1	
OBE	Oat bran ethanol extract	
RRM1	ribonucleotide reductase subunit M1	
RRM2	ribonucleotide reductase subunit M2	
AMPK	AMP-activated protein kinase	
CSCs	cancer stem-like cells	
EpCam+	epithelial cell adhesion molecule+	
BCL2L2	Bcl-2 like protein 2	
lncRNA	long non-coding RNAs	
HPNE	human pancreatic epithelial nestin-expressing	
CDk4	cyclin-dependent kinase 4	
DLTs	dose-limiting toxicities	
IQuS	Iscador Qu Spezial	

References

1. Oberstein, P.E.; Olive, K.P. Pancreatic cancer: Why is it so hard to treat? *Ther. Adv. Gastroenterol.* **2013**, *6*, 321–337. [CrossRef] [PubMed]
2. Tempero, M.A. NCCN Guidelines Updates: Pancreatic Cancer. *J. Natl. Compr. Canc. Netw.* **2019**, *17*, 603–605. [CrossRef]
3. Bray, F.; Ferlay, J.; Soerjomataram, I.; Siegel, R.L.; Torre, L.A.; Jemal, A. Global cancer statistics 2018: GLOBOCAN estimates of incidence and mortality worldwide for 36 cancers in 185 countries. *CA Cancer J. Clin.* **2018**, *68*, 394–424. [CrossRef] [PubMed]
4. McGuigan, A.; Kelly, P.; Turkington, R.C.; Jones, C.; Coleman, H.G.; McCain, R.S. Pancreatic cancer: A review of clinical diagnosis, epidemiology, treatment and outcomes. *World J. Gastroenterol.* **2018**, *24*, 4846–4861. [CrossRef] [PubMed]

5. Lumlerdkij, N.; Tantiwongse, J.; Booranasubkajorn, S.; Boonrak, R.; Akarasereenont, P.; Laohapand, T.; Heinrich, M. Understanding cancer and its treatment in Thai traditional medicine: An ethnopharmacological-anthropological investigation. *J. Ethnopharmacol.* **2018**, *216*, 259–273. [CrossRef]
6. Gokani, T. Ayurveda–the science of healing. *Headache* **2014**, *54*, 1103–1106. [CrossRef] [PubMed]
7. Leem, K.-H.; Park, H.-K. Traditional Korean medicine: Now and the future. *Neurol. Res.* **2007**, *29*, 3–4. [CrossRef] [PubMed]
8. Kang, Y.M.; Komakech, R.; Karigar, C.S.; Saqib, A. Traditional Indian medicine (TIM) and traditional Korean medicine (TKM): Aconstitutional-based concept and comparison. *Integr. Med. Res.* **2017**, *6*, 105–113. [CrossRef] [PubMed]
9. Xiang, Y.; Guo, Z.; Zhu, P.; Chen, J.; Huang, Y. Traditional Chinese medicine as a cancer treatment: Modern perspectives of ancient but advanced science. *Cancer Med.* **2019**, *8*, 1958–1975. [CrossRef] [PubMed]
10. Owen, H.C.; Appiah, S.; Hasan, N.; Ghali, L.; Elayat, G.; Bell, C. Phytochemical Modulation of Apoptosis and Autophagy: Strategies to Overcome Chemoresistance in Leukemic Stem Cells in the Bone Marrow Microenvironment. *Int. Rev. Neurobiol.* **2017**, *135*, 249–278. [CrossRef] [PubMed]
11. Xu, X.H.; Li, T.; Fong, C.M.; Chen, X.; Chen, X.J.; Wang, Y.T.; Huang, M.Q.; Lu, J.J. Saponins from Chinese Medicines as Anticancer Agents. *Molecules* **2016**, *21*, 1326. [CrossRef] [PubMed]
12. Nobili, S.; Lippi, D.; Witort, E.; Donnini, M.; Bausi, L.; Mini, E.; Capaccioli, S. Natural compounds for cancer treatment and prevention. *Pharm. Res* **2009**, *59*, 365–378. [CrossRef]
13. Abdel-Hafez, S.M.; Hathout, R.M.; Sammour, O.A. Attempts to enhance the anti-cancer activity of curcumin as a magical oncological agent using transdermal delivery. *Adv. Tradit. Med.* **2021**, *21*, 15–29. [CrossRef]
14. Buhrmann, C.; Yazdi, M.; Popper, B.; Shayan, P.; Goel, A.; Aggarwal, B.B.; Shakibaei, M. Resveratrol Chemosensitizes TNF-β-Induced Survival of 5-FU-Treated Colorectal Cancer Cells. *Nutrients* **2018**, *10*, 888. [CrossRef]
15. Buhrmann, C.; Yazdi, M.; Popper, B.; Kunnumakkara, A.B.; Aggarwal, B.B.; Shakibaei, M. Induction of the Epithelial-to-Mesenchymal Transition of Human Colorectal Cancer by Human TNF-β (Lymphotoxin) and its Reversal by Resveratrol. *Nutrients* **2019**, *11*, 704. [CrossRef] [PubMed]
16. Toden, S.; Okugawa, Y.; Jascur, T.; Wodarz, D.; Komarova, N.L.; Buhrmann, C.; Shakibaei, M.; Boland, C.R.; Goel, A. Curcumin mediates chemosensitization to 5-fluorouracil through miRNA-induced suppression of epithelial-to-mesenchymal transition in chemoresistant colorectal cancer. *Carcinogenesis* **2015**, *36*, 355–367. [CrossRef]
17. Kim, C.; Kim, B. Anti-Cancer Natural Products and Their Bioactive Compounds Inducing ER Stress-Mediated Apoptosis: A Review. *Nutrients* **2018**, *10*, 1021. [CrossRef] [PubMed]
18. Kaczanowski, S. Apoptosis: Its origin, history, maintenance and the medical implications for cancer and aging. *Phys. Biol.* **2016**, *13*, 031001. [CrossRef] [PubMed]
19. Wong, R.S.Y. Apoptosis in cancer: From pathogenesis to treatment. *J. Exp. Clin. Cancer Res. CR* **2011**, *30*, 87. [CrossRef] [PubMed]
20. Massagué, J.; Batlle, E.; Gomis, R.R. Understanding the molecular mechanisms driving metastasis. *Mol. Oncol.* **2017**, *11*, 3–4. [CrossRef] [PubMed]
21. Chatterjee, N.; Bivona, T.G. Polytherapy and Targeted Cancer Drug Resistance. *Trends Cancer* **2019**, *5*, 170–182. [CrossRef]
22. Elmore, S. Apoptosis: A review of programmed cell death. *Toxicol. Pathol.* **2007**, *35*, 495–516. [CrossRef]
23. Matsushita, Y.; Furutani, Y.; Matsuoka, R.; Furukawa, T. Hot water extract of Agaricus blazei Murrill specifically inhibits growth and induces apoptosis in human pancreatic cancer cells. *BMC Complement. Altern. Med.* **2018**, *18*, 319. [CrossRef] [PubMed]
24. Hu, W.; Jia, X.; Gao, Y.; Zhang, Q. Chaetospirolactone reverses the apoptotic resistance towards TRAIL in pancreatic cancer. *Biochem. Biophys. Res. Commun.* **2018**, *495*, 621–628. [CrossRef] [PubMed]
25. Koul, M.; Meena, S.; Kumar, A.; Sharma, P.R.; Singamaneni, V.; Riyaz-Ul-Hassan, S.; Hamid, A.; Chaubey, A.; Prabhakar, A.; Gupta, P.; et al. Secondary Metabolites from Endophytic Fungus Penicillium pinophilum Induce ROS-Mediated Apoptosis through Mitochondrial Pathway in Pancreatic Cancer Cells. *Planta Med.* **2016**, *82*, 344–355. [CrossRef] [PubMed]
26. Arora, D.; Sharma, N.; Singamaneni, V.; Sharma, V.; Kushwaha, M.; Abrol, V.; Guru, S.; Sharma, S.; Gupta, A.P.; Bhushan, S.; et al. Isolation and characterization of bioactive metabolites from Xylaria psidii, an endophytic fungus of the medicinal plant Aegle marmelos and their role in mitochondrial dependent apoptosis against pancreatic cancer cells. *Phytomedicine* **2016**, *23*, 1312–1320. [CrossRef]
27. Guzman, E.A.; Xu, Q.; Pitts, T.P.; Mitsuhashi, K.O.; Baker, C.; Linley, P.A.; Oestreicher, J.; Tendyke, K.; Winder, P.L.; Suh, E.M.; et al. Leiodermatolide, a novel marine natural product, has potent cytotoxic and antimitotic activity against cancer cells, appears to affect microtubule dynamics, and exhibits antitumor activity. *Int. J. Cancer* **2016**, *139*, 2116–2126. [CrossRef] [PubMed]
28. Lee, S.; Morita, H.; Tezuka, Y. Preferentially cytotoxic constituents of Andrographis paniculata and their preferential cytotoxicity against human pancreatic cancer cell lines. *Nat. Prod. Commun.* **2015**, *10*, 1934578X1501000704. [CrossRef]
29. Tuan, H.N.; Minh, B.H.; Tran, P.T.; Lee, J.H.; Oanh, H.V.; Ngo, Q.M.T.; Nguyen, Y.N.; Lien, P.T.K.; Tran, M.H. The Effects of 2′,4′-Dihydroxy-6′-methoxy-3′,5′-dimethylchalcone from Cleistocalyx operculatus Buds on Human Pancreatic Cancer Cell Lines. *Molecules* **2019**, *24*, 2538. [CrossRef]
30. LeJeune, T.M.; Tsui, H.Y.; Parsons, L.B.; Miller, G.E.; Whitted, C.; Lynch, K.E.; Ramsauer, R.E.; Patel, J.U.; Wyatt, J.E.; Street, D.S. Mechanism of action of two flavone isomers targeting cancer cells with varying cell differentiation status. *PLoS ONE* **2015**, *10*, e0142928. [CrossRef]
31. Zhang, Y.; Li, Z.; Min, Q.; Palida, A.; Zhang, Y.; Tang, R.; Chen, L.; Li, H. 8-Chrysoeriol, as a potential BCL-2 inhibitor triggers apoptosis of SW1990 pancreatic cancer cells. *Bioorg. Chem.* **2018**, *77*, 478–484. [CrossRef]

32. Tian, D.M.; Cheng, H.Y.; Jiang, M.M.; Shen, W.Z.; Tang, J.S.; Yao, X.S. Cardiac Glycosides from the Seeds of Thevetia peruviana. *J. Nat. Prod.* **2016**, *79*, 38–50. [CrossRef] [PubMed]
33. Rangarajan, P.; Dharmalingam Subramaniam, S.P.; Kwatra, D.; Palaniyandi, K.; Islam, S.; Harihar, S.; Ramalingam, S.; Gutheil, W.; Putty, S.; Pradhan, R. Crocetinic acid inhibits hedgehog signaling to inhibit pancreatic cancer stem cells. *Oncotarget* **2015**, *6*, 27661. [CrossRef] [PubMed]
34. Guo, W.; Chen, Y.; Gao, J.; Zhong, K.; Wei, H.; Li, K.; Tang, M.; Zhao, X.; Liu, X.; Nie, C.; et al. Diosgenin exhibits tumor suppressive function via down-regulation of EZH2 in pancreatic cancer cells. *Cell Cycle* **2019**, *18*, 1745–1758. [CrossRef] [PubMed]
35. Wang, W.; Luo, J.; Liang, Y.; Li, X. Echinacoside suppresses pancreatic adenocarcinoma cell growth by inducing apoptosis via the mitogen-activated protein kinase pathway. *Mol. Med. Rep.* **2016**, *13*, 2613–2618. [CrossRef] [PubMed]
36. Long, J.; Liu, Z.; Hui, L. Anti-tumor effect and mechanistic study of elemene on pancreatic carcinoma. *BMC Complement. Altern. Med.* **2019**, *19*, 133. [CrossRef]
37. Wang, W.; Zhan, L.; Guo, D.; Xiang, Y.; Tian, M.; Zhang, Y.; Wu, H.; Wei, Y.; Ma, G.; Han, Z. Grape seed proanthocyanidins inhibit proliferation of pancreatic cancer cells by modulating microRNA expression. *Oncol. Lett.* **2019**, *17*, 2777–2787. [CrossRef]
38. Guha Majumdar, A.; Subramanian, M. Hydroxychavicol from Piper betle induces apoptosis, cell cycle arrest, and inhibits epithelial-mesenchymal transition in pancreatic cancer cells. *Biochem. Pharm.* **2019**, *166*, 274–291. [CrossRef]
39. Boukes, G.J.; van de Venter, M. The apoptotic and autophagic properties of two natural occurring prodrugs, hyperoside and hypoxoside, against pancreatic cancer cell lines. *Biomed. Pharm.* **2016**, *83*, 617–626. [CrossRef]
40. Zheng, X.; Li, D.; Li, J.; Wang, B.; Zhang, L.; Yuan, X.; Li, C.; Cui, L.; Zhang, Q.; Yang, L.; et al. Optimization of the process for purifying icariin from Herba Epimedii by macroporous resin and the regulatory role of icariin in the tumor immune microenvironment. *Biomed. Pharm.* **2019**, *118*, 109275. [CrossRef] [PubMed]
41. Luo, B.; Wang, J.; Li, X.; Lu, W.; Yang, J.; Hu, Y.; Huang, P.; Wen, S. New mild and simple approach to isothiocyanates: A class of potent anticancer agents. *Molecules* **2017**, *22*, 773. [CrossRef]
42. Rahman, H.S. Phytochemical analysis and antioxidant and anticancer activities of mastic gum resin from Pistacia atlantica subspecies kurdica. *OncoTargets Ther.* **2018**, *11*, 4559. [CrossRef]
43. Akasaka, H.; Mizushina, Y.; Yoshida, K.; Ejima, Y.; Mukumoto, N.; Wang, T.; Inubushi, S.; Nakayama, M.; Wakahara, Y.; Sasaki, R. MGDG extracted from spinach enhances the cytotoxicity of radiation in pancreatic cancer cells. *Radiat. Oncol.* **2016**, *11*, 153. [CrossRef]
44. Wang, Y.; Wu, X.; Zhou, Y.; Jiang, H.; Pan, S.; Sun, B. Piperlongumine Suppresses Growth and Sensitizes Pancreatic Tumors to Gemcitabine in a Xenograft Mouse Model by Modulating the NF-kappa B Pathway. *Cancer Prev. Res.* **2016**, *9*, 234–244. [CrossRef]
45. Karki, K.; Hedrick, E.; Kasiappan, R.; Jin, U.-H.; Safe, S. Piperlongumine induces reactive oxygen species (ROS)-dependent downregulation of specificity protein transcription factors. *Cancer Prev. Res.* **2017**, *10*, 467–477. [CrossRef]
46. Zhang, L.; Wang, P.; Qin, Y.; Cong, Q.; Shao, C.; Du, Z.; Ni, X.; Li, P.; Ding, K. RN1, a novel galectin-3 inhibitor, inhibits pancreatic cancer cell growth in vitro and in vivo via blocking galectin-3 associated signaling pathways. *Oncogene* **2017**, *36*, 1297–1308. [CrossRef]
47. Su, J.; Wang, L.; Yin, X.; Zhao, Z.; Hou, Y.; Ye, X.; Zhou, X.; Wang, Z. Rottlerin exhibits anti-cancer effect through inactivation of S phase kinase-associated protein 2 in pancreatic cancer cells. *Am. J. Cancer Res.* **2016**, *6*, 2178–2191. [PubMed]
48. Hao, C.; Zhang, X.; Zhang, H.; Shang, H.; Bao, J.; Wang, H.; Li, Z. Sugiol (12?horbar;hydroxyabieta-8,11,13-trien-7-one) targets human pancreatic carcinoma cells (Mia-PaCa2) by inducing apoptosis, G2/M cell cycle arrest, ROS production and inhibition of cancer cell migration. *J. BUON* **2018**, *23*, 205–210. [PubMed]
49. Aliebrahimi, S.; Kouhsari, S.M.; Arab, S.S.; Shadboorestan, A.; Ostad, S.N. Phytochemicals, withaferin A and carnosol, overcome pancreatic cancer stem cells as c-Met inhibitors. *Biomed. Pharm.* **2018**, *106*, 1527–1536. [CrossRef] [PubMed]
50. Li, X.; Zhu, F.; Jiang, J.; Sun, C.; Zhong, Q.; Shen, M.; Wang, X.; Tian, R.; Shi, C.; Xu, M.; et al. Simultaneous inhibition of the ubiquitin-proteasome system and autophagy enhances apoptosis induced by ER stress aggravators in human pancreatic cancer cells. *Autophagy* **2016**, *12*, 1521–1537. [CrossRef] [PubMed]
51. Aamazadeh, F.; Ostadrahimi, A.; Rahbar Saadat, Y.; Barar, J. Bitter apricot ethanolic extract induces apoptosis through increasing expression of Bax/Bcl-2 ratio and caspase-3 in PANC-1 pancreatic cancer cells. *Mol. Biol. Rep.* **2020**, *47*, 1895–1904. [CrossRef]
52. Hii, L.W.; Lim, S.E.; Leong, C.O.; Chin, S.Y.; Tan, N.P.; Lai, K.S.; Mai, C.W. The synergism of Clinacanthus nutans Lindau extracts with gemcitabine: Downregulation of anti-apoptotic markers in squamous pancreatic ductal adenocarcinoma. *BMC Complement. Altern. Med.* **2019**, *19*, 257. [CrossRef] [PubMed]
53. Qian, Y.; Yang, B.; Xiong, Y.; Gu, M. Coix seed emulsion synergistically enhances the antitumor activity of gemcitabine in pancreatic cancer through abrogation of NF-κB signaling. *Oncol. Rep.* **2016**, *36*, 1517–1525. [CrossRef] [PubMed]
54. Luan, Y.P.; Li, Q.F.; Wu, S.G.; Mao, D.C.; Deng, Y.Y.; Chen, R.W. Tsoong induces apoptosis and inhibits proliferation, migration and invasion of pancreatic ductal adenocarcinoma cells. *Mol. Med. Rep.* **2018**, *17*, 3527–3536. [CrossRef] [PubMed]
55. Bhuyan, D.J.; Vuong, Q.V.; Bond, D.R.; Chalmers, A.C.; Bowyer, M.C.; Scarlett, C.J. Eucalyptus microcorys leaf extract derived HPLC-fraction reduces the viability of MIA PaCa-2 cells by inducing apoptosis and arresting cell cycle. *Biomed. Pharm.* **2018**, *105*, 449–460. [CrossRef]
56. Bhuyan, D.J.; Sakoff, J.; Bond, D.R.; Predebon, M.; Vuong, Q.V.; Chalmers, A.C.; van Altena, I.A.; Bowyer, M.C.; Scarlett, C.J. In vitro anticancer properties of selected Eucalyptus species. *Vitr. Cell. Dev. Biol. Anim.* **2017**, *53*, 604–615. [CrossRef] [PubMed]

57. Pak, P.J.; Kang, B.H.; Park, S.H.; Sung, J.H.; Joo, Y.H.; Jung, S.H.; Chung, N. Antitumor effects of herbal mixture extract in the pancreatic adenocarcinoma cell line PANC1. *Oncol. Rep.* **2016**, *36*, 2875–2883. [CrossRef]
58. Zhang, B.; Zeng, J.; Yan, Y.; Yang, B.; Huang, M.; Wang, L.; Zhang, Q.; Lin, N. Ethyl acetate extract from Inula helenium L. inhibits the proliferation of pancreatic cancer cells by regulating the STAT3/AKT pathway. *Mol. Med. Rep.* **2018**, *17*, 5440–5448. [CrossRef] [PubMed]
59. Hagoel, L.; Vexler, A.; Kalich-Philosoph, L.; Earon, G.; Ron, I.; Shtabsky, A.; Marmor, S.; Lev-Ari, S. Combined Effect of Moringa oleifera and Ionizing Radiation on Survival and Metastatic Activity of Pancreatic Cancer Cells. *Integr. Cancer Ther.* **2019**, *18*, 1534735419828829. [CrossRef]
60. Liu, Y.-H.; Weng, Y.-P.; Tsai, H.-Y.; Chen, C.-J.; Lee, D.-Y.; Hsieh, C.-L.; Wu, Y.-C.; Lin, J.-Y. Aqueous extracts of Paeonia suffruticosa modulates mitochondrial proteostasis by reactive oxygen species-induced endoplasmic reticulum stress in pancreatic cancer cells. *Phytomedicine* **2018**, *46*, 184–192. [CrossRef] [PubMed]
61. Tripathi, S.K.; Biswal, B.K. *Pterospermum acerifolium* (L.) wild bark extract induces anticarcinogenic effect in human cancer cells through mitochondrial-mediated ROS generation. *Mol. Biol. Rep.* **2018**, *45*, 2283–2294. [CrossRef] [PubMed]
62. Zhao, Q.; Huo, X.C.; Sun, F.D.; Dong, R.Q. Polyphenol-rich extract of Salvia chinensis exhibits anticancer activity in different cancer cell lines, and induces cell cycle arrest at the G(0)/G(1)-phase, apoptosis and loss of mitochondrial membrane potential in pancreatic cancer cells. *Mol. Med. Rep.* **2015**, *12*, 4843–4850. [CrossRef] [PubMed]
63. Bai, Y.; Chen, B.; Hong, W.; Liang, Y.; Zhou, M.; Zhou, L. Sedum sarmentosum Bunge extract induces apoptosis and inhibits proliferation in pancreatic cancer cells via the hedgehog signaling pathway. *Oncol. Rep.* **2016**, *35*, 2775–2784. [CrossRef] [PubMed]
64. Wang, Y.; Cao, H.J.; Sun, S.J.; Dai, J.Y.; Fang, J.W.; Li, Q.H.; Yan, C.; Mao, W.W.; Zhang, Y.Y. Total flavonoid aglycones extract in Radix scutellariae inhibits lung carcinoma and lung metastasis by affecting cell cycle and DNA synthesis. *J. Ethnopharmacol.* **2016**, *194*, 269–279. [CrossRef] [PubMed]
65. Liu, J.; Wang, H.; Wang, J.; Chang, Q.; Hu, Z.; Shen, X.; Feng, J.; Zhang, Z.; Wu, X. Total flavonoid aglycones extract in Radix Scutellariae induces cross-regulation between autophagy and apoptosis in pancreatic cancer cells. *J. Ethnopharmacol.* **2019**, *235*, 133–140. [CrossRef] [PubMed]
66. Yan, Y.; Zhang, Q.; Zhang, B.; Yang, B.; Lin, N. Active ingredients of Inula helenium L. exhibits similar anti-cancer effects as isoalantolactone in pancreatic cancer cells. *Nat. Prod. Res.* **2019**, *34*, 2539–2544. [CrossRef]
67. Steeg, P.S. Tumor metastasis: Mechanistic insights and clinical challenges. *Nat. Med.* **2006**, *12*, 895–904. [CrossRef] [PubMed]
68. Cheng, S.; Castillo, V.; Sliva, D. CDC20 associated with cancer metastasis and novel mushroom-derived CDC20 inhibitors with antimetastatic activity. *Int. J. Oncol.* **2019**, *54*, 2250–2256. [CrossRef]
69. Zhang, J.; Wang, W.; Zhou, Y.; Yang, J.; Xu, J.; Xu, Z.; Xu, Y.; Sun, L.; Cheng, X.D.; Li, M.; et al. Terphenyllin Suppresses Orthotopic Pancreatic Tumor Growth and Prevents Metastasis in Mice. *Front. Pharm.* **2020**, *11*, 457. [CrossRef] [PubMed]
70. Aravindan, S.; Ramraj, S.; Kandasamy, K.; Thirugnanasambandan, S.S.; Somasundaram, D.B.; Herman, T.S.; Aravindan, N. Hormophysa triquerta polyphenol, an elixir that deters CXCR4- and COX2-dependent dissemination destiny of treatment-resistant pancreatic cancer cells. *Oncotarget* **2017**, *8*, 5717–5734. [CrossRef]
71. Lee, S.Y.; Kim, W.; Lee, Y.G.; Kang, H.J.; Lee, S.H.; Park, S.Y.; Min, J.K.; Lee, S.R.; Chung, S.J. Identification of sennoside A as a novel inhibitor of the slingshot (SSH) family proteins related to cancer metastasis. *Pharm. Res.* **2017**, *119*, 422–430. [CrossRef]
72. Pei, Z.; Fu, W.; Wang, G. A natural product toosendanin inhibits epithelial-mesenchymal transition and tumor growth in pancreatic cancer via deactivating Akt/mTOR signaling. *Biochem. Biophys. Res. Commun.* **2017**, *493*, 455–460. [CrossRef]
73. Choi, H.S.; Lee, K.; Kim, M.K.; Lee, K.M.; Shin, Y.C.; Cho, S.G.; Ko, S.G. DSGOST inhibits tumor growth by blocking VEGF/VEGFR2-activated angiogenesis. *Oncotarget* **2016**, *7*, 21775–21785. [CrossRef] [PubMed]
74. Choi, H.S.; Kim, M.K.; Lee, K.; Lee, K.M.; Choi, Y.K.; Shin, Y.C.; Cho, S.G.; Ko, S.G. SH003 represses tumor angiogenesis by blocking VEGF binding to VEGFR2. *Oncotarget* **2016**, *7*, 32969–32979. [CrossRef]
75. Mizrahi, J.D.; Surana, R.; Valle, J.W.; Shroff, R.T. Pancreatic cancer. *Lancet* **2020**, *395*, 2008–2020. [CrossRef]
76. Qian, Y.; Xiong, Y.; Feng, D.; Wu, Y.; Zhang, X.; Chen, L.; Gu, M. Coix Seed Extract Enhances the Anti-Pancreatic Cancer Efficacy of Gemcitabine through Regulating ABCB1- and ABCG2-Mediated Drug Efflux: A Bioluminescent Pharmacokinetic and Pharmacodynamic Study. *Int. J. Mol. Sci.* **2019**, *20*, 5250. [CrossRef]
77. Shimada, T.; Nanimoto, Y.; Baron, B.; Kitagawa, T.; Tokuda, K.; Kuramitsu, Y. Enzyme-treated Asparagus Extract Down-regulates Heat Shock Protein 27 of Pancreatic Cancer Cells. *Vivo* **2018**, *32*, 759–763. [CrossRef]
78. Kim, M.; Mun, J.G.; Lee, H.J.; Son, S.R.; Lee, M.J.; Kee, J.Y. Inhibitory Effect of Oat Bran Ethanol Extract on Survival and Gemcitabine Resistance of Pancreatic Cancer Cells. *Molecules* **2019**, *24*, 3829. [CrossRef]
79. Li, L.; Zhao, S.L.; Yue, G.G.L.; Wong, T.P.; Pu, J.X.; Sun, H.D.; Fung, K.P.; Leung, P.C.; Han, Q.B.; Lau, C.B.S.; et al. Isodon eriocalyx and its bioactive component Eriocalyxin B enhance cytotoxic and apoptotic effects of gemcitabine in pancreatic cancer. *Phytomedicine* **2018**, *44*, 56–64. [CrossRef] [PubMed]
80. Shapira, S.; Pleban, S.; Kazanov, D.; Tirosh, P.; Arber, N. Terpinen-4-ol: A Novel and Promising Therapeutic Agent for Human Gastrointestinal Cancers. *PLoS ONE* **2016**, *11*, e0156540. [CrossRef] [PubMed]
81. Guzmán, E.A.; Pitts, T.P.; Diaz, M.C.; Wright, A.E. The marine natural product Scalarin inhibits the receptor for advanced glycation end products (RAGE) and autophagy in the PANC-1 and MIA PaCa-2 pancreatic cancer cell lines. *Investig. New Drugs* **2019**, *37*, 262–270. [CrossRef] [PubMed]

82. Somasagara, R.R.; Deep, G.; Shrotriya, S.; Patel, M.; Agarwal, C.; Agarwal, R. Bitter melon juice targets molecular mechanisms underlying gemcitabine resistance in pancreatic cancer cells. *Int. J. Oncol.* **2015**, *46*, 1849–1857. [CrossRef] [PubMed]
83. Dong, R.; Chen, P.; Chen, Q. Extract of the Medicinal Plant Pao Pereira Inhibits Pancreatic Cancer Stem-Like Cell In Vitro and In Vivo. *Integr Cancer Ther.* **2018**, *17*, 1204–1215. [CrossRef] [PubMed]
84. Chen, P.; Wang, M.; Wang, C. Qingyihuaji formula reverses gemcitabine resistant human pancreatic cancer through regulate lncRNA AB209630/miR-373/EphB2-NANOG signals. *Biosci. Rep.* **2019**, *39*, BSR20190610. [CrossRef] [PubMed]
85. Dong, R.; Chen, P.; Chen, Q. Inhibition of pancreatic cancer stem cells by Rauwolfia vomitoria extract. *Oncol. Rep.* **2018**, *40*, 3144–3154. [CrossRef] [PubMed]
86. UMIN-CTR. Phase 1/2 Study of gbs-01 in Patients with Gemcitabine-Refractory Advanced Pancreatic Cancer. Available online: https://upload.umin.ac.jp/cgi-open-bin/ctr/ctr.cgi?function=brows&action=brows&recptno=R000006430&type=summary&language=J (accessed on 16 August 2020).
87. Ikeda, M.; Sato, A.; Mochizuki, N.; Toyosaki, K.; Miyoshi, C.; Fujioka, R.; Mitsunaga, S.; Ohno, I.; Hashimoto, Y.; Takahashi, H. Phase I trial of GBS-01 for advanced pancreatic cancer refractory to gemcitabine. *Cancer Sci.* **2016**, *107*, 1818–1824. [CrossRef] [PubMed]
88. clinicalTrials.gov. Gemcitabine with Curcumin for Pancreatic Cancer. Available online: https://clinicaltrials.gov/ct2/show/NCT00192842?term=NCT00192842&draw=2&rank=1 (accessed on 1 June 2020).
89. ClinicalTrials.gov. Trial of Curcumin in Advanced Pancreatic Cancer. Available online: https://clinicaltrials.gov/ct2/show/NCT00094445?term=NCT00094445&draw=2&rank=1 (accessed on 1 June 2020).
90. ClinicalTrials.gov. Huachansu & Gemcitabine in Pancreatic Cancer. Available online: https://clinicaltrials.gov/ct2/show/NCT00837239?term=NCT00837239&draw=2&rank=1 (accessed on 15 May 2020).
91. Meng, Z.; Garrett, C.; Shen, Y.; Liu, L.; Yang, P.; Huo, Y.; Zhao, Q.; Spelman, A.; Ng, C.; Chang, D. Prospective randomised evaluation of traditional Chinese medicine combined with chemotherapy: A randomised phase II study of wild toad extract plus gemcitabine in patients with advanced pancreatic adenocarcinomas. *Br. J. Cancer* **2012**, *107*, 411–416. [CrossRef] [PubMed]
92. ClinicalTrials.gov. Safety and Exploratory Efficacy of Kanglaite Injection in Pancreatic Cancer. Available online: https://clinicaltrials.gov/ct2/show/NCT00733850?term=NCT00733850&draw=2&rank=1 (accessed on 15 May 2020).
93. Schwartzberg, L.S.; Arena, F.P.; Bienvenu, B.J.; Kaplan, E.H.; Camacho, L.H.; Campos, L.T.; Waymack, J.P.; Tagliaferri, M.A.; Chen, M.M.; Li, D. A randomized, open-label, safety and exploratory efficacy study of kanglaite injection (KLTi) plus gemcitabine versus gemcitabine in patients with advanced pancreatic cancer. *J. Cancer* **2017**, *8*, 1872. [CrossRef] [PubMed]
94. ISRCTNregistry. Mistletoe Therapy for Advanced Pancreatic Cancer. Available online: http://www.isrctn.com/ISRCTN70760582 (accessed on 1 June 2020).
95. Tröger, W.; Galun, D.; Reif, M.; Schumann, A.; Stankovic, N.; Milicevic, M. Quality of life of patients with advanced pancreatic cancer during treatment with mistletoe: A randomized controlled trial. *Dtsch. Ärzteblatt Int.* **2014**, *111*, 493.
96. clinicalTrials.gov. Mistletoe Therapy in Primary and Recurrent Inoperable Pancreatic Cancer (Mistral). Available online: https://clinicaltrials.gov/ct2/show/NCT02948309?term=Viscum+album&draw=3&rank=1 (accessed on 16 August 2020).
97. Fares, J.; Fares, M.Y.; Khachfe, H.H.; Salhab, H.A.; Fares, Y. Molecular principles of metastasis: A hallmark of cancer revisited. *Signal Transduct. Target. Ther.* **2020**, *5*, 1–17.
98. Qi, F.; Li, A.; Inagaki, Y.; Kokudo, N.; Tamura, S.; Nakata, M.; Tang, W. Antitumor activity of extracts and compounds from the skin of the toad Bufo bufo gargarizans Cantor. *Int. Immunopharmacol.* **2011**, *11*, 342–349. [CrossRef] [PubMed]
99. Enesel, M.B.; Acalovschi, I.; Grosu, V.; Sbarcea, A.; Rusu, C.; Dobre, A.; Weiss, T.; Zarkovic, N. Perioperative application of the Viscum album extract Isorel in digestive tract cancer patients. *Anticancer Res.* **2005**, *25*, 4583–4590.
100. Tezuka, Y.; Yamamoto, K.; Awale, S.; Li, F.; Yomoda, S.; Kadota, S. Anti-austeric activity of phenolic constituents of seeds of Arctium lappa. *Nat. Prod. Commun.* **2013**, *8*, 1934578X1300800414. [CrossRef]
101. Dhillon, N.; Aggarwal, B.B.; Newman, R.A.; Wolff, R.A.; Kunnumakkara, A.B.; Abbruzzese, J.L.; Ng, C.S.; Badmaev, V.; Kurzrock, R. Phase II trial of curcumin in patients with advanced pancreatic cancer. *Clin. Cancer Res.* **2008**, *14*, 4491–4499. [CrossRef] [PubMed]
102. Udenigwe, C.C.; Ramprasath, V.R.; Aluko, R.E.; Jones, P.J. Potential of resveratrol in anticancer and anti-inflammatory therapy. *Nutr. Rev.* **2008**, *66*, 445–454. [CrossRef] [PubMed]
103. Lin, C.-L.; Lin, J.-K. Curcumin: A potential cancer chemopreventive agent through suppressing NF-κB signaling. *J. Cancer Mol.* **2008**, *4*, 11–16.
104. Niu, Y.; Jin, Y.; Deng, S.-C.; Deng, S.-J.; Zhu, S.; Liu, Y.; Li, X.; He, C.; Liu, M.-L.; Zeng, Z. MiRNA-646-mediated reciprocal repression between HIF-1α and MIIP contributes to tumorigenesis of pancreatic cancer. *Oncogene* **2018**, *37*, 1743–1758. [CrossRef] [PubMed]
105. Yue, Q.; Gao, G.; Zou, G.; Yu, H.; Zheng, X. Natural products as adjunctive treatment for pancreatic cancer: Recent trends and advancements. *BioMed Res. Int.* **2017**, *2017*, 8412508. [CrossRef] [PubMed]

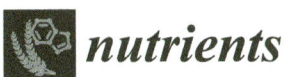

Article

Dracocephalum moldavica Ethanol Extract Suppresses LPS-Induced Inflammatory Responses through Inhibition of the JNK/ERK/NF-κB Signaling Pathway and IL-6 Production in RAW 264.7 Macrophages and in Endotoxic-Treated Mice

Kyeong-Min Kim [1], So-Yeon Kim [1], Tamanna Jahan Mony [2], Ho Jung Bae [2], Sang-Deok Han [1], Eun-Seok Lee [1], Seung-Hyuk Choi [1], Sun Hee Hong [3], Sang-Deok Lee [4,*] and Se Jin Park [1,2,*]

[1] Department of Food Biotechnology and Environmental Science, School of Natural Resources and Environmental Sciences, Kangwon National University, Chuncheon 24341, Korea; kasbai@kangwon.ac.kr (K.-M.K.); ykims95@kangwon.ac.kr (S.-Y.K.); 202016097@kangwon.ac.kr (S.-D.H.); dmstjr0806@kangwon.ac.kr (E.-S.L.); chltmdgur96@kangwon.ac.kr (S.-H.C.)

[2] Agriculture and Life Science Research Institute, Kangwon National University, Chuncheon 24341, Korea; tjmonycvasu@gmail.com (T.J.M.); baehj321@kangwon.ac.kr (H.J.B.)

[3] School of Applied Science in Natural Resources & Environment, Hankyong National University, Anseong 17579, Korea; shhong@hknu.ac.kr

[4] Division of Forest Science, Kangwon National University, Chuncheon 24341, Korea

* Correspondence: sdlee@kangwon.ac.kr (S.-D.L.); sejinpark@kangwon.ac.kr (S.J.P.)

Citation: Kim, K.-M.; Kim, S.-Y.; Mony, T.J.; Bae, H.J.; Han, S.-D.; Lee, E.-S.; Choi, S.-H.; Hong, S.H.; Lee, S.-D.; Park, S.J. *Dracocephalum moldavica* Ethanol Extract Suppresses LPS-Induced Inflammatory Responses through Inhibition of the JNK/ERK/NF-κB Signaling Pathway and IL-6 Production in RAW 264.7 Macrophages and in Endotoxic-Treated Mice. *Nutrients* **2021**, *13*, 4501. https://doi.org/10.3390/nu13124501

Academic Editor: Md Soriful Islam

Received: 11 November 2021
Accepted: 14 December 2021
Published: 16 December 2021

Publisher's Note: MDPI stays neutral with regard to jurisdictional claims in published maps and institutional affiliations.

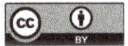

Copyright: © 2021 by the authors. Licensee MDPI, Basel, Switzerland. This article is an open access article distributed under the terms and conditions of the Creative Commons Attribution (CC BY) license (https://creativecommons.org/licenses/by/4.0/).

Abstract: The excessive synthesis of interleukin-6 (IL-6) is related to cytokine storm in COVID-19 patients. Moreover, blocking IL-6 has been suggested as a treatment strategy for inflammatory diseases such as sepsis. Sepsis is a severe systemic inflammatory response syndrome with high mortality. In the present study, we investigated the anti-inflammatory and anti-septic effects and the underlying mechanisms of *Dracocephalum moldavica* ethanol extract (DMEE) on lipopolysaccharide (LPS)-induced inflammatory stimulation in RAW 264.7 macrophages along with septic mouse models. We found that DMEE suppressed the release of inflammatory mediators NO and PGE$_2$ and inhibited both the mRNA and protein expression levels of iNOS and COX-2, respectively. In addition, DMEE reduced the release of proinflammatory cytokines, mainly IL-6 and IL-1β, in RAW 264.7 cells by inhibiting the phosphorylation of JNK, ERK and p65. Furthermore, treatment with DMEE increased the survival rate and decreased the level of IL-6 in plasma in LPS-induced septic shock mice. Our findings suggest that DMEE elicits an anti-inflammatory effect in LPS-stimulated RAW 264.7 macrophages and an anti-septic effect on septic mouse model through the inhibition of the ERK/JNK/NF-κB signaling cascades and production of IL-6.

Keywords: lipopolysaccharide; inflammation; interleukin-6; sepsis; *Dracocephalum moldavica*

1. Introduction

The inflammatory reaction (inflammation) is the foremost defense mechanism with a complex biological response from the body's tissues, after invasion of harmful stimuli. The inflammatory response is a multifactorial function accompanied by the activation of a signaling pathway that regulates inflammatory mediator levels in the host tissues [1]. The biological processes of the immune system are triggered by several factors, including pathogens, irritants, damaged cells and endotoxins such as lipopolysaccharide (LPS). LPS is the major glycoprotein that constitutes and acts as a highly immunogenic and the most important component of the outer cell wall of Gram-negative bacteria [2]. LPS binds with the binding protein (LBP) and is recognized by Toll-like receptors—most commonly by TLR4, which activates the immune system as part of the innate immune response [3]. The activated TLR4 complex signaling pathway, that includes the myeloid differentiation primary-response protein 88 (MyD88)-dependent pathway, can stimulate the upregulation of inflammatory gene expression [4]. The amino terminus of MyD88 recruits the IL-1 receptor-associated kinase (IRAK) family and then the phosphorylated MyD88/IRAK complex binds to TNF receptor-associated factor 6 (TRAF6) [5]. The transforming growth factor B-activated kinase (TAK1) complex is activated by TRAF6 and phosphorylated NF-κB, which translocate to the nucleus to initiate transcription and activate the gene expression of cytokines [6]. At the same time, TAK1 activates the MAPK family members, including JNK1/2, ERK1/2 and p38, which enter the nucleus and activate activator protein 1 (AP-1) [7].

Activated AP-1 and NF-κB signaling results in the secretion of proinflammatory cytokines, such as tumor necrosis factor-α (TNF-α), interleukin-6 (IL-6) and interleukin-1β (IL-1β), and chemokines. Excessive production of inflammatory cytokines and chemokines, which has been designated as a cytokine storm, leads to systemic inflammatory response syndromes such as COVID-19, rheumatoid arthritis and sepsis [8–10]. Sepsis is defined as a life-threatening organ dysfunction caused by the dysregulated host response to invading pathogens [11]. It is one of the typical diseases in systemic inflammatory response syndrome caused by a cytokine storm [12]. The main problem of sepsis is the high mortality due to the absence of distinct therapeutic strategies for increasing the survival rate [13,14]. The early administration of antibiotics is associated with decreased mortality, but patients who receive antibiotics such as vancomycin and piperacillin/tazobactam may have harmful outcomes, such as acute kidney injury [15,16]. Therefore, it is necessary to develop safe anti-septic therapies that positively increase the survival rate. Importantly, a number of patients with septic shock have increased IL-6 in their plasma levels, according to the ICU database [17]. Moreover, it has been reported that patients who had reduced IL-6 levels were 5.68 times more likely to survive than non-survivors [18]. Thus, blocking IL-6 levels may be an effective therapeutic strategy for reducing cytokine storm diseases.

Moldavian balm (*Dracocephalum moldavica*), known as Yixin Badi Ran Gibuya, is an annual herb that belongs to the family Lamiaceae [19]. *D. moldavica* is native in northern China, southeastern Xinjiang and eastern Europe. Furthermore, this herb has been used in traditional Uygur herbal drugs for headache, liver disorders and cardiovascular diseases, such as coronary heart disease, for many centuries [20]. This herbaceous plant has been reported to contain active components with anti-inflammatory and antioxidant effects, such as hydroxycinnamic acids, flavonoids and rosmarinic acid [21,22]. Rosmarinic acid (RA) has also been reported to significantly inhibit lung cell apoptosis and decrease the level of p53 in LPS-induced septic mice by inhibiting the activation of the GRP78/IRE1alpha/JNK pathway [23]. Additionally, RA has shown to downregulate the levels of TNF-a, IL-6 and HMGB-1 in LPS-induced RAW 264.7 cells by inhibiting the IkB kinase pathway [24]. Moreover, we confirmed that oleanolic acid (OA) was detected in *D. moldavica* ethanolic extract (DMEE), with an average level of approximately 4.32 ± 0.02 mg/g (Figure 1). OA has been reported to be useful as a therapeutic strategy for vascular inflammatory diseases by inhibiting hypermeability, the expression of cell adhesion molecules (CAMs) and the migration of leukocytes [25]. In addition, OA can regulate apoptosis and inflammation in spinal cord injury by blocking p38 and JNK [26].

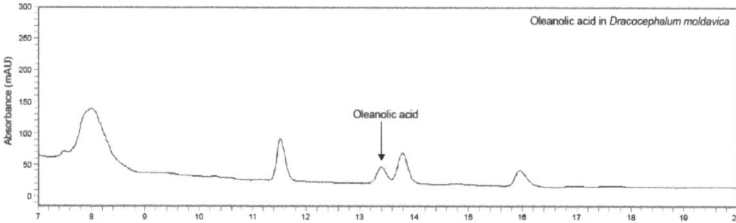

Figure 1. HPLC-UV chromatogram analysis of oleanolic acid in *D. moldavica* with detector responses at 210 nm.

Based on the anti-inflammatory effects of *D. moldavica* [27,28] and its ingredients, we speculated that DMEE may attenuate LPS-induced inflammatory responses and septic shocks in mice. In this study, we studied the anti-inflammatory effect and underlying mechanisms of DMEE on LPS-stimulated RAW 264.7 macrophages. Additionally, we further investigated the anti-septic effect of DMEE in LPS-induced septic shock mice.

2. Materials and Methods

2.1. Animals

Five-week-old male mice were supplied by Orient Bio (Seongnam, Korea). In each group, twelve mice were housed per cage with an optimized temperature of 21–25 °C and a 12 h light–dark cycle. Animals were provided with ad libitum food and water throughout the experimental period. All the animal experiments were conducted by following the ethical guidelines of the Institutional Animal Care and Use Committee of Kangwon National University (KW-200128-1).

2.2. Preparation of an Ethanolic Extract of D. moldavica

Dried leaves of *D. moldavica* were collected by Professor Xiang-Qian Liu (School of Pharmacy, Hunan University of Chinese Medicine, Changsha, China). We previously reported the preparation method of ethanolic extract of *D. moldavica* (DMEE) [29]. Briefly, dried *D. moldavica* leaves were mixed with 70% ethanol to extract DMEE, twice for 2 h by using an ultrasonic bath. After extracting, it was filtered and consequently concentrated in a water bath under vacuum pressure. Afterward, frozen and lyophilized phases were obtained. The obtained extract was stored at -20 °C until use.

2.3. High-Performance Liquid Chromatography (HPLC) Analysis

The HPLC analysis was performed to determine the levels of oleanolic acid in *D. moldavica* with a Perkin Elmer Flexar QUATERNARY Pump (PerkinElmer, Inc., Shelton, CT, USA) and a PDA LC detector (PerkinElmer, Inc., Shelton, CT, USA). The samples were separated by a YMC Pack-Pro C18 column (25 cm × 4.6 mm) in gradient elution mode. Two mobile phases were obtained that comprised 0.2% acetic acid in H_2O (A) and acetonitrile (B); the overall flow rate was 0.8 mL/min. The column temperature was 30 °C and the injection volume was 5 µL. The gradient conditions of oleanolic acid were 10% (A) and 90% (B) for 0–45 min. The test solution (*D. moldavica*) was weighed (60 mg) and dissolved at 20 mg/mL in MeOH. Then, the solution was sonicated for 30 min and filtered using a 0.45 µm PVDF membrane filter. Similarly, the standard solution (oleanolic acid) was weighed (1 mg) and dissolved at a concentration of 1 mg/mL in MeOH. The standard solution was sonicated and filtered under the same conditions as the test solution. The analysis of oleanolic acid in DMEE was detected at a 210 nm wavelength. The oleanolic acid composites were calculated by applying the following calibration curve equation: oleanolic acid, $y = 2567.7x + 23708$, $R^2 = 1$. The average level of oleanolic acid in *D. moldavica* was approximately 4.32 ± 0.02 mg/g (Figure 1).

2.4. Materials

Tetrazolium bromide (MTT), Dimethyl sulfoxide (DMSO), LPS, 3-(4,5-dimethylthiazol-2-yl)-2,5-diphenyl, Griess reagent and sodium nitrite were purchased from Sigma Chemical Co. (St. Louis, MO, USA). Penicillin–streptomycin (P/S), Dulbecco's phosphate buffered saline (DPBS), Dulbecco's modified Eagle's medium (DMEM) and DEPC water were purchased from Welgene (Gyeongsan, Korea). Fetal bovine serum (FBS) was provided by Atlas Biologicals (Fort Collins, CO, USA). RNAiso Plus was purchased from Takara Bio Inc. (Kusatsu, Japan). Chloroform, 2-propyl alcohol, acetone and olive oil were purchased from Daejung (Seongnam, Korea). Primers for cyclooxygenase-2 (COX-2), inducible nitric oxide synthase (iNOS), TNF-α, IL-1β, IL-6 and β-actin oligonucleotide were purchased from Integrated DNA Technologies (Coralville, IA, USA). We used enzyme-linked immunosorbent assay (ELISA) kits for prostagladin E_2 (PGE_2) from R&D Systems

(Minneapolis, MN, USA) and IL-6 and IL-1β from Abcam (Cambridge, UK). TransScript® All-in-One First-Strand cDNA Synthesis SuperMix for qPCR (One-Step gDNA Removal) was obtained from TransGen Biotech Co. (Beijing, China). PowerSYBR® Green PCR Master Mix from Applied Biosystems was purchased from Thermo Fisher Scientific (Rockford, IL, USA). Antibodies against p38, JNK, ERK, p65, phosphorylated p38 (p-p38), phosphorylated JNK (p-JNK), phosphorylated ERK (p-ERK) and phosphorylated p65 (p-p65) were supplied by Cell Signaling Technology, Inc. (Danvers, MA, USA). Other materials were purchased from usual commercial sources and ensured the highest available grade.

2.5. Cell Culture

Raw 264.7 cells—mouse-originated macrophages (RAW 264.7)—were supplied by the Korean Cell Line Bank (KCLB, Seoul, Korea). For cell culture, DMEM (100 units/Ml), P/S and 10% FBS were used as media. The cultured cells were incubated at 37 °C and 5% CO_2 and subsequently subcultured every two days.

2.6. Analysis of Cell Viability

The MTT assay was performed to measure the cell viability. First, DMEE-treated cells were incubated for 24 h; subsequently, the MTT assay was conducted. After incubation with MTT solution (5 mg/mL), the cells were mixed with PBS and incubated at 37 °C for 4 h. After that, the MTT solution was removed and the produced purple formazan crystals were solubilized in DMSO (100 μL/well) as described by [30]. The optical density was measured at 540 nm with a microplate spectrophotometer (SpectraMax, Molecular Devices, Sunnyvale, CA, USA).

2.7. Determination of Nitric Oxide Production

RAW 264.7 cells were pretreated with different concentrations of DMEE (50, 100, 200 and 400 μg/mL) for 1 h; later, they were stimulated with LPS at a concentration of 1 μg/mL for 24 h. Nitrite accumulation in the culture medium was considered as an indicator of nitric oxide (NO) production. The total NO production was measured with Griess reagent. Equal volumes of 100 μL of the supernatant and Griess reagent were mixed for 10 min [31]. The optical density was determined using a microplate reader (SpectraMax, molecular Devices, Sunnyvale, CA, USA) at 540 nm. The total of nitrite in the samples was determined based on a sodium nitrite standard curve.

2.8. PGE_2, IL-6 and IL-1β Assays

The expression levels of PGE_2, IL-6 and IL-1β, both in macrophage culture medium and plasma, were measured using commercial ELISA kits. The cells were pretreated with DMEE at various concentrations (from 50 μg/mL to 400 μg/mL) for 1 h; afterwards, they were treated with LPS (1 μg/mL) for 24 h. Cytokine expression in the cell was determined by ELISA, referring to the manufacturer's given protocol.

2.9. RNA Extraction and Real Time-Quantative PCR (RT-PCR)

The mRNA expressions of iNOS, COX-2, IL-6 and IL-1β were detected by performing RT-PCR. Total RNA was extracted using RNAiso PLUS (Takara, Otsu, Japan). From 1 μg of total RNA, cDNA was synthesized using the All-in-One FirstStrand cDNA Synthesis SuperMix, as previously described by [32]. The synthesized cDNAs were used as template for qRT-PCR using a QuantStudio 3 (Applied Biosystems, Foster City, CA, USA) system with POWER SYBR Green PCR master mix and gene-specific primers (Table 1). A dissociation curve analysis of iNOS, COX-2, IL-6, IL-1β and β-actin demonstrated a single peak. The expression levels of target genes were quantified by duplicate measurements and normalized with the $2^{-\Delta\Delta CT}$ method relative to control β-actin. The PCR analyses were performed under the following conditions: 40 cycles of 95 °C for 15 s; 57 °C for 20 s; and 72 °C for 40 s.

Table 1. Primer sequences used in the RT-PCR analyses.

Target Gene		Primer Sequence
iNOS	F	5′-CATGCTACTGGAGGTGGGTG-3′
	R	5′-CATTGATCTCCGTGACAGCC-3′
COX-2	F	5′-TGCTGTACAAGCAGTGGCAA-3
	R	5′-GCAGCCATTTCCTTCTCTCC-3′
IL-6	F	5′-GAGGATACCACTCCCAACAGACC-3′
	R	5′-AAGTGCATCATCGTTGTTCATACA-3′
IL-1β	F	5′-ACCTGCTGGTGTGTGACGTT-3′
	R	5′-TCGTTGCTTGGTTCTCCTTG-3′
β-actin	F	5′-ATCACTATTGGCAACGAGCG-3′
	R	5′-TCAGCAATGCCTGGGTACAT-3′

2.10. Western Blot Analysis

For immunoblot analysis, LPS-stimulated cells were washed twice with ice-cold PBS. Total proteins were isolated from the cells using a lysis buffer with cocktails of protein inhibitors and then harvested with a cell scraper [33]. Total cellular protein was quantified using the Bradford assay. The protein (20 μg/well protein) was loaded to 10% SDS-PAGE and then transferred to PVDF membranes [34]. The membranes were blocked with 5% skimmed milk for 2 h and then incubated with primary antibodies against p-JNK (Cell Signaling Technology (Danvers, MA, USA), 1:1000), p-ERK (Cell Signaling Technology, 1:1000), p-p65 (Cell Signaling Technology, 1:1000), JNK (Cell Signaling Technology, 1:1000), ERK (Cell Signaling Technology, 1:1000), p65 (Cell Signaling Technology, 1:1000), iNOS (Cell Signaling Technology, 1:500), COX-2 (Cell Signaling Technology, 1:1000), or β-actin (Cell Signaling Technology, 1:500) at 4 °C overnight. After washing, the membranes were again incubated for 2 h at room temperature with a secondary antibody (Cell signaling, 1:1000). The probed membranes were developed with enhanced chemiluminescence. The immunoblots were imaged using an LAS-500 mini-imager (General Electric, Boston, MA, USA) and analyzed with the ImageJ program. The phosphorylation level was determined by calculating the ratio of phosphorylated protein to the total protein on the same membrane; this was measured to determine the level of phosphorylation.

2.11. LPS-Induced Septic Shock Mice

To examine the effect of DMEE on LPS-induced modality changes in septic shock mice (n = 12 per group), the mice were orally treated with DMEE (50, 100 and 200 mg/kg body weight) or vehicle (0.9% saline) for 7 days. To induce septic shock in the mouse models, LPS at 25 mg/kg was injected intraperitoneally to mice and the survival of the mice was monitored for 3 days. In the satellite study (n = 4 per group), the mice were sacrificed at 12 h after LPS injection and a blood sample was collected to determine proinflammatory cytokine levels in the plasma.

2.12. Statistical Analyses

The statistical analyses were performed using GraphPad Prism Version 8.0 (GraphPad, La Jolla, CA, USA). All data are expressed as the mean ± S.E.M. The data were analyzed by a one-way analysis of variance (ANOVA), followed by a Student–Newman–Keuls test for multiple comparisons. A $p < 0.05$ was considered as a significant statistical value.

3. Results

3.1. HPLC-UV Chromatograms Analysis of Oleanolic Acid in DMEE

Based on the reported anti-inflammatory property of oleanolic acid, we performed the HPLC-UV detector analysis of oleanolic acid in DMEE. We confirmed that the average level of oleanolic acid in DMEE was approximately 4.32 ± 0.02 mg/g (Figure 1).

3.2. DMEE Inhibits the LPS-Stimulated Production of Inflammatory Mediators and iNOS and COX-2 Expression in RAW 264.7 Cells

We conducted an MTT assay to exhibit the effect of DMEE on the viability of RAW 264.7 macrophages. No cytotoxicity of DMEE was observed at any tested concentration (50, 100, 200 and 400 µg/mL) (Figure 2A). Moreover, DMEE blocked cell death stimulated with LPS at concentrations above 100 µg/mL (Figure 2B). To determine the effect of DMEE on LPS-stimulated NO and PGE$_2$ production, the cells were pretreated with DMEE for 1 h and then treated with LPS (1 µg/mL) for 24 h. We observed that DMEE suppressed the LPS-induced NO and PGE$_2$ production in a dose-dependent manner (Figure 2C,D). Furthermore, we found that the mRNA expression of iNOS and COX-2, which synthesize NO and PGE$_2$, was significantly reduced at the DMEE concentrations of 200 and 400 µg/mL (Figure 2E,F). We also observed that the protein expression of iNOS and COX-2 were decreased by DMEE treatment in RAW 264.7 cells (Figure 2G,H). These results indicate that DMEE moderates the production of proinflammatory mediators NO and PGE$_2$ via the suppression of iNOS and COX-2 expression.

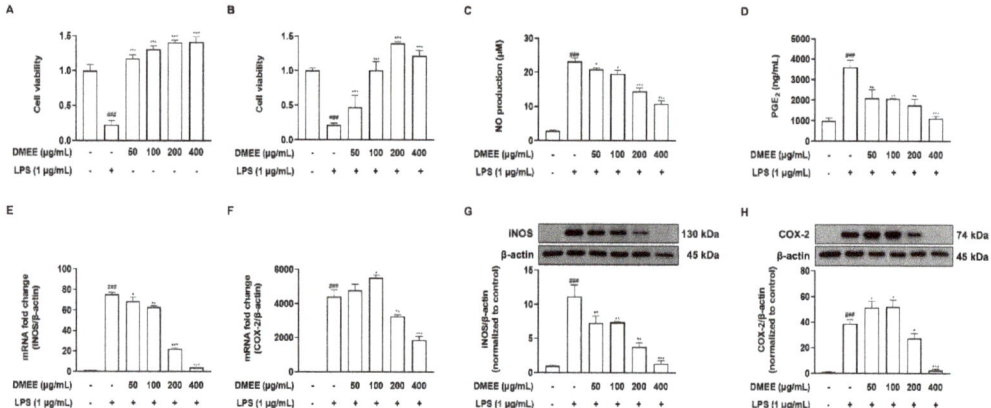

Figure 2. Effects of *D. moldavica* on LPS-induced inflammatory response in RAW 264.7 cells. Cells were pretreated with *D. moldavica* for 1 h and then treated with LPS (1 µg/mL) for 24 h. Cell viability was determined by MTT assay (*n* = 5) (**A,B**). The production of NO was measured by Griess reaction (*n* = 3) (**C**). The level of PGE$_2$ was measured by PGE$_2$ ELISA kit (*n* = 3) (**D**). The mRNA expression of iNOS and COX-2 was determined by RT-PCR (*n* = 3) (**E,F**). The protein levels of iNOS and COX-2 were measured by Western blotting and the quantification of iNOS and COX-2 was normalized to the control (*n* = 3) (**G,H**). The data shown are representative of three independent experiments and indicate mean ± S.E.M. $^{\#\#\#}$ $p < 0.001$ versus the vehicle-treated controls; * $p < 0.05$, ** $p < 0.01$ and *** $p < 0.001$ versus the LPS-treated group.

3.3. DMEE Reduced the Secretion of Proinflammatory Cytokines in LPS-Stimulated RAW 264.7 Cells

During inflammatory responses, immune cells such as macrophages secrete the proinflammatory cytokines that induce various inflammation reactions and the production of NO and PGE$_2$ [35]. Thus, inflammatory cytokines are pleiotropic molecules that play a pivotal role in inflammatory reactions [36]. For that reason, we investigated the inhibitory effects of DMEE on the release of proinflammatory cytokines such as IL-6 and IL-1β in RAW 264.7 cells. Macrophages were pretreated with DMEE for 1 h and consequently stimulated with LPS (1 µg/mL) for 24 h. The mRNA expression level of proinflammatory cytokines was determined in the collected medium by RT-PCR analysis. As shown in Figure 3A,B, the mRNA expression levels of IL-6 and IL-1β were significantly increased in LPS-stimulated macrophages compared to the control, which were dose-dependently inhibited by DMEE. We further determined whether treatment with DMEE downregulated the protein levels of IL-6 and IL-1β by using ELISA. Similar to the mRNA expression, the protein expression of IL-6 and IL-1β was also significantly reduced at 400 µg/mL DMEE (Figure 3C,D).

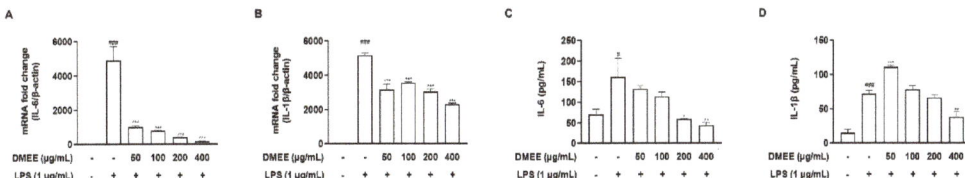

Figure 3. Effects of *D. moldavica* on LPS-induced proinflammatory cytokine expression in RAW 264.7 cells. Cells were pretreated with *D. moldavica* for 1 h and then treated with LPS (1 µg/mL) for 24 h. The mRNA expression of IL-6 and IL-1β was determined by RT-PCR (*n* = 3) (**A,B**) and the secretion of IL-6 and IL-1β was measured by IL-6 and IL-1β ELISA kit (*n* = 3) (**C,D**). The data shown are representative of three independent experiments and indicate mean ± S.E.M. # $p < 0.05$, ### $p < 0.001$ versus the vehicle-treated controls; * $p < 0.05$, ** $p < 0.01$ and *** $p < 0.001$ versus the LPS-treated group.

3.4. DMEE Suppresses the MAPK/NF-κB Pathway

After LPS binds to TLR4, it activates the phosphorylation of transcription inducers, for example the MAPK and NF-κB pathways. It is known that the expression of inflammatory cytokines in LPS-induced RAW 264.7 macrophages is associated with the MAPK/NF-κB phosphorylation pathway [37]. Therefore, we investigated whether DMEE inhibited the phosphorylation of p65, a subunit of NF-κB. The phosphorylation of p65 was increased by LPS treatment, but DMEE significantly reduced LPS-stimulated phosphorylation of p65 in RAW 264.7 cells (Figure 4A). Next, we wanted to identify which kinase was involved in the regulation of NF-κB activity. Our results demonstrate that the phosphorylation of JNK 1/2 and ERK 1/2 was increased by LPS stimulation, but DMEE inhibited the phosphorylation of JNK 1/2 and ERK 1/2 (Figure 4B,C). These results indicate that the anti-inflammatory effects of DMEE may be associated with its inhibitory properties on JNK- and ERK-mediated NF-κB activation.

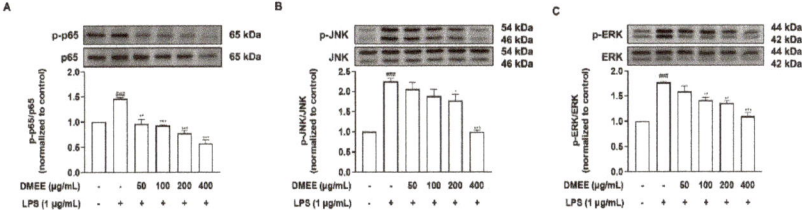

Figure 4. Effects of *D. moldavica* on the MAPK/NF-κB pathway in RAW 264.7 cells. Cells were pretreated with *D. moldavica* for 1 h and then treated with LPS (1 µg/mL) for 30 min. The phosphorylation activity was normalized to the untreated control group. The expression of phospho-JNK, JNK, phospho-ERK, ERK, phosphor-p65, p65 and β-actin was determined by Western blotting (*n* = 3) (**A–C**). The data shown are representative of three independent experiments and indicate mean ± S.E.M. ### $p < 0.001$ versus the vehicle-treated controls; * $p < 0.05$, ** $p < 0.01$ and *** $p < 0.001$ versus the LPS-treated group.

3.5. DMEE Enhances the Survival Rate and Reduces the Level of IL-6 in Plasma in LPS-Stimulated Septic Shock in Mice

Based on the anti-inflammatory activity of DMEE in vitro, we examined the anti-septic effects of DMEE on LPS-induced septic shock mice (Figure 5A). We orally treated mice with DMEE at the different concentrations of 50, 100 and 200 mg/kg for seven days and then septic shock was induced by LPS (25 mg/kg, i.p.). At 3 days after LPS injection, the survival rate of the LPS-only injected group was the lowest (38%) and the survival rates of the septic shock mice in the group treated with DMEE increased dose-dependently (from 42% to 75%) (Figure 5B). At 12 h after LPS injection, blood samples were collected to measure proinflammatory cytokines, such as IL-6 and IL-1β, in the plasma (Figure 5A). The level of IL-6 in plasma was significantly reduced, but the level of IL-1β was unchanged in LPS-induced septic shock mice (Figure 5C,D). These results indicate that DMEE attenuates LPS-induced septic shock in mice via inhibition of IL-6 production.

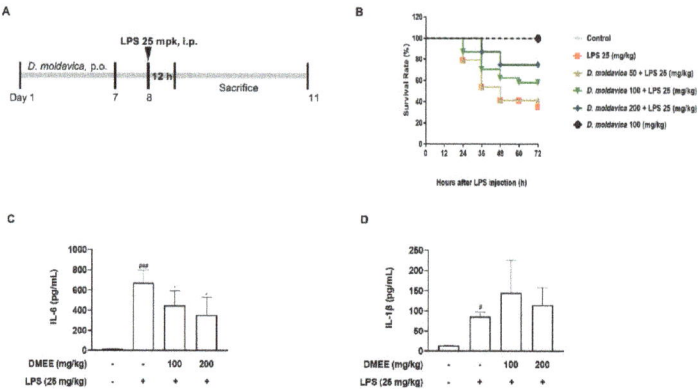

Figure 5. Effect of *D. moldavica* on the survival rate and level of IL-6 in plasma in LPS-induced septic shock mice. Mice were administered with *D. moldavica* (50, 100 and 200 mg/kg p.o.) or vehicle (0.9% saline) for 7 days and then injected with LPS (25 mg/kg, i.p.). The survival rate was measured for 3 days and blood samples were collected 12 h after LPS injection. Timetable of the LPS-induced septic shock mouse model (**A**). Survival rate of the group injected with *D. moldavica* or LPS (control *D. moldavica* 100 mpk, 100%; LPS 25 mpk, 38%; *D. moldavica* 50 mpk + LPS, 42%; *D. moldavica* 100 mpk + LPS, 58%; *D. moldavica* 200 mpk + LPS, 75%) (n = 8/group) (**B**). The levels of IL-6 and IL-1β in plasma were determined by ELISA kit (n = 4/group) (**C,D**). The data shown are representative of three independent experiments and indicate mean ± S.E.M. # $p < 0.05$ and ### $p < 0.001$ versus the vehicle-treated controls; * $p < 0.05$ versus the LPS-treated group.

4. Discussion

Sepsis is considered as a systemic inflammatory response syndrome triggered by an immoderate cytokine expression to counter infections [38]. When the septic response is activated by augmented levels of inflammatory mediators and cytokines, such as NO, TNF-α, IL-1β, COX-2 and IL-6, this causes septic shock in terms of tissue damage and multisystem organ dysfunction, which leads to death [39,40]. Although the analysis of septic shock with cytokine storm with the target treatment of TNF and IL-1 showed promising results in reducing morbidity and mortality in septic shock models, no beneficial results were found in clinical trials [41]. Because of the complex biological responses, there are no effective therapeutic strategies for septic shock. Thus, it is important to impede the excessive expression of inflammatory mediators and cytokines known as cytokine storms [42]. Previous studies reported that IL-6 was determined to be a promising target molecule for systemic inflammatory response syndromes such as sepsis. Moreover, IL-6R antagonists may provide improved results for patients with infectious diseases such as COVID-19 or sepsis [43]. Therefore, blockade of IL-6 suggests that it can regulate cytokine storm diseases [44]. In this study, we observed that the administration of *D. moldavica* increased the survival rate up to 75% in LPS-triggered septic shock mice by inhibiting the secretion level of IL-6 in plasma. Therefore, we suggest that *D. moldavica* would be a promising preventive option for cytokine storm in sepsis or COVID-19.

Moldavian balm is an herb plant (*Dracocephalum moldavica*) of the Lamiaceae family used for traditional Uygur medicine. Uygur people have used *Dracocephalum moldavica* as a therapy for cardiovascular diseases such as myocardial ischemia, hypertension and coronary heart diseases [45]. Moreover, total flavonoids isolated from *D. moldavica* have been demonstrated to inhibit the proliferation and migration of intercellular adhesion molecule-1 and vascular cell adhesion molecule-1 in vascular smooth muscle cells by inhibiting NF-κB expression [46]. In addition, *D. moldavica* has been reported to markedly improve on rat cerebral ischemia reperfusion injury by reducing the levels of IL-6, IL-8 and TNF-α and elevating the activities of superoxide dismutase (SOD) and glutathione peroxidase (GSH-Px) [47]. Notably, we found that the DMEE used in this study contained the active component oleanolic acid. Previous studies reported that oleanolic acid exerts anti-inflammatory effects through inhibited the phosphorylation of ERK1/2, p38, JNK1/2 and p65 in LPS-stimulated RAW 264.7 cells [48–50]. Other studies also reported that DMEE contains rosmarinic acid and chlorogenic acid that inhibit the inflammatory mediators and inflammatory symptoms in LPS-stimulated RAW 264.7 cells [51,52]. Altogether, we speculate that the terpenoids and phenolic acids contained in DMEE collectively exhibit anti-inflammatory effects.

NO and PGE_2 production, which plays key roles in the modulation of immune responses, mediates inflammatory responses, including pain and hypersensitivity [53,54]. Our experimental data showed that DMEE significantly inhibited the production and accumulation of the inflammatory mediators NO and PGE_2 by decreasing the expression of iNOS and COX-2. We also found that DMEE was related to ameliorating nociception in the formalin test (data not shown). Moreover, DMEE significantly downregulated the phosphorylation of JNK1/2, ERK1/2 and p65 (Figure 6). However, DMEE did not reduce the phosphorylation of p38 in LPS-induced RAW 264.7 cells, since oleanolic acid may facilitate the phosphorylation of p38 [55]. As a result, DMEE reduced the expression of IL-6 and IL-1β in LPS-triggered RAW 264.7 cells by inhibiting the activation of the JNK, ERK and NF-κB pathways. Although the expression of IL-1β in LPS-stimulated RAW 264.7 cells was reduced, it could not be reduced in LPS-induced septic mice. Therefore, we suggest that further research to verify the changes on various inflammatory cytokines in septic mice by DMEE is needed. In addition, we observed that DMEE protected against LPS-induced cell death in RAW 264.7 cells (Figure 2B). However, we cannot rule out that DMEE may enhance cell proliferation but has no protective effects. Therefore, in a future study, we will examine whether the effect of DMEE on LPS-induced cell death is due to its protection or cell proliferation.

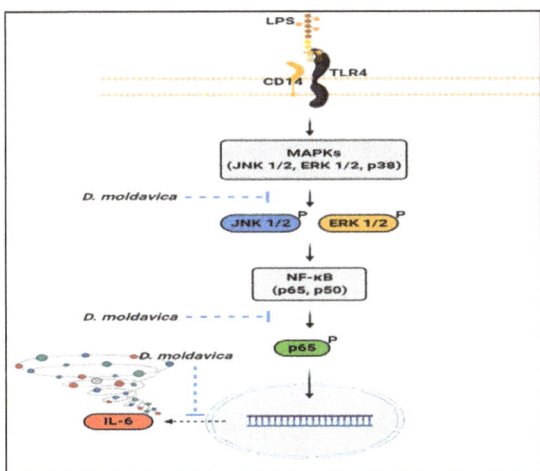

Figure 6. The anti-inflammatory pathways of *D. moldavica* in LPS-stimulated RAW 264.7 macrophages.

In conclusion, our data demonstrated that DMEE elicits an anti-inflammatory effect by inhibiting the JNK/ERK/NF-κB signaling pathway in LPS-stimulated RAW 264.7 macrophages and has an anti-septic effect by blocking IL-6, which was found in the plasma of LPS-stimulated septic shock mice. Because of the anti-inflammatory properties of DMEE, it could be an effective therapeutic strategy in systemic inflammatory response syndromes such as septic shock or COVID-19.

Author Contributions: Methodology, S.H.H.; formal analysis, S.-Y.K., T.J.M., H.J.B., S.-D.H., E.-S.L. and S.-H.C.; investigation, K.-M.K.; data curation, S.-Y.K., T.J.M., H.J.B., S.-D.H., E.-S.L. and S.-H.C.; writing—original draft preparation, K.-M.K.; writing—review and editing, S.-D.L. and S.J.P.; supervision, S.J.P.; project administration, S.J.P. All authors have read and agreed to the published version of the manuscript.

Funding: This research study was supported by the Korean Ministry of Environment (2018002270002), the National Research Foundation of Korea (NRF) grant funded by the Ministry of Science, ICT and Future Planning (NRF-2020R1C1C1004911) and the Basic Science Research Program through the National Research Foundation of Korea (NRF) founded by the Ministry of Education (NRF-2021R1A6A1A03044242).

Institutional Review Board Statement: The study was approved by the Institutional Animal Care and Use Committee (IACUC) of the Laboratory Animal Research Center at Kangwon National University (KW-200128-1).

Informed Consent Statement: Not applicable.

Data Availability Statement: Data is contained within the article.

Conflicts of Interest: The authors declare that there are no conflict of interest.

References

1. Chen, L.; Deng, H.; Cui, H.; Fang, J.; Zuo, Z.; Deng, J.; Li, Y.; Wang, X.; Zhao, L. Inflammatory responses and inflammation-associated diseases in organs. *Oncotarget* **2018**, *9*, 7204–7218. [CrossRef] [PubMed]
2. Iwasaki, A.; Medzhitov, R. Control of adaptive immunity by the innate immune system. *Nat. Immunol.* **2015**, *16*, 343–353. [CrossRef]
3. Joh, E.H.; Gu, W.; Kim, D.H. Echinocystic acid ameliorates lung inflammation in mice and alveolar macrophages by inhibiting the binding of LPS to TLR4 in NF-kappaB and MAPK pathways. *Biochem. Pharmacol.* **2012**, *84*, 331–340. [CrossRef] [PubMed]
4. Su, Y.; Xiong, S.; Lan, H.; Xu, L.; Wei, X. Molecular mechanism underlying anti-inflammatory activities of lirioresinol B dimethyl ether through suppression of NF-kappaB and MAPK signaling in in vitro and in vivo models. *Int. Immunopharmacol.* **2019**, *73*, 321–332. [CrossRef]
5. Neumann, D.; Lienenklaus, S.; Rosati, O.; Martin, M.U. IL-1beta-induced phosphorylation of PKB/Akt depends on the presence of IRAK-1. *Eur. J. Immunol.* **2002**, *32*, 3689–3698. [CrossRef]
6. Balan, I.; Beattie, M.C.; O'Buckley, T.K.; Aurelian, L.; Morrow, A.L. Endogenous Neurosteroid (3alpha,5alpha)3-Hydroxypregnan-20-one Inhibits Toll-like-4 Receptor Activation and Pro-inflammatory Signaling in Macrophages and Brain. *Sci. Rep.* **2019**, *9*, 1220. [CrossRef]
7. Park, S.H.; Kwak, J.A.; Jung, S.H.; Ahn, B.; Cho, W.J.; Yun, C.Y.; Na, C.S.; Hwang, B.Y.; Hong, J.T.; Han, S.B.; et al. Piperidyl-methyloxychalcone improves immune-mediated acute liver failure via inhibiting TAK1 activity. *Exp. Mol. Med.* **2017**, *49*, e392. [CrossRef] [PubMed]
8. Kotch, C.; Barrett, D.; Teachey, D.T. Tocilizumab for the treatment of chimeric antigen receptor T cell-induced cytokine release syndrome. *Expert Rev. Clin. Immunol.* **2019**, *15*, 813–822. [CrossRef] [PubMed]
9. Gupta, K.K.; Khan, M.A.; Singh, S.K. Constitutive Inflammatory Cytokine Storm: A Major Threat to Human Health. *J. Interferon Cytokine Res.* **2020**, *40*, 19–23. [CrossRef]
10. Kim, J.S.; Lee, J.Y.; Yang, J.W.; Lee, K.H.; Effenberger, M.; Szpirt, W.; Kronbichler, A.; Shin, J.I. Immunopathogenesis and treatment of cytokine storm in COVID-19. *Theranostics* **2021**, *11*, 316–329. [CrossRef] [PubMed]
11. Keeley, A.; Hine, P.; Nsutebu, E. The recognition and management of sepsis and septic shock: A guide for non-intensivists. *Postgrad. Med. J.* **2017**, *93*, 626–634. [CrossRef] [PubMed]
12. Cecconi, M.; Evans, L.; Levy, M.; Rhodes, A. Sepsis and septic shock. *Lancet* **2018**, *392*, 75–87. [CrossRef]
13. Weisberg, A.; Park, P.; Cherry-Bukowiec, J.R. Early Goal-Directed Therapy: The History and Ongoing Impact on Management of Severe Sepsis and Septic Shock. *Surg. Infect.* **2018**, *19*, 142–146. [CrossRef] [PubMed]
14. Arens, C.; Bajwa, S.A.; Koch, C.; Siegler, B.H.; Schneck, E.; Hecker, A.; Weiterer, S.; Lichtenstern, C.; Weigand, M.A.; Uhle, F. Sepsis-induced long-term immune paralysis—Results of a descriptive, explorative study. *Crit. Care* **2016**, *20*, 93. [CrossRef] [PubMed]
15. Thompson, K.; Venkatesh, B.; Finfer, S. Sepsis and septic shock: Current approaches to management. *Intern. Med. J.* **2019**, *49*, 160–170. [CrossRef]

16. Allison, M.G.; Heil, E.L.; Hayes, B.D. Appropriate Antibiotic Therapy. *Emerg. Med. Clin. N. Am.* **2017**, *35*, 25–42. [CrossRef]
17. Molano Franco, D.; Arevalo-Rodriguez, I.; Roque, I.F.M.; Montero Oleas, N.G.; Nuvials, X.; Zamora, J. Plasma interleukin-6 concentration for the diagnosis of sepsis in critically ill adults. *Cochrane Database Syst. Rev.* **2019**, *4*, CD011811. [CrossRef]
18. Thao, P.T.N.; Tra, T.T.; Son, N.T.; Wada, K. Reduction in the IL-6 level at 24 h after admission to the intensive care unit is a survival predictor for Vietnamese patients with sepsis and septic shock: A prospective study. *BMC Emerg. Med.* **2018**, *18*, 39. [CrossRef]
19. Tan, M.E.; He, C.H.; Jiang, W.; Zeng, C.; Yu, N.; Huang, W.; Gao, Z.G.; Xing, J.G. Development of solid lipid nanoparticles containing total flavonoid extract from *Dracocephalum moldavica* L. and their therapeutic effect against myocardial ischemia-reperfusion injury in rats. *Int. J. Nanomed.* **2017**, *12*, 3253–3265. [CrossRef]
20. Miernisha, A.; Bi, C.W.; Cheng, L.K.; Xing, J.G.; Liu, J.; Maiwulanjiang, M.; Aisa, H.A.; Dong, T.T.; Lin, H.; Huang, Y.; et al. Badiranji Buya Keli, a Traditional Uyghur Medicine, Induces Vasodilation in Rat Artery: Signaling Mediated by Nitric Oxide Production in Endothelial Cells. *Phytother. Res.* **2016**, *30*, 16–24. [CrossRef]
21. Wojtowicz, A.; Oniszczuk, A.; Oniszczuk, T.; Kocira, S.; Wojtunik, K.; Mitrus, M.; Kocira, A.; Widelski, J.; Skalicka-Wozniak, K. Application of Moldavian dragonhead (*Dracocephalum moldavica* L.) leaves addition as a functional component of nutritionally valuable corn snacks. *J. Food Sci. Technol.* **2017**, *54*, 3218–3229. [CrossRef] [PubMed]
22. Rahmati, E.; Sharifian, F.; Fattahi, M. Process optimization of spray-dried Moldavian balm (*Dracocephalum moldavica* L.) extract powder. *Food Sci. Nutr.* **2020**, *8*, 6580–6591. [CrossRef] [PubMed]
23. Zhang, Z.K.; Zhou, Y.; Cao, J.; Liu, D.Y.; Wan, L.H. Rosmarinic acid ameliorates septic-associated mortality and lung injury in mice via GRP78/IRE1alpha/JNK pathway. *J. Pharm. Pharmacol.* **2021**, *73*, 916–921. [CrossRef]
24. Jiang, W.L.; Chen, X.G.; Qu, G.W.; Yue, X.D.; Zhu, H.B.; Tian, J.W.; Fu, F.H. Rosmarinic acid protects against experimental sepsis by inhibiting proinflammatory factor release and ameliorating hemodynamics. *Shock* **2009**, *32*, 608–613. [CrossRef]
25. Lee, W.; Yang, E.J.; Ku, S.K.; Song, K.S.; Bae, J.S. Anti-inflammatory effects of oleanolic acid on LPS-induced inflammation in vitro and in vivo. *Inflammation* **2013**, *36*, 94–102. [CrossRef] [PubMed]
26. Wang, J.L.; Ren, C.H.; Feng, J.; Ou, C.H.; Liu, L. Oleanolic acid inhibits mouse spinal cord injury through suppressing inflammation and apoptosis via the blockage of p38 and JNK MAPKs. *Biomed. Pharmacother.* **2020**, *123*, 109752. [CrossRef]
27. Nie, L.; Li, R.; Huang, J.; Wang, L.; Ma, M.; Huang, C.; Wu, T.; Yan, R.; Hu, X. Abietane diterpenoids from *Dracocephalum moldavica* L. and their anti-inflammatory activities in vitro. *Phytochemistry* **2021**, *184*, 112680. [CrossRef]
28. Shen, W.; Anwaier, G.; Cao, Y.; Lian, G.; Chen, C.; Liu, S.; Tuerdi, N.; Qi, R. Atheroprotective Mechanisms of Tilianin by Inhibiting Inflammation Through Down-Regulating NF-kappaB Pathway and Foam Cells Formation. *Front. Physiol.* **2019**, *10*, 825. [CrossRef]
29. Deepa, P.; Bae, H.J.; Park, H.B.; Kim, S.Y.; Choi, J.W.; Kim, D.H.; Liu, X.Q.; Ryu, J.H.; Park, S.J. Dracocephalum moldavica attenuates scopolamine-induced cognitive impairment through activation of hippocampal ERK-CREB signaling in mice. *J. Ethnopharmacol.* **2020**, *253*, 112651. [CrossRef]
30. Chiu, H.F.; Wang, H.M.; Shen, Y.C.; Venkatakrishnan, K.; Wang, C.K. Anti-inflammatory properties of fermented pine (*Pinus morrisonicola* Hay.) needle on lipopolysaccharide-induced inflammation in RAW 264.7 macrophage cells. *J. Food Biochem.* **2019**, *43*, e12994. [CrossRef]
31. Park, Y.; Yoo, S.A.; Kim, W.U.; Cho, C.S.; Woo, J.M.; Yoon, C.H. Anti-inflammatory effects of essential oils extracted from Chamaecyparis obtusa on murine models of inflammation and RAW 264.7 cells. *Mol. Med. Rep.* **2016**, *13*, 3335–3341. [CrossRef]
32. Ko, W.K.; Lee, S.H.; Kim, S.J.; Jo, M.J.; Kumar, H.; Han, I.B.; Sohn, S. Anti-inflammatory effects of ursodeoxycholic acid by lipopolysaccharide-stimulated inflammatory responses in RAW 264.7 macrophages. *PLoS ONE* **2017**, *12*, e0180673. [CrossRef]
33. Baek, H.S.; Min, H.J.; Hong, V.S.; Kwon, T.K.; Park, J.W.; Lee, J.; Kim, S. Anti-Inflammatory Effects of the Novel PIM Kinase Inhibitor KMU-470 in RAW 264.7 Cells through the TLR4-NF-kappaB-NLRP3 Pathway. *Int. J. Mol. Sci.* **2020**, *21*, 5138. [CrossRef]
34. Hirai, S.; Horii, S.; Matsuzaki, Y.; Ono, S.; Shimmura, Y.; Sato, K.; Egashira, Y. Anti-inflammatory effect of pyroglutamyl-leucine on lipopolysaccharide-stimulated RAW 264.7 macrophages. *Life Sci.* **2014**, *117*, 1–6. [CrossRef]
35. Chang, C.T.; Huang, S.S.; Lin, S.S.; Amagaya, S.; Ho, H.Y.; Hou, W.C.; Shie, P.H.; Wu, J.B.; Huang, G.J. Anti-inflammatory activities of tormentic acid from suspension cells of Eriobotrya Japonicaex vivo and in vivo. *Food Chem.* **2011**, *127*, 1131–1137. [CrossRef]
36. Kim, Y.K.; Na, K.S.; Myint, A.M.; Leonard, B.E. The role of pro-inflammatory cytokines in neuroinflammation, neurogenesis and the neuroendocrine system in major depression. *Prog. Neuro-Psychopharmacol. Biol. Psychiatry* **2016**, *64*, 277–284. [CrossRef] [PubMed]
37. Nyati, K.K.; Masuda, K.; Zaman, M.M.; Dubey, P.K.; Millrine, D.; Chalise, J.P.; Higa, M.; Li, S.; Standley, D.M.; Saito, K.; et al. TLR4-induced NF-kappaB and MAPK signaling regulate the IL-6 mRNA stabilizing protein Arid5a. *Nucleic. Acids Res.* **2017**, *45*, 2687–2703. [CrossRef] [PubMed]
38. Huet, O.; Chin-Dusting, J.P. Septic shock: Desperately seeking treatment. *Clin. Sci.* **2014**, *126*, 31–39. [CrossRef]
39. Perner, A.; Gordon, A.C.; De Backer, D.; Dimopoulos, G.; Russell, J.A.; Lipman, J.; Jensen, J.U.; Myburgh, J.; Singer, M.; Bellomo, R.; et al. Sepsis: Frontiers in diagnosis, resuscitation and antibiotic therapy. *Intensive Care Med.* **2016**, *42*, 1958–1969. [CrossRef] [PubMed]
40. Cohen, J. The immunopathogenesis of sepsis. *Nature* **2002**, *420*, 885–891. [CrossRef] [PubMed]
41. Dinarello, C.A. The proinflammatory cytokines interleukin-1 and tumor necrosis factor anf treatment of the septic shock syndrome. *J. Infect. Dis.* **1991**, *163*, 1177–1184. [CrossRef]
42. Chen, L.; Lin, X.; Xiao, J.; Tian, Y.; Zheng, B.; Teng, H. Sonchus oleraceus Linn protects against LPS-induced sepsis and inhibits inflammatory responses in RAW264.7 cells. *J. Ethnopharmacol.* **2019**, *236*, 63–69. [CrossRef]

43. Jones, S.A.; Hunter, C.A. Is IL-6 a key cytokine target for therapy in COVID-19? *Nat. Rev. Immunol.* **2021**, *21*, 337–339. [CrossRef] [PubMed]
44. Tanaka, T.; Narazaki, M.; Kishimoto, T. Immunotherapeutic implications of IL-6 blockade for cytokine storm. *Immunotherapy* **2016**, *8*, 959–970. [CrossRef]
45. Cao, W.; Hu, N.; Yuan, Y.; Cheng, J.; Guo, X.; Wang, Y.; Wang, X.; Hu, P. Effects of Tilianin on Proliferation, Migration and TGF-beta/Smad Signaling in Rat Vascular Smooth Muscle Cells Induced with Angiotensin II. *Phytother. Res.* **2017**, *31*, 1240–1248. [CrossRef] [PubMed]
46. Xing, J.; Peng, K.; Cao, W.; Lian, X.; Wang, Q.; Wang, X. Effects of total flavonoids from Dracocephalum moldavica on the proliferation, migration, and adhesion molecule expression of rat vascular smooth muscle cells induced by TNF-alpha. *Pharm. Biol.* **2013**, *51*, 74–83. [CrossRef]
47. Jia, J.X.; Zhang, Y.; Wang, Z.L.; Yan, X.S.; Jin, M.; Huo, D.S.; Wang, H.; Yang, Z.J. The inhibitory effects of *Dracocephalum moldavica* L. (DML) on rat cerebral ischemia reperfusion injury. *J. Toxicol. Environ. Health A* **2017**, *80*, 1206–1211. [CrossRef] [PubMed]
48. Han, Y.; Yuan, C.; Zhou, X.; Han, Y.; He, Y.; Ouyang, J.; Zhou, W.; Wang, Z.; Wang, H.; Li, G. Anti-Inflammatory Activity of Three Triterpene from *Hippophae rhamnoides* L. in Lipopolysaccharide-Stimulated RAW264.7 Cells. *Int. J. Mol. Sci.* **2021**, *22*, 12009. [CrossRef]
49. Hwang, Y.J.; Song, J.; Kim, H.R.; Hwang, K.A. Oleanolic acid regulates NF-kappaB signaling by suppressing MafK expression in RAW 264.7 cells. *BMB Rep.* **2014**, *47*, 524–529. [CrossRef]
50. Suh, S.J.; Jin, U.H.; Kim, K.W.; Son, J.K.; Lee, S.H.; Son, K.H.; Chang, H.W.; Lee, Y.C.; Kim, C.H. Triterpenoid saponin, oleanolic acid 3-O-beta-D-glucopyranosyl(1→3)-alpha-L-rhamnopyranosyl(1→2)-alpha-L-arabinopy ranoside (OA) from *Aralia elata* inhibits LPS-induced nitric oxide production by down-regulated NF-kappaB in raw 264.7 cells. *Arch. Biochem. Biophys.* **2007**, *467*, 227–233. [CrossRef] [PubMed]
51. So, Y.; Lee, S.Y.; Han, A.R.; Kim, J.B.; Jeong, H.G.; Jin, C.H. Rosmarinic Acid Methyl Ester Inhibits LPS-Induced NO Production via Suppression of MyD88- Dependent and -Independent Pathways and Induction of HO-1 in RAW 264.7 Cells. *Molecules* **2016**, *21*, 1083. [CrossRef] [PubMed]
52. Zhao, X.L.; Yu, L.; Zhang, S.D.; Ping, K.; Ni, H.Y.; Qin, X.Y.; Zhao, C.J.; Wang, W.; Efferth, T.; Fu, Y.J. Cryptochlorogenic acid attenuates LPS-induced inflammatory response and oxidative stress via upregulation of the Nrf2/HO-1 signaling pathway in RAW 264.7 macrophages. *Int. Immunopharmacol.* **2020**, *83*, 106436. [CrossRef]
53. Guzik, T.J.; Korbut, R.; Adamek-Guzik, T. Nitric oxide and superoxide in inflammation and immune regulation. *J. Physiol. Pharmacol.* **2003**, *54*, 469–487. [PubMed]
54. Aoki, T.; Narumiya, S. Prostaglandins and chronic inflammation. *Trends Pharmacol. Sci.* **2012**, *33*, 304–311. [CrossRef] [PubMed]
55. Chen, J.Y.; Zhang, L.; Zhang, H.; Su, L.; Qin, L.P. Triggering of p38 MAPK and JNK signaling is important for oleanolic acid-induced apoptosis via the mitochondrial death pathway in hypertrophic scar fibroblasts. *Phytother. Res.* **2014**, *28*, 1468–1478. [CrossRef]

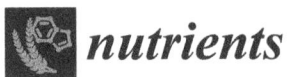

Article

Lactoferrin Prevents Hepatic Injury and Fibrosis via the Inhibition of NF-κB Signaling in a Rat Non-Alcoholic Steatohepatitis Model

Yoshinaga Aoyama [1,2], Aya Naiki-Ito [1,*], Kuang Xiaochen [1], Masayuki Komura [1], Hiroyuki Kato [1], Yuko Nagayasu [1], Shingo Inaguma [1], Hiroyuki Tsuda [3], Mamoru Tomita [4], Yoichi Matsuo [2], Shuji Takiguchi [2] and Satoru Takahashi [1]

[1] Department of Experimental Pathology and Tumor Biology, Nagoya City University Graduate School of Medical Sciences, 1-Kawasumi, Mizuho-cho, Mizuho-ku, Nagoya 467-8601, Japan; yoshinaga52@gmail.com (Y.A.); kuangxiaochen094@hotmail.com (K.X.); komura@med.nagoya-cu.ac.jp (M.K.); h.kato@med.nagoya-cu.ac.jp (H.K.); nagap1113@gmail.com (Y.N.); inaguma@med.nagoya-cu.ac.jp (S.I.); sattak@med.nagoya-cu.ac.jp (S.T.)
[2] Department of Gastroenterological Surgery, Nagoya City University Graduate School of Medical Sciences, 1-Kawasumi, Mizuho-cho, Mizuho-ku, Nagoya 467-8601, Japan; matsuo@med.nagoya-cu.ac.jp (Y.M.); takiguch@med.nagoya-cu.ac.jp (S.T.)
[3] Nanotoxicology Project, Nagoya City University, Nagoya 467-8603, Japan; htsuda@phar.nagoya-cu.ac.jp
[4] Dairy Techno Inc., Tokyo 105-0014, Japan; m-tomita@dairytechno.co.jp
* Correspondence: ayaito@med.nagoya-cu.ac.jp; Tel.: +81-52-853-8156; Fax: +81-52-842-0817

Abstract: Non-alcoholic steatohepatitis (NASH) can cause liver cirrhosis and hepatocellular carcinoma (HCC), with cases increasing worldwide. To reduce the incidence of liver cirrhosis and HCC, NASH is targeted for the development of treatments, along with viral hepatitis and alcoholic hepatitis. Lactoferrin (LF) has antioxidant, anti-cancer, and anti-inflammatory activities. However, whether LF affects NASH and fibrosis remains unelucidated. We aimed to clarify the chemopreventive effect of LF on NASH progression. We used a NASH model with metabolic syndrome established using connexin 32 (Cx32) dominant negative transgenic (Cx32ΔTg) rats. Cx32ΔTg rats (7 weeks old) were fed a high-fat diet and intraperitoneally injected with dimethylnitrosamine (DMN). Rats were divided into three groups for LF treatment at 0, 100, or 500 mg/kg/day for 17 weeks. Lactoferrin significantly protected steatosis and lobular inflammation in Cx32ΔTg rat livers and attenuated bridging fibrosis or liver cirrhosis induced by DMN. By quantitative RT–PCR, LF significantly down-regulated inflammatory (*Tnf-α*, *Il-6*, *Il-18*, and *Il-1β*) and fibrosis-related (*Tgf-β1*, *Timp2*, and *Col1a1*) cytokine mRNAs. Phosphorylated nuclear factor (NF)-κB protein decreased in response to LF, while phosphorylated JNK protein was unaffected. These results indicate that LF might act as a chemopreventive agent to prevent hepatic injury, inflammation, and fibrosis in NASH via NF-κB inactivation.

Keywords: NASH; lactoferrin; fibrosis; hepatocarcinogenesis; connexin

Citation: Aoyama, Y.; Naiki-Ito, A.; Xiaochen, K.; Komura, M.; Kato, H.; Nagayasu, Y.; Inaguma, S.; Tsuda, H.; Tomita, M.; Matsuo, Y.; et al. Lactoferrin Prevents Hepatic Injury and Fibrosis via the Inhibition of NF-κB Signaling in a Rat Non-Alcoholic Steatohepatitis Model. *Nutrients* 2022, 14, 42. https://doi.org/10.3390/nu14010042

Academic Editor: Md Soriful Islam

Received: 18 November 2021
Accepted: 20 December 2021
Published: 23 December 2021

Publisher's Note: MDPI stays neutral with regard to jurisdictional claims in published maps and institutional affiliations.

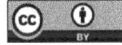

Copyright: © 2021 by the authors. Licensee MDPI, Basel, Switzerland. This article is an open access article distributed under the terms and conditions of the Creative Commons Attribution (CC BY) license (https://creativecommons.org/licenses/by/4.0/).

1. Introduction

The development of non-alcoholic fatty liver disease (NAFLD) is associated with obesity and disorders of lipid metabolism in patients with metabolic syndrome. With a global increase in recent years of the obese population, the number of cases of NAFLD has also increased [1,2]. A global meta-analysis describes the prevalence of NAFLD worldwide, which is approximately 25%, with the highest rates of 31% and 32% occurring in South America and the Middle East, respectively [3]. The concept of NAFLD is a broad spectrum of disease, ranging from simple steatosis without inflammation to non-alcoholic steatohepatitis (NASH) with chronic progressive inflammation and fibrosis. Continuous inflammation produces abundant inflammatory cytokines and accumulates reactive oxygen species (ROS) in the liver, leading to fibrosis. Once fibrosis develops to bridge cirrhosis, they are irreversible and can develop into hepatocellular carcinoma (HCC), as occurs in various chronic liver diseases, such as alcohol-induced injury and viral hepatitis [1,4].

Connexin (Cx) is a component of gap junctions, which exist between cells and is responsible for the transfer of small molecules less than 1 kDa, such as second messengers, ions, and cell metabolites [5,6]. This cellular interaction is called gap junctional intercellular communication (GJIC) and contributes to maintain tissue homeostasis and control cell growth and differentiation [7,8]. Within the liver, Cx32 exists as a major gap junction protein of hepatocytes [9,10]. In particular, decreased expression of Cx32 is followed by the continued progression of chronic liver diseases, such as liver cirrhosis and HCC [11].

We previously assessed the function of Cx32 in liver diseases via the establishment of Cx32 dominant negative transgenic (Cx32ΔTg) rats with a dominant negative mutant of Cx32 controlled by an albumin (Alb) promoter [12]. Cx32ΔTg rats showed greatly decreased Cx32 expression localized at the membrane and depressed GJIC capacity in their hepatocytes, as well as a high susceptibility to chemical-induced hepatocarcinogenesis compared to wild-type (Wt) rats [13,14]. Cx32 is involved in not only carcinogenesis but also NASH. There was no difference in susceptibilities to hepatotoxicity and hepatocarcinogenesis in the Cx32ΔTg as compared to Wt rats in basal diet feeding without any chemical treatment [14]. However, dysfunction of Cx32 in Cx32ΔTg rats exacerbated hepatocyte injury, steatohepatitis, and fibrosis due to increased ROS levels in the NASH induced by the methionine-choline deficient diet (MCDD) [10]. The acceleration of NASH development by Cx32 inactivation was also observed in another model that was induced by a combination of a high-fat diet (HFD) plus dimethylnitrosamine (DMN) in Cx32ΔTg rats [15]. Comparing the two models, nuclear factor (NF)-κB was commonly activated with the up-regulation of inflammatory cytokines, such as tumor necrosis factor (TNF)-α and transforming growth factor (TGF)-β1 in NASH induced by Cx32 dysfunction. Therefore, NF-κB is one of the key contributors to the progression of NASH.

Lactoferrin (LF) is an 80-kDa iron-binding glycoprotein found in all exocrine fluids, including tears, sweat, and saliva, and is especially abundant in milk. It was first isolated and purified in 1960 and was involved in the promotion of iron absorption and lipid metabolism. LF has various physiological functions, including anti-bacterial, anti-fungal, anti-viral, anti-oxidant, anti-cancer, anti-inflammatory effects, which have been reported. We focused on LF as a suppressor of inflammation. A previous study indicated that bovine LF inhibited chronic inflammation in the lungs in a mouse cystic fibrosis model. Tanaka et al. reported that bovine LF improved colitis in a dextran sulfate sodium-induced colitis model in rats and mice due to a reduction in the inflammation level by LF correlated with a decrease in proinflammatory cytokines, such as TNF-α, IL-1β, and interleukin (IL)-6 [16,17]. With regard to the liver, decreased IL-1β by LF leads to the inhibition of carbon tetrachloride-induced hepatitis in a rat model [18]. Another report suggests that LF reduced the expression of TGF-β1, IL-1β, and TNF-α and suppressed liver fibrosis in a rat systemic lupus erythematosus model [19]. The anti-tumor abilities of LF have also been described in various cancer cell lines, such as those of the breast [20], stomach [21], head, and neck [22]. A randomized placebo-controlled clinical trial indicated that the growth of colorectal adenomatous polyp was significantly retarded by intake of 3 g LF without any adverse events related to the intervention [23]. However, the effects of LF on hepatotoxicity, as well as fibrosis and carcinogenesis on NASH, have not been clearly established as yet.

In this study, we aimed to determine the chemopreventive effect of dietary LF on NASH development and hepatocarcinogenesis using a Cx32ΔTg–HFD–DMN NASH model.

2. Materials and Methods

2.1. Chemicals

A HFD (HFD-60) was bought from Oriental BioService, Inc. (Kyoto, Japan). DMN was supplied by Tokyo Kasei Kogyo Co. Ltd. (Tokyo, Japan). Bovine LF was provided by the Dairy Techno Inc. (Tokyo, Japan).

2.2. Development and Screening of Transgenic Rats

Cx32ΔTg rats were bred and screened as previously described [12]. Rats were housed in cages containing hardwood chips under specific pathogen-free conditions at 22 ± 2 °C and 50% humidity using a 12 h light/12 h dark cycle. Rats ate food and tap water that were available ad libitum. Protocols for animal experiments were approved by the Institutional Animal Care and Use Committee of Nagoya City University School of Medical Sciences (no. 19-025, approved on 24 September 2019).

2.3. Animal Treatments and Biochemical Analysis

A total of 48 male Cx32ΔTg rats (7 weeks old) ate a HFD for 17 weeks. After 5 weeks, DMN was injected intraperitoneally six times once every 2 weeks. DMN was used at 15 mg/kg (injections 1 and 2), 10 mg/kg (injections 3 and 4), and 5 mg/kg (injections 5 and 6). Rats were randomly divided into three groups ($n = 16$ each). One group of rats received tap water (Control), and the other two groups of rats continuously received either 100 or 500 mg/kg/day LF (LF100 or LF500) in drinking water for 17 weeks. During animal experiments, one rat in the control group unexpectedly died at week 10. Therefore, we analyzed 47 rats in total (Control: 15 rats, LF100: 16 rats, and LF500: 16 rats) once the experiment was completed. All rats were sacrificed under deep anesthesia, and samples of blood were taken from the abdominal aorta. Total adipose tissues around spermatic ducts were weighed to assess visceral fat.

The serum levels of Alb, total protein, alkaline phosphatase, aspartate aminotransferase (AST), alanine aminotransferase, high-density lipoprotein cholesterol, low-density lipoprotein cholesterol (LDL-C), total cholesterol, and glucose were assessed and measured at the DIMS Institute of Medical Science, Inc. (Aichi, Japan).

2.4. Histology of NASH

Rat livers were surgically excised and sliced into 3–4 mm thick sections. After fixing with 10% buffered formalin, sections were embedded in paraffin for histological evaluation (thickness 2–3 μm). Histological sections were stained with Azan or hematoxylin and eosin (H&E), as well as immunohistochemically stained with antibody against α-smooth muscle actin (α-SMA; Dako, Tokyo, Japan). Steatohepatitis and fibrosis were evaluated using a non-alcoholic fatty liver disease activity score (NAS), as previously described in detail [10,24]. The NAS and fibrosis scores were evaluated by three very experienced pathologists (A.N.-I., M.K., and S.Takahashi).

2.5. Evaluation of Preneoplastic Foci in the Liver

The glutathione S-transferase placental form (GST-P) was immunohistochemically stained, as previously described [25]. Averages of GST-P–positive foci that were >80 μm in diameter in the entire liver section were evaluated using an image analyzer (Keyence, Osaka, Japan).

2.6. Western Blotting

Protein samples were extracted from frozen liver tissues using radioimmunoprecipitation buffer (Thermo Fisher Scientific, Rockford, IL, USA) with added protease and phosphatase inhibitors (Thermo Fisher Scientific). The protein concentration of samples was quantified by a Bradford assay. Protein samples (30 μg per lane) were separated in 12% polyacrylamide gels and transferred onto nitrocellulose membranes (Hybond-ECL; GE Healthcare UK Ltd., Buckinghamshire, UK). Membranes were probed with primary antibodies against: Cdc42, IκB-α, NF-κB, phosphorylated (p) NF-κB (Ser536), Mkk4, pMkk4 (Thr261), Jnk, pJnk (Thr183/Tyr185) (Cell Signaling Technology, Danvers, MA, USA), and β-actin (Sigma-Aldrich, St. Louis, MI, USA). Anti–β-actin was used at a 1:5000 dilution, and all other antibodies were used at 1:1000. ImageJ software, ver.1.52 (National Cancer Institute, Bethesda, MD, USA), was used to quantify bands from blots.

2.7. Quantitative Reverse Transcription PCR

RNA samples were extracted, and quantitative reverse transcription (qRT)–PCR was performed, as previously described [15]. Phenol–chloroform was used to isolate total RNA from liver tissue (Isogen, Nippon Gene Co., Ltd., Tokyo, Japan) and then converted to cDNA with Moloney murine leukemia virus reverse transcriptase (Takara, Otsu, Japan). Quantitative reverse transcription was performed using an AriaMx Real-Time PCR system (g8830a, Agilent, Santa Clara, CA, USA). The sequences of primers used in this study were provided in a previous study [15].

2.8. Selection of a Candidate Reference Gene

In order to select a reference gene that is stably expressed and has low variability in the present experiment system, the stability of the five candidate housekeeping genes (Table 1) was validated using NormFinder (MOMA, Aarhus, Denmark). The relative quantification for qRT-PCR was performed by standard curve method.

Table 1. Sequence of primers for housekeeping genes tested with quantitative reverse transcription PCR.

Symbol	Gene Name	Accession Number	Primers (5′-3′)
Gapdh	Glyceraldehyde-3-phosphate dehydrogenase	NM_017008.4	GCATCCTGCACCACCAACTG GCCTGCTTCACCACCTTCTT
B2m	Beta-2 microglobulin	NM_012512.2	CCTTCAGCAAGGACTGGTCT TACATGTCTCGGTCCCAGGT
Actb	Actin, beta	NM_031144.3	GCGAGTACAACCTTCTTGCAG CATACCCACCATCACACCCTG
Ppia	Peptidylprolyl isomerase A	NM_017101.1	TGCTGGACCAAACACAATG GAAGGGGAATGAGGAAAATA
Gusb	Glucuronidase, beta	NM_017015.3	CCGACAGGAGAGTGGTGTTG GCTTGGTGATGTCAGCCTCA

2.9. Statistical Analysis

Data are presented as the mean ± standard deviation (SD), and one-way ANOVA and Tukey multiple comparison tests were used to compare differences between groups using the software package, Graph Pad Prism 8 (GraphPad Software, Inc., La Jolla, CA, USA). $p < 0.05$ was considered significant.

3. Results

3.1. LF Prevents Steatohepatitis and Fibrosis in Cx32ΔTg Rats

We initially investigated the safety and chemopreventive effect of LF on NASH in a Cx32ΔTg–HFD–DMN rat NASH model. The dosage of LF in previous clinical studies was to reflect the selection of dosages in the present study [23]. A significant difference in body weights between control and LF-treated groups was not found. A dose-dependent change in organ weights was not noted, although liver weights were significantly increased in the LF100 compared to control group (Table 2).

Histological observation by H&E staining also indicated that LF did not induce any changes in kidneys. In the liver, treatments of a HFD and DMN induced diffuse deposits of fat droplets with hepatocellular ballooning and neutrophil infiltration in the lobule (Figure 1a). Lactoferrin treatment significantly reduced fat deposition, lobular inflammation, and ballooning injury of hepatocytes in a dose-dependent manner (Figure 1a–d and Table S1), resulting in decreased NAS (Figure 1e and Table S1). Bridging fibrosis and activated hepatic stellate cells (HSC) were visualized by Azan staining and α-SMA immunohistochemical staining, respectively, in a Cx32ΔTg–HFD–DMN rat NASH model (Figure 2a). The histological fibrosis score, percentages of the Azan-positive area (collagen), and percentages of the α-SMA-positive area (activated HSCs) were significantly reduced by LF in the NASH model (Figure 2a–d and Table S1).

Table 2. Body and various organ weights in connexin 32 dominant negative transgenic rats fed a high-fat diet and dimethylnitrosamine with or without lactoferrin (100 or 500 mg/kg/day) at week 17.

	No. of rats	Body Weight (g)	Liver		Kidney		Visceral Fat	
			Absolute (g)	Relative (%)	Absolute (g)	Relative (%)	Absolute (g)	Relative (%)
Control	15	564.7 ± 67.9	12.22 ± 2.70	2.14 ± 0.33	2.59 ± 0.15	0.48 ± 0.09	15.34 ± 4.68	2.65 ± 0.64
LF100	16	607.9 ± 63.2	14.59 ± 1.91 **	2.40 ± 0.18 *	2.67 ± 0.16	0.44 ± 0.04	16.90 ± 4.56	2.74 ± 0.53
LF500	16	585.8 ± 33.3	13.37 ± 1.79	2.28 ± 0.22	2.66 ± 0.18	0.46 ± 0.03	14.98 ± 3.15	2.54 ± 0.44

LF100, lactoferrin 100 mg/kg/day; LF500, lactoferrin 500 mg/kg/day. Dunnett's test *: $p < 0.05$, **: $p < 0.01$ vs. Control.

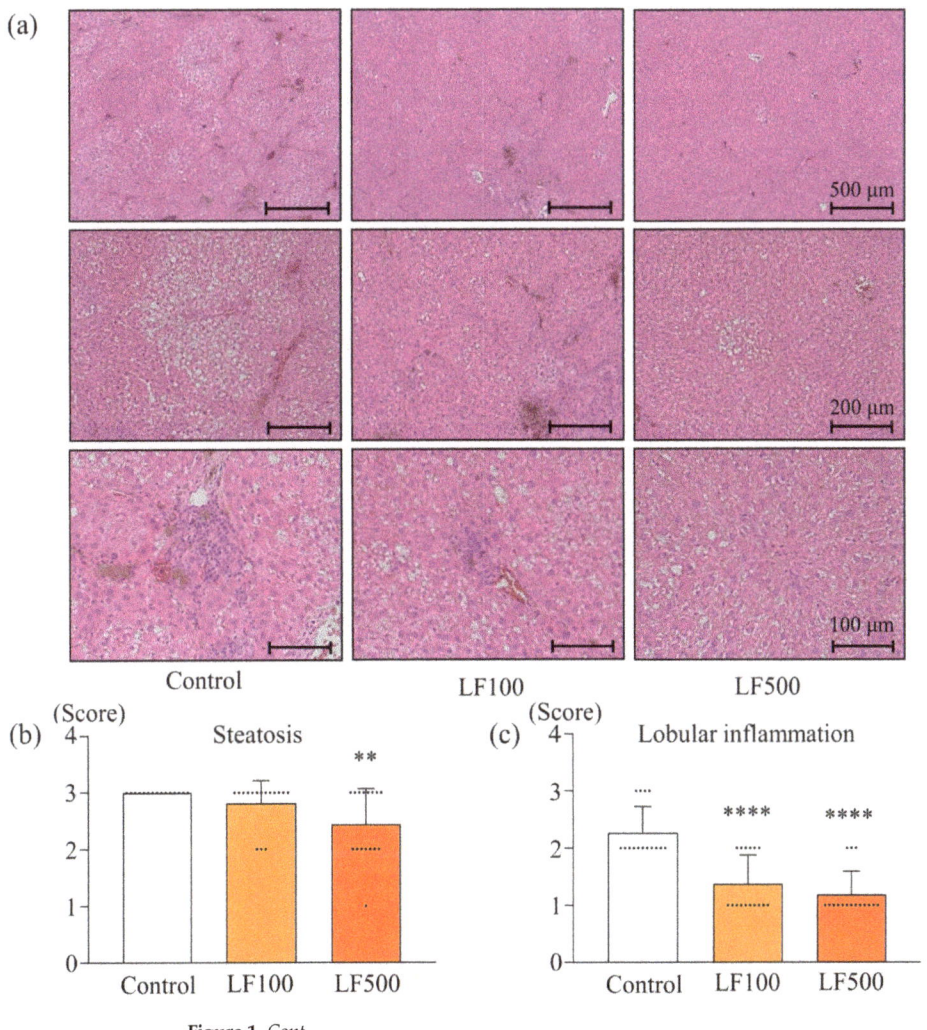

Figure 1. Cont.

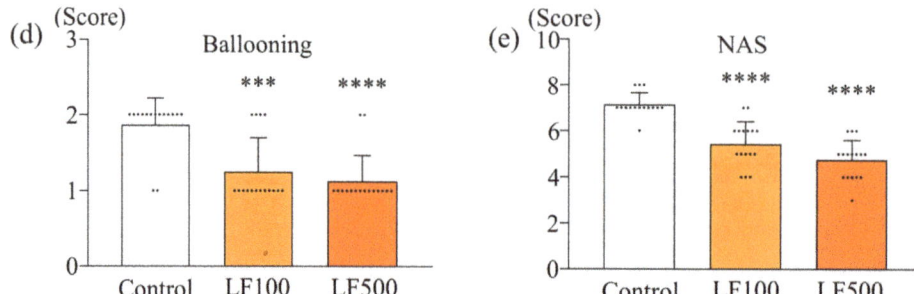

Figure 1. Preventive effect of lactoferrin on nonalcoholic steatohepatitis in rats. Connexin 32 dominant negative transgenic (Cx32ΔTg) rats were fed a high-fat diet (HFD), given an intraperitoneal injection of dimethylnitrosamine (DMN), and treated with lactoferrin (LF) for 17 weeks. (**a**) Representative histological findings of hematoxylin and eosin (H&E) stains in liver sections taken from Control, LF 100 mg/kg/day (LF100) or LF 500 mg/kg/day (LF500) rat groups. (**b–e**) Histopathological analysis of non-alcoholic steatohepatitis (NASH) was evaluated by severity scores for (**b**) steatosis, (**c**) lobular inflammation, (**d**) hepatocellular ballooning, and (**e**) a non-alcoholic fatty liver disease activity score (NAS). Data is shown as the mean ± SD, n = 15–16 per group, ** $p < 0.01$, *** $p < 0.001$, **** $p < 0.0001$ compared to the Control group.

Biochemical analysis of serum indicated that the level of AST, T-chol, and LDL-C in the LF–treated groups was lower than that in the control group and the level of glucose of the LF100 was significantly higher than that of the control group. However, there was no dose-dependent change in serum hepatic enzymes, proteins, glucose, or lipids (Table 3). These results indicated that LF administration prevented the development of steatohepatitis and fibrosis without any adverse effects observed in a rat NASH model.

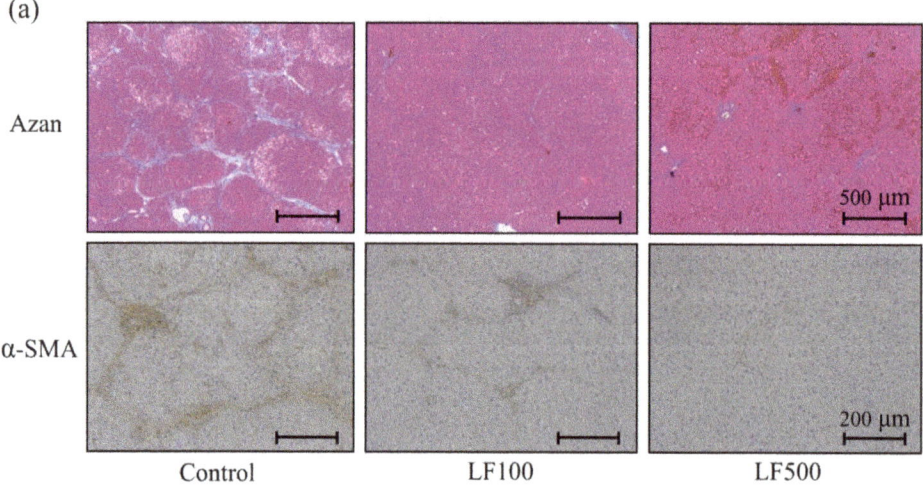

Figure 2. *Cont.*

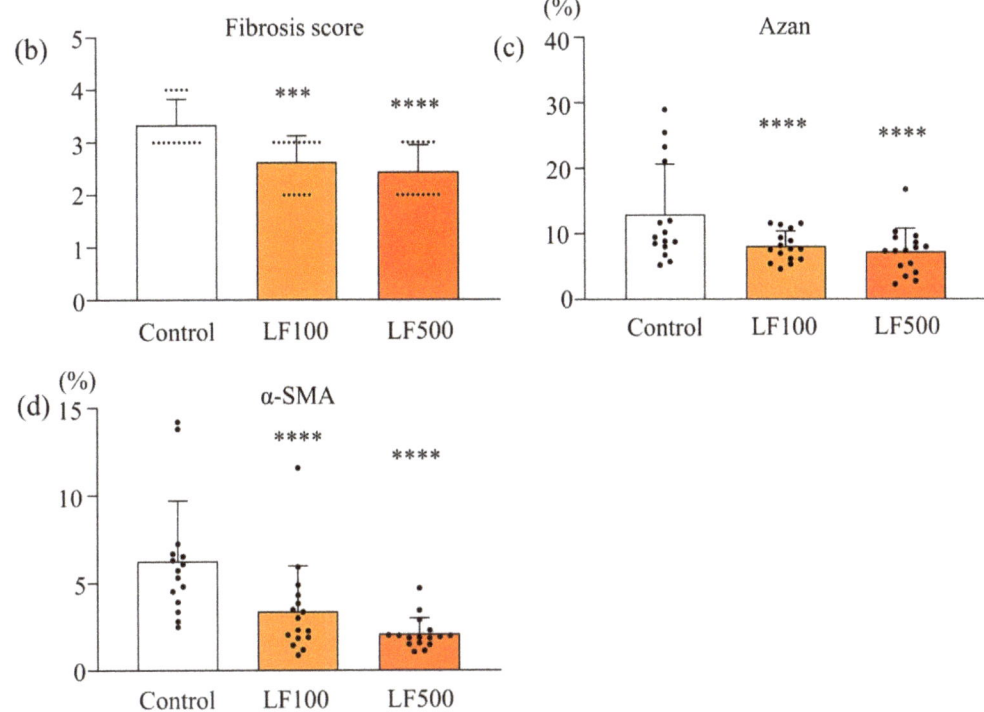

Figure 2. Attenuation effect of lactoferrin on fibrosis in rat nonalcoholic steatohepatitis. Connexin 32 dominant negative transgenic (Cx32ΔTg) rats were fed a high-fat diet (HFD), given an intraperitoneal injection of dimethylnitrosamine (DMN), and treated with lactoferrin (LF) for 17 weeks. (**a**) Azan staining (upper panels) and α-smooth muscle actin (α-SMA; lower panels) immunohistochemical stains of liver sections from Control, LF 100 mg/kg/day (LF100), or LF 500 mg/kg/day (LF500) rat groups. (**b**) Azan staining was used to evaluate the fibrosis score and (**c**) percentage of fibrosis area. (**d**) α-SMA–positive area. Data is shown as the mean ± SD, n = 15–16 per group, *** $p < 0.001$, **** $p < 0.0001$ compared to the Control group.

Table 3. Hepatic enzyme serum levels in connexin 32 dominant negative transgenic rats fed a high-fat diet and dimethylnitrosamine with or without lactoferrin (100 or 500 mg/kg/day) at week 17.

	No. of rats	TP (g/dL)	ALB (g/dL)	AST (U/L)	ALT (U/L)	ALP (U/L)	GLU (mg/dL)	T-chol (mg/dL)	LDL-C (mg/dL)	HDL-C (mg/dL)
Control	15	5.9 ± 0.6	4.1 ± 0.2	117.0 ± 86.6	45.5 ± 11.8	1249.9 ± 516.2	136.0 ± 18.2	91.1 ± 68.9	16.9 ± 15.0	46.8 ± 11.4
LF100	16	6.1 ± 0.2	4.1 ± 0.2	88.9 ± 21.5	47.4 ± 14.6	922.6 ± 286.9	161.2 ± 29.2 *	74.4 ± 14.4	10.6 ± 2.7	51.6 ± 11.4
LF500	16	6.0 ± 0.3	4.1 ± 0.2	91.2 ± 21.0	45.4 ± 9.7	1061.7 ± 437.1	153.0 ± 33.0	72.2 ± 13.3	11.1 ± 2.9	48.6 ± 9.3

Alb, albumin; ALP, alkaline phosphatase; ALT, alanine aminotransferase; GLU, glucose; HDL-C, high-density lipoprotein cholesterol; LDL-C, low-density lipoprotein cholesterol; LF100, lactoferrin 100 mg/kg/day; LF500, lactoferrin 500 mg/kg/day; T-chol, total cholesterol; TP, total protein. Dunnett's test *: $p < 0.05$ vs. Control.

3.2. LF Tends to Decrease the Induction of Preneoplastic Lesions in Cx32ΔTg Rats

To explore the effect of LF on carcinogenic potential during the development of NASH, the formation of preneoplastic hepatic foci, namely GST-P–positive foci, was quantitated by immunohostochemistry. A combination of HFD and DMN treatment increased both the number and area of GST-P–positive foci in Cx32ΔTg rats, although the carcinogenic potential was weaker than that induced by MCDD plus diethylnitrosamine (DEN; Figure 3a–c) [10,15]. In contrast, both the number and area of GST-P–positive lesions tended to be decreased by LF intake (Figure 3a–c and Table S1). In accordance with these results, LF may have the potential to reduce hepatocarcinogenesis in NASH.

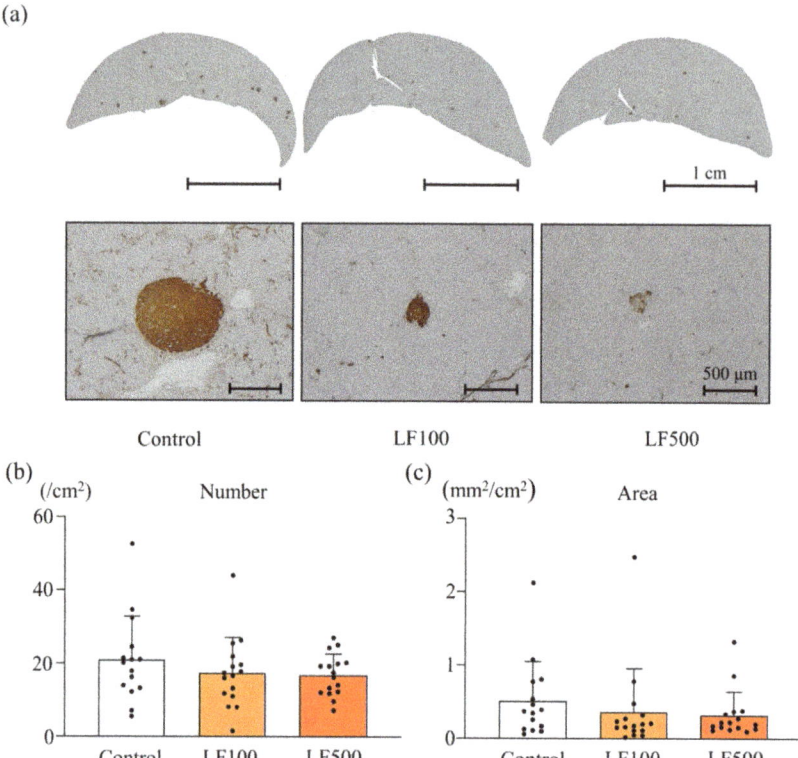

Figure 3. Effect of lactoferrin on hepatocarcinogenesis in rat nonalcoholic steatohepatitis. Connexin 32 dominant negative transgenic (Cx32ΔTg) rats were fed a high-fat diet (HFD), given an intraperitoneal injection of dimethylnitrosamine (DMN), and treated with lactoferrin (LF) for 17 weeks. (a) Liver sections showing representative foci positive for glutathione S-transferase placental form (GST-P) from Control, LF 100 mg/kg/day (LF100), or LF 500 mg/kg/day (LF500) rat groups. (b) The number and (c) area of GST-P–positive hepatic foci. Data is shown as the mean ± SD, n = 15–16 per group.

3.3. LF Down-Regulates mRNA Expression of Inflammatory Cytokines in Cx32ΔTg Rats

Previous studies, including ours, strongly indicated that expression of inflammatory cytokines associated with inflammation (*Tnf-α*, *Il-6*, *Il-18*, *Ifn-γ*, and *Il-1β*) and fibrosis (*Tgf-β1*, *Timp1*, *Timp2*, *Col1a1*, and *Ctgf*) correlated with histological NASH activity in human and rodent models [15,26–28]. Thus, we further quantitated their mRNA expression level using qRT–PCR. NormFinder analysis revealed that the stability value of *Gapdh* was the smallest among examined candidate housekeeping genes (Figure 4a). Therefore, we concluded *Gapdh* as the most stable gene and used it as a reference. As shown in Figure 4b, the inflammatory cytokines, *Il-6*, *Tnf-α*, *Il-18*, and *Il-1β*, were significantly down-regulated by LF compared with the control, and a dose-dependency was observed with *Il-6*, *Il-18*, and *Il-1β*. While not significant, *Ifn-γ* mRNA expression also tended to be decreased by LF (Figure 4b and Table S2). The mRNA expression of *Tgf-β1*, *Col1a1*, *Timp1*, *Timp2*, and *Ctgf* as fibrosis-related cytokines was also measured; *Timp2*, *Col1a1*, and *Tgf-β1* were significantly down-regulated by LF (Figure 4c and Table S2). These results suggests that down-regulation of inflammatory cytokines by LF was involved in the attenuation of steatohepatitis and hepatic fibrosis in a Cx32ΔTg–HFD–DMN rat NASH model.

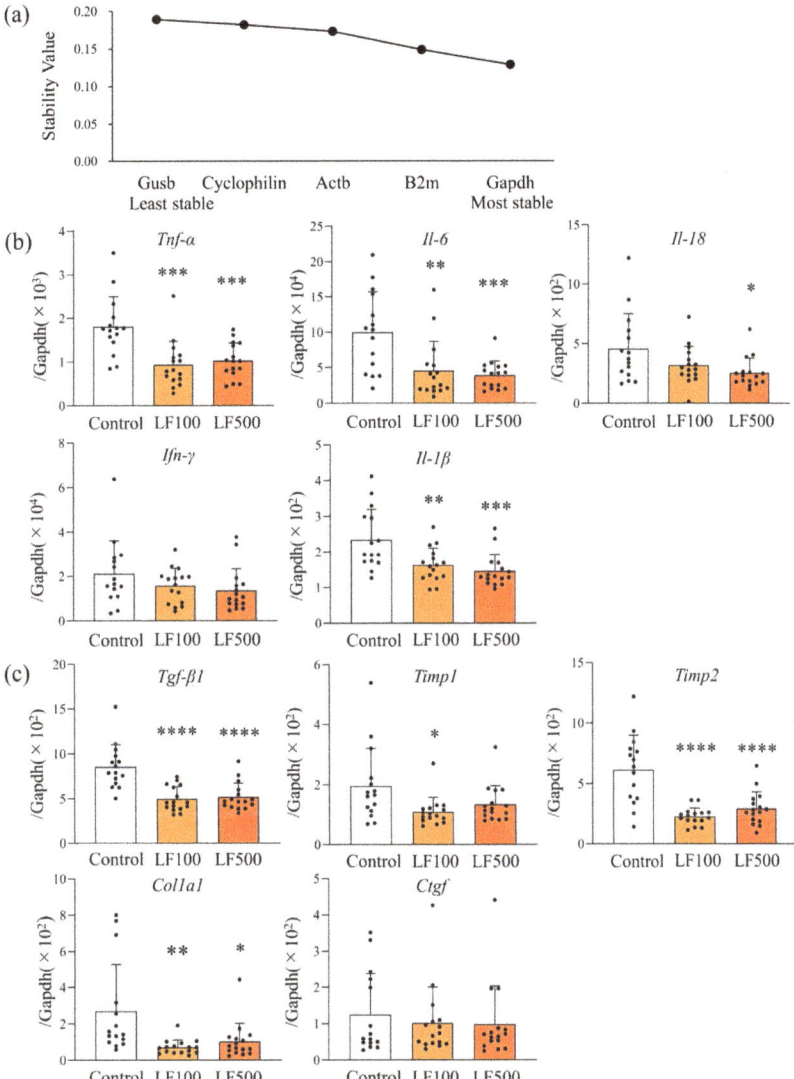

Figure 4. Down-regulation of inflammatory cytokines by lactoferrin in rat nonalcoholic steatohepatitis. Connexin 32 dominant negative transgenic (Cx32ΔTg) rats were fed a high-fat diet (HFD), given an intraperitoneal injection of dimethylnitrosamine (DMN), and treated with lactoferrin (LF) for 17 weeks. (**a**) NormFinder stability values for candidate housekeeping genes (*Gapdh*, *B2m*, *Actb*, *Ppia*, and *Gusb*). (**b**,**c**) mRNA levels of (**b**) pro-inflammatory cytokines (*Tnf-α*, *Il-6*, *Il-18*, *Ifn-γ*, and *Il-1β*) and (**c**) pro-fibrotic cytokines (*Tgf-β1*, *Timp1*, *Timp2*, *Col1a1*, and *Ctgf*) in Control, LF 100 mg/kg/day (LF100), or LF 500 mg/kg/day (LF500) rat groups were measured using quantitative reverse transcription (RT)–PCR. Data is shown as the mean ± SD, n = 15–16 per group, * $p < 0.05$, ** $p < 0.01$, *** $p < 0.001$, **** $p < 0.0001$ compared to the Control group.

3.4. LF Administration Reduces NF-κB Signaling in Cx32ΔTg Rats

Previous studies showed that NF-κB and JNK/SAPK signaling were switched on in a rat NASH model mediated by MCDD or HFD and DMN combined [10,15]. Therefore, we investigated how such signal transduction was altered by the administration of LF. Western blotting showed that elevated pNF-κB protein expression in NASH was significantly decreased by the administration of LF in a dose-dependent manner. In contrast, phosphorylated Mkk4 and Jnk, which belong to JNK/SAPK signaling, were not affected by LF, even though their upstream protein, Cdc42, was significantly reduced in LF–treated groups (Figure 5). Such results indicate that the inactivation of NF-κB, but not JNK/SAPK signaling, is involved in the preventive effect of LF against NASH development in rats.

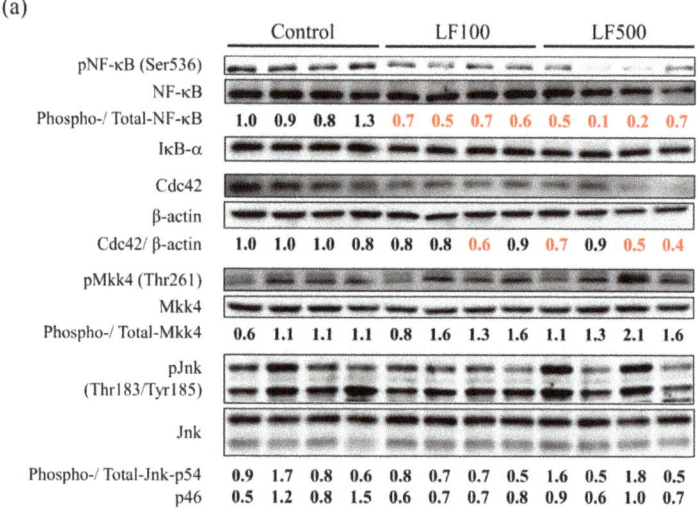

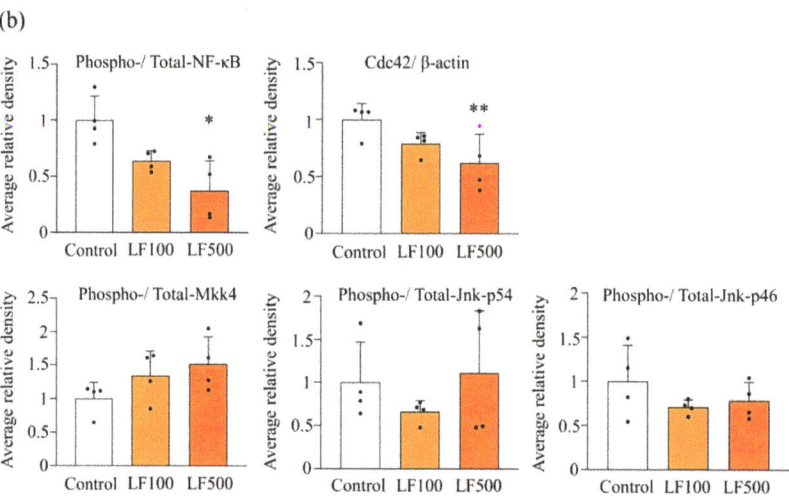

Figure 5. Down-regulation of inflammatory cytokines and deactivation of NF-κB and JNK signaling after the administration of lactoferrin in nonalcoholic steatohepatitis induced in Cx32 dominant negative transgenic rats. Connexin 32 dominant negative transgenic (Cx32ΔTg) rats were fed a high-fat diet (HFD),

given an intraperitoneal injection of dimethylnitrosamine (DMN), and treated with lactoferrin (LF) for 17 weeks. (**a**) Protein levels of nuclear factor (NF)-κB-related (NF-κB, phosphorylated (p)NF-κB, IκB-α) and SAPK/JNK (Cdc42, Mkk4, pMkk4, Jnk, and pJnk) signaling proteins in Control, LF 100 mg/kg/day (LF100), or LF 500 mg/kg/day (LF500) rat groups were assessed by western blotting. Each lane represents a protein sample from an individual rat. Phospho, phosphorylated. (**b**) Data is shown as the mean ± SD. * $p < 0.05$, ** $p < 0.01$ compared to the Control group.

4. Discussion

In this study, we examined the chemopreventive effect of LF on NASH in a Cx32ΔTg–HFD–DMN rat NASH model. NASH is an internationally prevalent chronic liver disease that shows fatty accumulations in the liver, ballooning, and inflamed hepatocyte. Non-alcoholic fatty liver disease often occurs in adults as a complication of lifestyle-related diseases, although it has also been found in children and is increasing all over the world regardless of a country's industrialization level [3,29]. Eventually, continuous inflammation leads to fibrosis and progresses to cirrhosis and HCC. It is known that nearly 20% of NASH cases progress to liver cirrhosis and HCC, with or without liver cirrhosis [30,31]. Therefore, NASH is one of the most crucial targets for deterring liver cirrhosis and HCC.

Currently, the main treatments for NASH include an improvement in life-style, represented by diet and exercise therapies. In addition, existing drugs for other diseases might also be effective for countering NASH. For instance, for drug repositioning, insulin sensitizers, such as pioglitazone, improved hepatocyte injury and fibrosis in a randomized, placebo-controlled trial [32]. Ratziu et al. reported that rosiglitazone decreased liver steatosis, but an improvement in hepatocyte injury and fibrosis was not found [33]. Vitamin E [34,35] and drugs for hypercholesterolemia [36] have also been used as drug therapies for NASH but have not been established as standard treatments due to their less potent medicinal effects and possible side effects after long-term use [33,37,38]. Consequently, daily intervention with functional supplements, along with lifestyle modification, is considered essential in preventing NASH progression. Considering the pathogenesis of NASH, we hypothesized that the anti-inflammatory effects of LF would prevent this disease. Previous studies proposed that LF expression in the liver was decreased in high-fructose, high-fat, or MCD-induced mouse NAFLD models [39]. In contrast, LF ameliorated HFD-induced hepatic steatosis and elevated the triglyceride level in mouse models [40–42]. In addition, the levels of hepatic triglycerides and visceral fat were decreased by LF and were positively correlated in ICR mice [43], indicating that LF has the potential to reduce fat accumulation in the liver.

In the present study, for the first time, the effect of LF on histological features of NASH, including steatosis, hepatocyte injury, and inflammation, was quantitated using scoring systems originally designed for humans [24,44]. Lactoferrin significantly improved steatosis in the liver but did not affect visceral fat weight in the rat NASH model. These findings indicated that LF might protect hepatic steatosis by moderating fatty acid metabolism in the liver or in adipose tissue. The balance of lipid metabolism in a whole body may determine the effect on the lipid environment in each organ. Hepatocyte injury and inflammation in NASH were also decreased in LF–treated groups. It is well-known that the inflammation-associated cytokines, *Il-6*, *Tnf-α*, and *Il-1β*, were up-regulated and involved in the evocation of chronic inflammation in the colon and liver [15,17]. As already demonstrated in the colon, down-regulation of these cytokines by LF was also induced in NASH in the present study. Altogether, LF may prevent steatohepatitis via a decrease of inflammatory cytokines.

Persistent chronic inflammation in NASH leads to increased fibrosis; similar to other chronic hepatitis diseases, the irreversible alteration of liver structure due to progressive fibrosis eventually leads to cirrhosis [45]. Therefore, fibrosis is one of the most important prognostic factors for patients with NASH. In accordance with previous studies, LF has the potential to suppress liver fibrosis induced by thioacetamide [46,47]; however, the effect on fibrosis during NASH has not yet been established. This is due to the fact that it is not easy to induce fibrosis with NASH over a short time period in an animal model. As shown in Figure 3a, advanced fibrosis when bridging between lobules, or a lobule and portal vein, was induced by LF in a Cx32ΔTg–HFD–DMN rat NASH model. Lactoferrin significantly decreased not only steatohepatitis but also the histological score and area of fibrosis in the model. The numbers of hepatic stellate cells with an active phenotype were increased in NASH and decreased in the livers of LF–treated rats. These novel findings indicate that LF prevents the liver fibrosis of NASH via the inactivation of HSC.

To date, the anti-tumor effect of LF on HCC was described in previous studies using a DEN-induced HCC model in rats or mice [48,49], but effects of LF on NASH-related hepatocarcinogenesis have not been established. The glutathione S-transferase placental form is a well-known marker for preneoplastic lesions in rat liver. Therefore, carcinogenic potentials in the liver can be measured by GST-P immunohistochemistry in the early phase of hepatocarcinogenesis [25]. The number and area of GST-P-positive foci in the liver tended to decrease in LF-treated groups, although a significant difference was not found (Figure 4). We previously induced GST-P-positive foci in a NASH model using DEN [10] or DMN [15]. Both the number and area of GST-P-positive foci induced by DMN were decreased compared to those induced by DEN, which might influence the lack of significant difference by LF in this study. The chemopreventive effect of LF on NASH-related hepatocarcinogenesis should be investigated in a future study.

Nuclear factor-κB signaling plays central roles in inflammation and fibrosis during NASH progression. Especially in regard to fibrosis, activation of NF-κB stimulates parenchymal cells, including Kupffer cells [50] and enhanced TGF-β1 signaling that is essential as a profibrogenic mediator [51]. Transforming growth factor-β1 signaling modulates HSC as an active phenotype [27,52]. However, other reports indicated that TGF-β1 induced NF-κB activation [53]. In the present study, LF treatment decreased activated HSC and prevented fibrosis in a rat NASH model. Furthermore, NF-κB activation and TGF-β1 up-regulation in the model were attenuated by LF. However, JNK, which is also an important signaling pathway for fibrosis, was not altered by LF administration. These results suggest that LF protected the development of fibrosis by inhibiting NF-κB and TGF-β1 signaling.

5. Conclusions

This study demonstrated that LF prevents steatohepatitis and fibrosis without any adverse effects in a Cx32ΔTg–HFD–DMN rat NASH model. Therefore, LF may be a potential preventive or therapeutic application for this disease.

Supplementary Materials: The following supporting information can be downloaded at: https://www.mdpi.com/article/10.3390/nu14010042/s1, Table S1: Histopathology of NASH, fibrosis, and hepatocarcinogenesis in connexin 32 dominant negative transgenic rats fed a high-fat diet and dimethylnitrosamine with or without lactoferrin (100 or 500 mg/kg/day) at week 17; Table S2: mRNA level of inflammatory cytokines using quantitative reverse transcription PCR.

Author Contributions: Conceptualization and methodology: A.N.-I. and S.T. (Satoru Takahashi); validation, formal analysis, and investigation: Y.A., A.N.-I., K.X., M.K., H.K., Y.N., S.I., Y.M., S.T. (Shuji Takiguchi) and S.T. (Satoru Takahashi); data curation, writing of original draft preparation: Y.A. and A.N.-I.; writing by reviewing and editing: A.N.-I. and S.T. (Satoru Takahashi); resources: H.T., M.T. and S.T. (Satoru Takahashi); project administration, funding acquisition, visualization, and supervision: A.N.-I. and S.T. (Satoru Takahashi). All authors have read and agreed to the published version of the manuscript.

Funding: This work was supported by JSPS KAKENHI Grant Number 26460492 and 19K07509 to A.N-I.

Institutional Review Board Statement: The study was conducted according to the guidelines of the Declaration of Helsinki and approved by the Animal Care and Use Committee (ethic code: no. 19-025, approved on 24 September 2019) at Nagoya City University Graduate School of Medical Sciences.

Informed Consent Statement: Not applicable.

Data Availability Statement: The data presented in this study are available on request from the corresponding author.

Acknowledgments: The authors are sincerely grateful to Koji Kato and Junko Takekawa for excellent technical assistance with preparing tissue sections and immunohistochemical staining.

Conflicts of Interest: The authors declare that they have no conflict of interest.

Abbreviations

The following abbreviations are used in this manuscript:

Alb	Albumin
AST	Aspartate aminotransferase
Bex1	Brain expressed, X-linked 1
Cx	Connexin
Cx32ΔTg	Cx32 dominant negative transgenic
DEN	Diethylnitrosamine
DMN	Dimethylnitrosamine
GST-P	Glutathione S-transferase placental form
HCC	Hepatocellular carcinoma
HFD	High-fat diet
HSC	Hepatic stellate cell
IL	Interleukin
LDL-C	Low-density lipoprotein cholesterol
LF	Lactoferrin
MCDD	Methionine choline-deficient diet
NAFLD	Non-alcoholic fatty liver disease
NAS	Non-alcoholic fatty liver disease activity score
NASH	Non-alcoholic steatohepatitis
NF-κB	Nuclear factor-κB
ROS	Reactive oxygen species
TGF	Transforming growth factor
TNF	Tumor necrosis factor
Wt	Wild-type

References

1. Chalasani, N.; Younossi, Z.; Lavine, J.E.; Diehl, A.M.; Brunt, E.M.; Cusi, K.; Charlton, M.; Sanyal, A.J. The diagnosis and management of non-alcoholic fatty liver disease: Practice guideline by the American Gastroenterological Association, American Association for the Study of Liver Diseases, and American College of Gastroenterology. *Gastroenterology* **2012**, *142*, 1592–1609. [CrossRef] [PubMed]
2. Younossi, Z.M. Non-alcoholic fatty liver disease—A global public health perspective. *J. Hepatol.* **2019**, *70*, 531–544. [CrossRef] [PubMed]
3. Younossi, Z.; Anstee, Q.M.; Marietti, M.; Hardy, T.; Henry, L.; Eslam, M.; George, J.; Bugianesi, E. Global burden of NAFLD and NASH: Trends, predictions, risk factors and prevention. *Nat. Rev. Gastroenterol. Hepatol.* **2018**, *15*, 11–20. [CrossRef]
4. Anstee, Q.M.; Targher, G.; Day, C.P. Progression of NAFLD to diabetes mellitus, cardiovascular disease or cirrhosis. *Nat. Rev. Gastroenterol. Hepatol.* **2013**, *10*, 330–344. [CrossRef] [PubMed]
5. Evans, W.H.; Martin, P.E. Gap junctions: Structure and function (Review). *Mol. Membr. Biol.* **2002**, *19*, 121–136. [CrossRef]
6. Loewenstein, W.R. Junctional intercellular communication: The cell-to-cell membrane channel. *Physiol. Rev.* **1981**, *61*, 829–913. [CrossRef]
7. Yamasaki, H. Gap junctional intercellular communication and carcinogenesis. *Carcinogenesis* **1990**, *11*, 1051–1058. [CrossRef]
8. Trosko, J.E.; Chang, C.C. Role of stem cells and gap junctional intercellular communication in human carcinogenesis. *Radiat. Res.* **2001**, *155*, 175–180. [CrossRef]
9. Paul, D.L. Molecular cloning of cDNA for rat liver gap junction protein. *J. Cell Biol.* **1986**, *103*, 123–134. [CrossRef]
10. Sagawa, H.; Naiki-Ito, A.; Kato, H.; Naiki, T.; Yamashita, Y.; Suzuki, S.; Sato, S.; Shiomi, K.; Kato, A.; Kuno, T.; et al. Connexin 32 and luteolin play protective roles in non-alcoholic steatohepatitis development and its related hepatocarcinogenesis in rats. *Carcinogenesis* **2015**, *36*, 1539–1549. [CrossRef]
11. Nakashima, Y.; Ono, T.; Yamanoi, A.; El-Assal, O.N.; Kohno, H.; Nagasue, N. Expression of gap junction protein connexin32 in chronic hepatitis, liver cirrhosis, and hepatocellular carcinoma. *J. Gastroenterol.* **2004**, *39*, 763–768. [CrossRef]
12. Asamoto, M.; Hokaiwado, N.; Murasaki, T.; Shirai, T. Connexin 32 dominant-negative mutant transgenic rats are resistant to hepatic damage by chemicals. *Hepatology* **2004**, *40*, 205–210. [CrossRef] [PubMed]
13. Hokaiwado, N.; Asamoto, M.; Ogawa, K.; Shirai, T. Transgenic disruption of gap junctional intercellular communication enhances early but not late stage hepatocarcinogenesis in the rat. *Toxicol. Pathol.* **2005**, *33*, 695–701. [CrossRef] [PubMed]

14. Hokaiwado, N.; Asamoto, M.; Futakuchi, M.; Ogawa, K.; Takahashi, S.; Shirai, T. Both early and late stages of hepatocarcinogenesis are enhanced in Cx32 dominant negative mutant transgenic rats with disrupted gap junctional intercellular communication. *J. Membr. Biol.* **2007**, *218*, 101–106. [CrossRef] [PubMed]
15. Naiki-Ito, A.; Kato, H.; Naiki, T.; Yeewa, R.; Aoyama, Y.; Nagayasu, Y.; Suzuki, S.; Inaguma, S.; Takahashi, S. A novel model of non-alcoholic steatohepatitis with fibrosis and carcinogenesis in connexin 32 dominant-negative transgenic rats. *Arch. Toxicol.* **2020**, *94*, 4085–4097. [CrossRef] [PubMed]
16. Tanaka, H.; Gunasekaran, S.; Saleh, D.M.; Alexander, W.T.; Alexander, D.B.; Ohara, H.; Tsuda, H. Effects of oral bovine lactoferrin on a mouse model of inflammation associated colon cancer. *Biochem. Cell Biol.* **2021**, *99*, 159–165. [CrossRef]
17. Togawa, J.; Nagase, H.; Tanaka, K.; Inamori, M.; Nakajima, A.; Ueno, N.; Saito, T.; Sekihara, H. Oral administration of lactoferrin reduces colitis in rats via modulation of the immune system and correction of cytokine imbalance. *J. Gastroenterol. Hepatol.* **2002**, *17*, 1291–1298. [CrossRef]
18. Farid, A.S.; El Shemy, M.A.; Nafie, E.; Hegazy, A.M.; Abdelhiee, E.Y. Anti-inflammatory, anti-oxidant and hepatoprotective effects of lactoferrin in rats. *Drug Chem. Toxicol.* **2021**, *44*, 286–293. [CrossRef]
19. Chen, H.A.; Chiu, C.C.; Huang, C.Y.; Chen, L.J.; Tsai, C.C.; Hsu, T.C.; Tzang, B.S. Lactoferrin Increases Antioxidant Activities and Ameliorates Hepatic Fibrosis in Lupus-Prone Mice Fed with a High-Cholesterol Diet. *J. Med. Food* **2016**, *19*, 670–677. [CrossRef]
20. Duarte, D.C.; Nicolau, A.; Teixeira, J.A.; Rodrigues, L.R. The effect of bovine milk lactoferrin on human breast cancer cell lines. *J. Dairy Sci.* **2011**, *94*, 66–76. [CrossRef]
21. Xu, X.X.; Jiang, H.R.; Li, H.B.; Zhang, T.N.; Zhou, Q.; Liu, N. Apoptosis of stomach cancer cell SGC-7901 and regulation of Akt signaling way induced by bovine lactoferrin. *J. Dairy Sci.* **2010**, *93*, 2344–2350. [CrossRef] [PubMed]
22. Xiao, Y.; Monitto, C.L.; Minhas, K.M.; Sidransky, D. Lactoferrin down-regulates G1 cyclin-dependent kinases during growth arrest of head and neck cancer cells. *Clin. Cancer Res.* **2004**, *10*, 8683–8686. [CrossRef] [PubMed]
23. Kozu, T.; Iinuma, G.; Ohashi, Y.; Saito, Y.; Akasu, T.; Saito, D.; Alexander, D.B.; Iigo, M.; Kakizoe, T.; Tsuda, H. Effect of orally administered bovine lactoferrin on the growth of adenomatous colorectal polyps in a randomized, placebo-controlled clinical trial. *Cancer Prev. Res.* **2009**, *2*, 975–983. [CrossRef] [PubMed]
24. Kleiner, D.E.; Brunt, E.M.; Van Natta, M.; Behling, C.; Contos, M.J.; Cummings, O.W.; Ferrell, L.D.; Liu, Y.C.; Torbenson, M.S.; Unalp-Arida, A.; et al. Design and validation of a histological scoring system for nonalcoholic fatty liver disease. *Hepatology* **2005**, *41*, 1313–1321. [CrossRef]
25. Naiki-Ito, A.; Kato, H.; Asamoto, M.; Naiki, T.; Shirai, T. Age-dependent carcinogenic susceptibility in rat liver is related to potential of gap junctional intercellular communication. *Toxicol. Pathol.* **2012**, *40*, 715–721. [CrossRef]
26. Dela Pena, A.; Leclercq, I.; Field, J.; George, J.; Jones, B.; Farrell, G. NF-kappaB activation, rather than TNF, mediates hepatic inflammation in a murine dietary model of steatohepatitis. *Gastroenterology* **2005**, *129*, 1663–1674. [CrossRef]
27. Seki, E.; De Minicis, S.; Osterreicher, C.H.; Kluwe, J.; Osawa, Y.; Brenner, D.A.; Schwabe, R.F. TLR4 enhances TGF-beta signaling and hepatic fibrosis. *Nat. Med.* **2007**, *13*, 1324–1332. [CrossRef]
28. Wieckowska, A.; Papouchado, B.G.; Li, Z.; Lopez, R.; Zein, N.N.; Feldstein, A.E. Increased hepatic and circulating interleukin-6 levels in human nonalcoholic steatohepatitis. *Am. J. Gastroenterol.* **2008**, *103*, 1372–1379. [CrossRef]
29. Nobili, V.; Alisi, A.; Valenti, L.; Miele, L.; Feldstein, A.E.; Alkhouri, N. NAFLD in children: New genes, new diagnostic modalities and new drugs. *Nat. Rev. Gastroenterol. Hepatol.* **2019**, *16*, 517–530. [CrossRef]
30. Bullock, R.E.; Zaitoun, A.M.; Aithal, G.P.; Ryder, S.D.; Beckingham, I.J.; Lobo, D.N. Association of non-alcoholic steatohepatitis without significant fibrosis with hepatocellular carcinoma. *J. Hepatol.* **2004**, *41*, 685–686. [CrossRef]
31. Marrero, J.A.; Fontana, R.J.; Su, G.L.; Conjeevaram, H.S.; Emick, D.M.; Lok, A.S. NAFLD may be a common underlying liver disease in patients with hepatocellular carcinoma in the United States. *Hepatology* **2002**, *36*, 1349–1354. [CrossRef]
32. Aithal, G.P.; Thomas, J.A.; Kaye, P.V.; Lawson, A.; Ryder, S.D.; Spendlove, I.; Austin, A.S.; Freeman, J.G.; Morgan, L.; Webber, J. Randomized, placebo-controlled trial of pioglitazone in nondiabetic subjects with nonalcoholic steatohepatitis. *Gastroenterology* **2008**, *135*, 1176–1184. [CrossRef] [PubMed]
33. Ratziu, V.; Giral, P.; Jacqueminet, S.; Charlotte, F.; Hartemann-Heurtier, A.; Serfaty, L.; Podevin, P.; Lacorte, J.M.; Bernhardt, C.; Bruckert, E.; et al. Rosiglitazone for nonalcoholic steatohepatitis: One-year results of the randomized placebo-controlled Fatty Liver Improvement with Rosiglitazone Therapy (FLIRT) Trial. *Gastroenterology* **2008**, *135*, 100–110. [CrossRef] [PubMed]
34. Sanyal, A.J.; Chalasani, N.; Kowdley, K.V.; McCullough, A.; Diehl, A.M.; Bass, N.M.; Neuschwander-Tetri, B.A.; Lavine, J.E.; Tonascia, J.; Unalp, A.; et al. Pioglitazone, vitamin E, or placebo for nonalcoholic steatohepatitis. *N. Engl. J. Med.* **2010**, *362*, 1675–1685. [CrossRef] [PubMed]
35. Harrison, S.A.; Torgerson, S.; Hayashi, P.; Ward, J.; Schenker, S. Vitamin E and vitamin C treatment improves fibrosis in patients with nonalcoholic steatohepatitis. *Am. J. Gastroenterol.* **2003**, *98*, 2485–2490. [CrossRef] [PubMed]
36. Athyros, V.G.; Tziomalos, K.; Gossios, T.D.; Griva, T.; Anagnostis, P.; Kargiotis, K.; Pagourelias, E.D.; Theocharidou, E.; Karagiannis, A.; Mikhailidis, D.P. Safety and efficacy of long-term statin treatment for cardiovascular events in patients with coronary heart disease and abnormal liver tests in the Greek Atorvastatin and Coronary Heart Disease Evaluation (GREACE) Study: A post-hoc analysis. *Lancet* **2010**, *376*, 1916–1922. [CrossRef]
37. Nissen, S.E.; Wolski, K. Effect of rosiglitazone on the risk of myocardial infarction and death from cardiovascular causes. *N. Engl. J. Med.* **2007**, *356*, 2457–2471. [CrossRef]

38. Filozof, C.; Goldstein, B.J.; Williams, R.N.; Sanyal, A. Non-Alcoholic Steatohepatitis: Limited Available Treatment Options but Promising Drugs in Development and Recent Progress Towards a Regulatory Approval Pathway. *Drugs* **2015**, *75*, 1373–1392. [CrossRef]
39. Lee, S.; Son, B.; Jeon, J.; Park, G.; Kim, H.; Kang, H.; Youn, H.; Jo, S.; Song, J.Y.; Youn, B. Decreased Hepatic Lactotransferrin Induces Hepatic Steatosis in Chronic Non-Alcoholic Fatty Liver Disease Model. *Cell Physiol. Biochem.* **2018**, *47*, 2233–2249. [CrossRef]
40. Min, Q.Q.; Qin, L.Q.; Sun, Z.Z.; Zuo, W.T.; Zhao, L.; Xu, J.Y. Effects of Metformin Combined with Lactoferrin on Lipid Accumulation and Metabolism in Mice Fed with High-Fat Diet. *Nutrients* **2018**, *10*, 1628. [CrossRef]
41. Xiong, L.; Ren, F.; Lv, J.; Zhang, H.; Guo, H. Lactoferrin attenuates high-fat diet-induced hepatic steatosis and lipid metabolic dysfunctions by suppressing hepatic lipogenesis and down-regulating inflammation in C57BL/6J mice. *Food Funct.* **2018**, *9*, 4328–4339. [CrossRef] [PubMed]
42. Li, Y.C.; Hsieh, C.C. Lactoferrin dampens high-fructose corn syrup-induced hepatic manifestations of the metabolic syndrome in a murine model. *PLoS ONE* **2014**, *9*, e97341. [CrossRef] [PubMed]
43. Morishita, S.; Ono, T.; Fujisaki, C.; Ishihara, Y.; Murakoshi, M.; Kato, H.; Hosokawa, M.; Miyashita, K.; Sugiyama, K.; Nishino, H. Bovine lactoferrin reduces visceral fat and liver triglycerides in ICR mice. *J. Oleo Sci.* **2013**, *62*, 97–103. [CrossRef] [PubMed]
44. Brunt, E.M.; Janney, C.G.; Di Bisceglie, A.M.; Neuschwander-Tetri, B.A.; Bacon, B.R. Nonalcoholic steatohepatitis: A proposal for grading and staging the histological lesions. *Am. J. Gastroenterol.* **1999**, *94*, 2467–2474. [CrossRef]
45. Tsuchida, T.; Friedman, S.L. Mechanisms of hepatic stellate cell activation. *Nat. Rev. Gastroenterol. Hepatol.* **2017**, *14*, 397–411. [CrossRef]
46. Rizk, F.H.; Sarhan, N.I.; Soliman, N.A.; Ibrahim, M.A.A.; Abd-Elsalam, M.; Abd-Elsalam, S. Heat shock protein 47 as indispensible participant in liver fibrosis: Possible protective effect of lactoferrin. *IUBMB Life* **2018**, *70*, 795–805. [CrossRef]
47. Hessin, A.; Hegazy, R.; Hassan, A.; Yassin, N.; Kenawy, S. Lactoferrin Enhanced Apoptosis and Protected Against Thioacetamide-Induced Liver Fibrosis in Rats. *Open Access Maced. J. Med. Sci.* **2015**, *3*, 195–201. [CrossRef]
48. Hegazy, R.R.; Mansour, D.F.; Salama, A.A.; Abdel-Rahman, R.F.; Hassan, A.M. Regulation of PKB/Akt-pathway in the chemopreventive effect of lactoferrin against diethylnitrosamine-induced hepatocarcinogenesis in rats. *Pharmacol. Rep.* **2019**, *71*, 879–891. [CrossRef]
49. Mohammed, M.M.; Ramadan, G.; Zoheiry, M.K.; El-Beih, N.M. Antihepatocarcinogenic activity of whey protein concentrate and lactoferrin in diethylnitrosamine-treated male albino mice. *Environ. Toxicol.* **2019**, *34*, 1025–1033. [CrossRef]
50. Sun, B.; Karin, M. NF-kappaB signaling, liver disease and hepatoprotective agents. *Oncogene* **2008**, *27*, 6228–6244. [CrossRef]
51. Yu, Y.; Liu, Y.; An, W.; Song, J.; Zhang, Y.; Zhao, X. STING-mediated inflammation in Kupffer cells contributes to progression of nonalcoholic steatohepatitis. *J. Clin. Investig.* **2019**, *129*, 546–555. [CrossRef] [PubMed]
52. Okina, Y.; Sato-Matsubara, M.; Matsubara, T.; Daikoku, A.; Longato, L.; Rombouts, K.; Thanh Thuy, L.T.; Ichikawa, H.; Minamiyama, Y.; Kadota, M.; et al. TGF-beta-driven reduction of cytoglobin leads to oxidative DNA damage in stellate cells during non-alcoholic steatohepatitis. *J. Hepatol.* **2020**, *73*, 882–895. [CrossRef] [PubMed]
53. Liu, C.; Yuan, X.; Tao, L.; Cheng, Z.; Dai, X.; Sheng, X.; Xue, D. Xia-yu-xue decoction (XYXD) reduces carbon tetrachloride (CCl4)-induced liver fibrosis through inhibition hepatic stellate cell activation by targeting NF-kappaB and TGF-beta1 signaling pathways. *BMC Complement. Altern. Med.* **2015**, *15*, 201. [CrossRef] [PubMed]

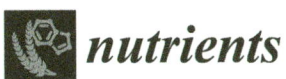

Article

Sargassum plagiophyllum Extract Enhances Colonic Functions and Modulates Gut Microbiota in Constipated Mice

Pissared Khuituan [1,2], Nawiya Huipao [1,2], Nilobon Jeanmard [2,3], Sitthiwach Thantongsakul [2,3], Warittha Promjun [2,3], Suwarat Chuthong [2,3], Chittipong Tipbunjong [1,2] and Saranya Peerakietkhajorn [2,3,*]

1. Division of Health and Applied Sciences, Faculty of Science, Prince of Songkla University, Songkhla 90110, Thailand; pissared.k@psu.ac.th (P.K.); nawiya.h@psu.ac.th (N.H.); chittipong.t@psu.ac.th (C.T.)
2. Gut Biology and Microbiota Research Unit, Prince of Songkla University, Songkhla 90110, Thailand; nilo.jean18@gmail.com (N.J.); 5910210317@psu.ac.th (S.T.); waritthapj@gmail.com (W.P.); suwarat1041@gmail.com (S.C.)
3. Division of Biological Science, Faculty of Science, Prince of Songkla University, Songkhla 90110, Thailand
* Correspondence: saranya.pe@psu.ac.th

Abstract: Constipation is a symptom that is widely found in the world's population. Various dietary supplementations are used to relieve and prevent constipation. Seaweed is widely used for its health benefits. In this study, we aimed to investigate the effects of *Sargassum plagiophyllum* extract (SPE) on functions of the gastrointestinal tract and gut microbiota. The results show that SPE pretreatment increased the frequency of gut contraction, leading to reduce gut transit time. SPE pretreatment also significantly increased the secretion of Cl^- and reduced Na^+ absorption, increasing fecal water content in constipated mice ($p < 0.05$). In addition, the Bifidobacteria population in cecal contents was significantly higher in constipated mice pretreated with 500 mg/kg SPE for 14 days than in untreated constipated mice ($p < 0.05$). Our findings suggest that SPE can prevent constipation in loperamide-induced mice. This study may be useful for the development of human food supplements from *S. plagiophyllum*, which prevent constipation.

Keywords: brown algae; *Sargassum plagiophyllum*; constipation; gastrointestinal transit; gut microbiota; transepithelial transport

Citation: Khuituan, P.; Huipao, N.; Jeanmard, N.; Thantongsakul, S.; Promjun, W.; Chuthong, S.; Tipbunjong, C.; Peerakietkhajorn, S. *Sargassum plagiophyllum* Extract Enhances Colonic Functions and Modulates Gut Microbiota in Constipated Mice. *Nutrients* 2022, 14, 496. https://doi.org/10.3390/nu14030496

Academic Editor: Md Soriful Islam

Received: 14 December 2021
Accepted: 21 January 2022
Published: 24 January 2022

Publisher's Note: MDPI stays neutral with regard to jurisdictional claims in published maps and institutional affiliations.

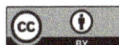

Copyright: © 2022 by the authors. Licensee MDPI, Basel, Switzerland. This article is an open access article distributed under the terms and conditions of the Creative Commons Attribution (CC BY) license (https://creativecommons.org/licenses/by/4.0/).

1. Introduction

Constipation is a health symptom that has been reported to affect approximately 8.2–32.9% of the world's population [1,2]. Constipation is often defined as infrequent and/or difficult bowel movements with a hard, dry stool [3,4], and it can be brought on by reduced physical activity, insufficient fluid intake, medication, and depression [5]. The condition is associated with gut microbiota imbalances involving decreased numbers of Bifidobacteria and Lactobacilli, increased numbers of pathogens, and suppressed intestinal motility [6]. Bifidobacteria, Lactobacilli, and Enterococci were effectively used in the treatment of constipation [7–9], and previous studies revealed that the levels of these bacteria were decreased in irritable bowel syndrome with constipation [10,11]. Several studies also showed that Enterobacteriaceae were increased in the condition of chronic constipation [10,12]. The recommended treatments for constipation include osmotic laxatives, generally lactulose, magnesium oxide, or polyethylene glycol [13], but the overuse of osmotic laxatives can result in dehydration and electrolyte imbalance. Clearly, these laxatives, which are available over the counter, can be harmful if patients incorrectly use them.

Alternative treatments emphasize dietary management to ensure a sufficient intake of dietary fiber and fluids [14–16]. Moreover, some nutritional plant products have been reported to aid the management of constipation. The extracts of *Aloe ferox* Mill, agarwood (*Aquilaria sinensis* and *Aquilaria crasna*), *Liriope platyphylla*, and prunes can increase intestinal motility, as well as the frequency and weight of stools. In Japan, the consumption of the seaweed *Ulva prolifera* gives effective relief to constipation sufferers [17]. The nutritional and pharmaceutical benefits of algae have been known for many centuries. Algae contain compounds that exert anti-inflammatory, antimicrobial, and antioxidant effects [18]. They also contain high amounts of dietary fiber, which has been widely used for the treatment of gastrointestinal disorders, including constipation, diarrhea, and ulcerative colitis [17–21]. Usually, the fiber component of algae principally comprises structural polysaccharides. A recent study reported that algal polysaccharides increased the populations of Bifidobacteria and Lactobacilli both in vivo and in vitro [22–24]. The large group of brown algae includes the macroalgal genus *Sargassum*, which is widely distributed along the coasts of the Gulf of Thailand and the Andaman Sea [25]. In the *Sargassum* species, the dominant polysaccharides include alginate, laminarin, and fucoidan [26]. The polysaccharides in *Sargassum* have been widely studied in pharmacological research, such as research on anti-obesity, anticancer, anti-inflammatory, antibacterial, and antiviral activities [27,28]. A previous study revealed that the components of *Sargassum plagiophyllum* were 68.69% carbohydrates (including 22.24% fiber), 9.05% protein, 0.88% lipid and 21.38% ash [29]. Fucoidan is a long-chain-sulfated polysaccharide found in *S. plagiophyllum*, which potentially reduces inflammation, and has antioxidant, antitumor, and anti-cholesterol activities [30,31]. Moreover, several studies revealed that *S. plagiophyllum* extract contains phenolic compounds and fucoxanthin, which have therapeutic activity, such as antioxidant, anti-inflammatory, anticancer, anti-obesity, and antidiabetic activities [32,33]. A recent study revealed that *S. plagiophyllum* extract also has antioxidant activity [34].

The present study aimed to investigate the effects of *Sargassum plagiophyllum* extract (SPE) on the changes in colonic functions and gut microbiota in a constipation model of mice. The gut transit time, colonic motility patterns, colonic smooth muscle contractility, electrolyte transport across cell membranes in the colon, and colonic microbiota composition were investigated.

2. Materials and Methods

2.1. Sargassum plagiophyllum Extract (SPE) Preparation

Adult-stage *Sargassum plagiophyllum* was collected from Lanta Island, Krabi, Thailand. The preparation of SPE followed the method of a previously described extraction of an algal sample [35]. Briefly, 1 g of finely ground dried *S. plagiophyllum* was added to 100 mL of distilled water and autoclaved at 121 °C for 20 min. The autoclaved *S. plagiophyllum* was centrifuged at 2220× g for 10 min, and the supernatant was collected and freeze dried to obtain SPE powder.

2.2. Animals and Experimental Design

Adult male ICR/Mlac mice (4–5 weeks old, 25–30 g) were obtained from the National Laboratory Animal Center, Mahidol University, Thailand. The mice were reared in a humidity- and temperature-controlled room (50–55% humidity and 25 ± 2 °C) and under 12 h light: 12 h dark photoperiod at the Southern Laboratory Animal Facility, Prince of Songkla University, Thailand. All mice had free access to food and water. All experiments were approved and guided by the Animal Ethics Committee of the Prince of Songkla University, Thailand (Project license number: MOE 0521.11/1555, Ref.68/2018).

The mice were divided into six groups (n = 5–6 in each group): a normal control, a constipation control, a positive control, and three treatments of SPE. The normal and constipation control groups were supplemented with 0.2 mL of distilled water. The positive control group was supplemented with 0.2 mL of 500 mg lactulose /kg of body weight, and the treatment groups were supplemented with 0.2 mL of SPE at 100, 500, and 1000 mg/kg of body weight. Lactulose and SPE were administered daily by oral gavage for two weeks. To prepare SPE and lactulose solutions for daily administration, SPE powder was freshly dissolved in distilled water. In all mice, except mice in the normal control group, constipation was induced by injection of 5 mg/kg loperamide (Lop) on day 12, day 13, and day 14 [34,36]. The body weight of each mouse was recorded every day.

On day 14, fecal pellets were collected for 4 h and then weighed and dried to calculate fecal water content. Gastrointestinal transit was also measured. The mice were anesthetized with 70 mg/kg thiopental sodium, and the small intestine, caecum, and colon were collected and dissected to study upper gut transit, colonic motility patterns, colonic smooth muscle contractility, epithelial transport in distal colon, and the composition of microbiota in cecal contents.

2.3. Measurement of Gastrointestinal Transit

To evaluate total gut transit time, mice were given a 0.1 mL Evans blue marker meal containing 5% Evans blue in 1.5% methylcellulose, and the time of the first blue pellet expulsion was recorded. A 3 mm glass bead was inserted into the colon (approximately 2 cm) using a plastic tip lubricated with petroleum jelly, and then the time to bead expulsion was recorded to observe the distal colonic transit time. For small intestinal transit, mice were gavage fed a 0.3 mL charcoal meal containing 10% w/v charcoal in 5% w/v gum arabic at 30 min before euthanasia. The euthanized mice were dissected, and transit (%) was calculated from the following equation [37]:

$$\text{Small intestinal transit } (\%) = \frac{\text{the distance of charcoal meal}}{\text{total length of the small intestine}} \times 100$$

2.4. Colonic Motility Pattern

After dissection, the whole colon with natural fecal pellets was collected and placed in ice-cold Krebs solution (pH 7.4 with an osmolality of 289–292 mmol/kg H_2O) in an organ bath with a Gastrointestinal Motility Monitor (GIMM) (Catamount Research and Development, St. Albans, VT, USA) and then continuously perfused at 10 mL/min with fresh oxygenated Krebs solution. The colon was allowed to equilibrate for 30 min in Krebs solution at 37 °C. The movement of fecal pellets was recorded using a video camera above the chamber, and then the images from each individual run were analyzed, and we constructed the spatiotemporal maps of motility using GIMM software [20]. The contraction patterns comprised propagating contractions and non-propagating contractions. The total number of spontaneous contractions was defined as the sum of propagating and non-propagating contractions.

2.5. Colonic Smooth Muscle Contractility

To observe colonic smooth muscle contractility, the colon was first cleared of luminal content, and 1 cm colonic segments of proximal and distal colon were used and suspended in the direction of longitudinal smooth muscle fibers in a 10 mL organ bath containing oxygenated Krebs solution at 37 °C. To stimulate contraction, carbachol (Tocris Bioscience, Bristol, UK) was added to the Krebs solution in the organ bath in a cumulative fashion. The concentrations of carbachol progressed from 0.1 to 1 to 10 μM, without washing between increments. The amplitude of contraction (g) and frequency of contraction (times/min) were recorded with the PowerLab® System (AD Instruments, New South Wales, Australia) and analyzed with LabChart7 program software [20,37].

2.6. Transepithelial Transport of Electrolytes across Cell Membranes in Distal Colon

To observe the transport of Na^+ and Cl^- across the epithelial cell membrane, 1 cm of distal colon tissue was opened and oriented as a flat sheet on an Ussing slider, which was placed in an Ussing chamber (Physiologic Instruments, San Diego, CA, USA) containing Krebs solution at 37 °C [21]. Carbogen was also included in this system to maintain the buffer at the physiological pH of 7.4 during the experiment. After that, transepithelial voltage (V_t) was recorded for 30 min as an equilibration period by injection of external current pulses (3 μA). To investigate Na^+ absorption by distal colon, 10 μM amiloride was added to the chamber at the apical membrane to inhibit Na^+ absorption by the epithelial sodium channel (ENaC), and the change in V_t was then recorded for 10 min. Cl^- secretion of Ca^{2+}-activated Cl^- channels (CaCC) was then induced by adding 100 µM of carbachol to the chamber at the basolateral membrane, and the change in V_t was again recorded for 10 min. Cl^- secretion of the cystic fibrosis transmembrane conductance regulator (CFTR) was then induced by adding 10 µM forskolin at the basolateral membrane, and the changes in V_t were recorded for 10 min. Following Ohm's law, the transepithelial potential difference (V_{te}), transepithelial resistance (R_{te}), and equivalent short-circuit current (I_{sc}) were calculated to represent the transepithelial transport of electrolytes in the collected distal colon [38,39].

2.7. Composition of Colonic Microbiota Analyses

Bacterial DNA of all samples were extracted from collected cecal content [40]. To amplify and detect bacterial 16S rRNA genes, qPCR was performed using LineGene 9600 Plus System (BIOER, Hangzhou, China) and SensiFAST™ SYBR® No-ROX Kit (Bioline). The following primer sets were used: FW 5'-CGATGAGTGCTAGGTGTTGGA-3' and RV 5'-CAAGATGTCAAGACCTGGTAAG-3' for total bacteria, LM26 5'-GATTCTGGCTCAGGAT GAACGC-3' and Bif228 5'-CTGATAGGACGCGACCCCAT-3' for Bifidobacteria, FW 5'-CGATGAGTGCTAGGTGTTGGA-3' and RV 5'-CAAGATGTCAAGACCTGGTAAG-3' for Lactobacilli, F-ent 5'- ATGGCTGTCGTCAGCTCGT-3' and R-ent 5'-CCTACTTCTTTTGCAA CCCACTC-3' for Enterobacteriaceae, and ECF 5'-AGAAATTCCAAACGAACTTG-3' and ECR 5'-CAGTGCTCTACCTCCATCATT-3' for Enterococci [41–45]. The following thermal cycling condition was used for all amplifications: 3 min at 95 °C, followed by 40 cycles of a two-step PCR reaction (5 s at 95 °C and 30 s at 60 °C) [40].

2.8. Statistical Analysis

All data are presented as means ± standard error (SE). The differences between groups were tested using one-way or two-way analysis of variance (ANOVA), followed by Bonferroni's test at $\alpha = 0.05$ using GraphPad Prism 5 (version 5.01).

3. Results

3.1. Effect of SPE Pretreatment on Body Weight, Fecal Water Content, and Gut Transit in Constipated Mice

On day 14, the body weight of the mice in all treatment groups was not significantly different (Figure 1A, $p > 0.05$). Fecal water content was significantly lower in the constipation control group than in the normal control group (Figure 1B, $p < 0.05$). Fecal water content was significantly higher in the lactulose and SPE treatment groups than in the constipation control group ($p < 0.05$).

The effects of SPE treatment on gut transit were determined using the total gut transit time, small intestinal transit time, and evacuation time (Figure 2). The total gut transit time in the constipation control group was 503.60 ± 19.78 min. The total gut transit time in the normal control group was significantly shorter at 240.20 ± 26.59 min (Figure 2A, $p < 0.001$). The total gut transit time was also shorter in all three SPE treatment groups, and it was the shortest in the 1000 mg/kg SPE group ($p < 0.001$). The small intestinal transit time was not significantly different among all groups (Figure 2B). The evacuation time was slightly longer in the constipation control group (26.01 ± 3.40 min) than in the normal control group (25.02 ± 2.13 min), but it was not significantly different (Figure 2C, $p > 0.05$). However, the evacuation times were significantly shorter in the positive control (Lactulose + Lop) group and the 1000 mg/kg SPE treatment group than in the constipation control group ($p < 0.05$). Our results suggest that SPE pretreatment could shorten total gut transit time and evacuation time.

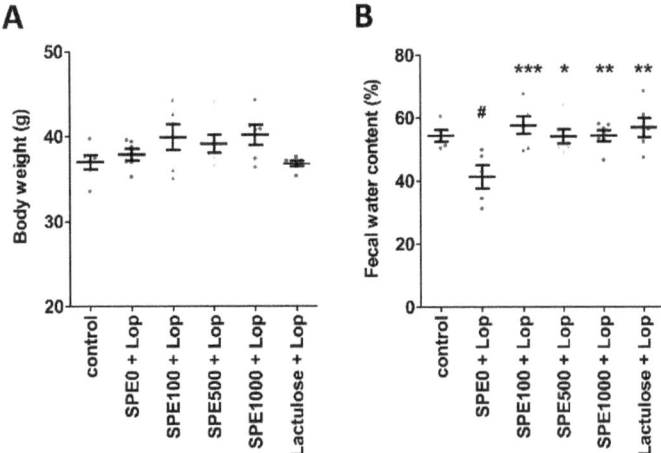

Figure 1. Effects of *Sargassum plagiophyllum* extract (SPE) pretreatment on body weight and fecal water content of constipated mice. (**A**) Body weight and (**B**) fecal water content of normal control group (control); constipation control group (SPE0 + Lop); 100, 500, and 1000 mg/kg SPE treatment groups (SPE100 + Lop, SPE500 + Lop, and SPE1000 + Lop, respectively); and positive control group (Lactulose + Lop). Symbols above the bars indicate significant differences from normal control or constipation control (# means $p < 0.05$ when compared with normal control group, and *, **, and *** mean $p < 0.05$, 0.01, and 0.001, respectively, when compared with constipation control group).

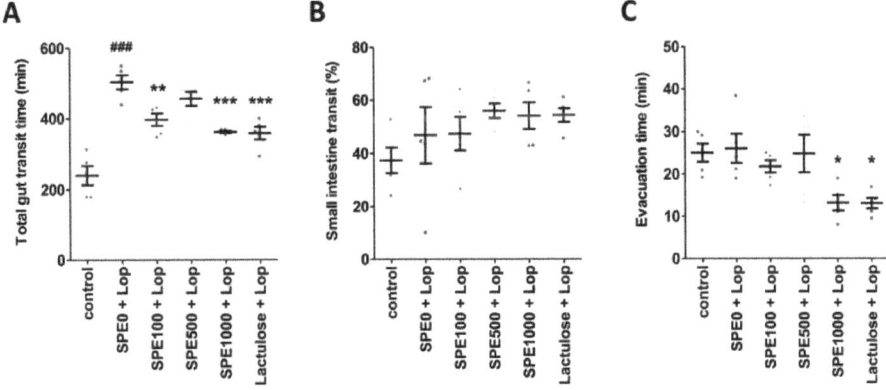

Figure 2. Effects of *Sargassum plagiophyllum* extract (SPE) pretreatment on gut transit of constipated mice. (**A**) Total gut transit time, (**B**) small intestine transit, and (**C**) evacuation time of normal control group (control); constipation control group (SPE0 + Lop); 100, 500, and 1000 mg/kg SPE treatment groups (SPE100 + Lop, SPE500 + Lop, and SPE1000 + Lop, respectively); and positive control group (Lactulose + Lop). Symbols above the bars indicate significant differences from normal control or constipation control (### means $p < 0.001$ when compared with the normal control group, and *, **, and *** mean $p < 0.05$, 0.01, and 0.001, respectively, when compared with the constipation control group).

3.2. Effect of SPE Pretreatment on Colonic Motility Pattern in Constipated Mice

The colonic motility pattern was investigated by determining the total number of contractions, the number of propagation contractions (peristalsis), and the number of non-propagation contractions (segmentation). Spatiotemporal maps were produced from an analysis of the contraction data using GIMM software (Figure 3). The total number of contractions was insignificantly higher in the normal control group than in the constipation control group (Figure 3A, $p > 0.05$), but the total number of contractions was significantly higher in the 500 mg/kg SPE treatment group than in the constipation control group ($p < 0.05$). Moreover, the number of propagation contractions was also significantly higher in the 500 and 1000 mg/kg SPE treatment groups than in the constipation control group (Figure 3B, $p < 0.01$). Non-propagation contractions were not significantly different among the groups (Figure 3C, $p > 0.05$).

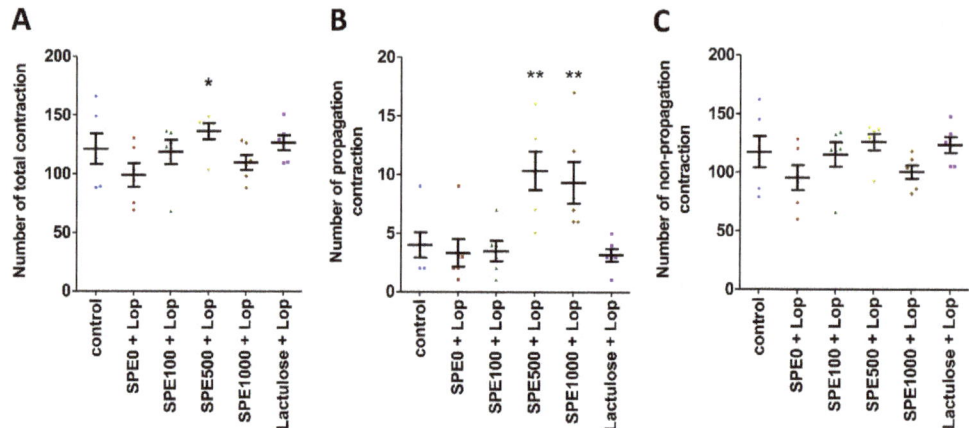

Figure 3. Effects of *Sargassum plagiophyllum* extract (SPE) pretreatment on the colonic motility pattern of constipated mice. (**A**) Number of total contractions, (**B**) number of propagation contractions, and (**C**) number of non-propagation contractions of normal control group (control); constipation control group (SPE0 + Lop); 100, 500, and 1000 mg/kg SPE treatment groups (SPE100 + Lop, SPE500 + Lop, and SPE1000 + Lop, respectively); and positive control group (Lactulose + Lop). Symbols above the bars indicate significant differences from constipation control (* and ** mean $p < 0.05$ and 0.01, respectively, when compared with the constipation control group).

3.3. Effect of SPE Pretreatment on Colonic Smooth Muscle Contractility in Constipated Mice

The amplitude and frequency of the contractions of the longitudinal smooth muscle fibers of the proximal and distal colon were observed to investigate the colonic smooth muscle contractility (Figure 4). The results revealed that the contractions of both the proximal and distal colon tended to be more frequent in the positive control (Lactulose + Lop) and SPE treatment groups. After adding 10 μM of carbachol, proximal colonic contractions occurred significantly less frequently in the constipation control (SPE0 + Lop) group (7.00 ± 0.73 times/min) than in the 500 mg/kg SPE treatment group (11.00 ± 1.63 times/min) (Figure 4A, $p < 0.05$). Distal colonic contractions were also significantly less frequent in the constipation control group (SPE0 + Lop) (9.33 ± 1.54 times/min) than in the normal control group (13.67 ± 1.12 times/min) (Figure 4B, $p < 0.05$). Even at 0.1 μM, contractions in the distal colon were significantly less frequent (6.83 ± 0.95 times/min) in the constipation control group than in the normal control group (11.83 ± 1.05 times/min) ($p < 0.05$).

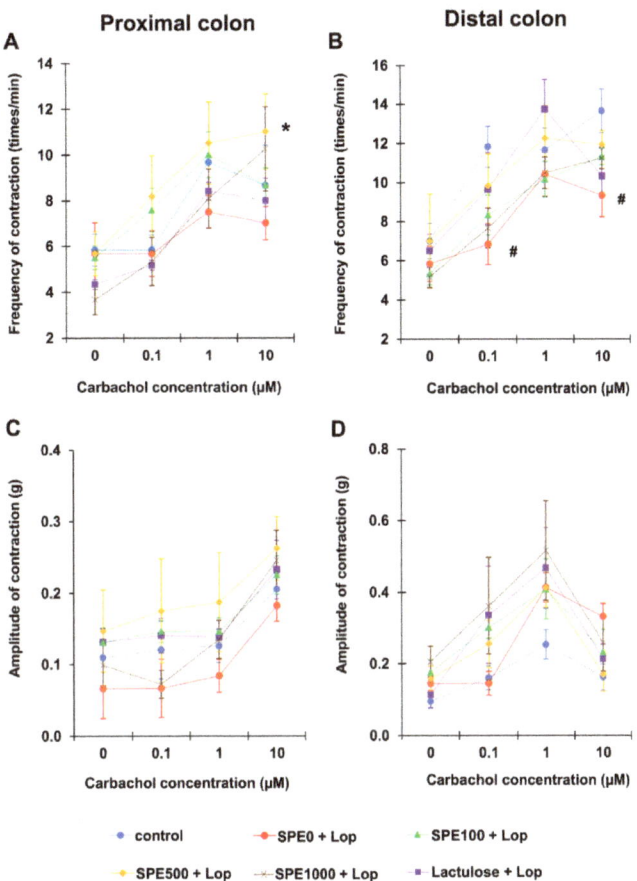

Figure 4. Effects of *Sargassum plagiophyllum* extract (SPE) pretreatment on colonic smooth muscle contractility of constipated mice. Frequency and amplitude of contractions of (**A,C**) proximal colon and (**B,D**) distal colon of normal control group (control); constipation control group (SPE0 + Lop); 100, 500, and 1000 mg/kg SPE treatment groups (SPE100 + Lop, SPE500 + Lop, and SPE1000 + Lop, respectively); and positive control group (Lactulose + Lop). Symbols indicate significant differences from normal control or constipation control (# means $p < 0.05$ when compared with the normal control group, and * means $p < 0.05$ when compared with the constipation control group).

The amplitude of the proximal colonic contractions showed a similar trend in all groups in that the amplitude of the contractions was highest at 10 μM of carbachol (Figure 4C). The amplitude of the proximal colonic contractions was lower in the constipation control group than in the normal control and positive control groups, as well as the 100, 500, and 1000 mg/kg SPE treatment groups, but there was no significant difference among all groups at all concentrations of carbachol ($p > 0.05$). The amplitude of the distal colonic contractions was highest at 1 μM of carbachol, but there was, again, no significant difference among all groups at all concentrations of carbachol (Figure 4D, $p > 0.05$).

3.4. Effect of SPE Pretreatment on Transport of Electrolytes across Cell Membranes in Distal Colon of Constipated Mice

The basal transport values (V_{te}, R_{te}, and I_{sc}) of the distal colon were not significantly different among the groups (Table 1). However, these values did show significant differences when the distal colon was exposed to amiloride, carbachol, and forskolin. The amiloride-induced I_{sc} of the distal colon in the constipation control group (62.95 ± 1.77 μAm/cm^2) was significantly higher than the amiloride-induced I_{sc} of the distal colon in the normal control ($p < 0.001$), positive control ($p < 0.01$), and SPE treatment ($p < 0.001$) groups (Figure 5A). In contrast, the carbachol-induced I_{sc} of the distal colon in the constipation control group (19.46 ± 3.13 μAm/cm^2) was significantly lower than the carbachol-induced I_{sc} of the distal colon in the normal control, positive control, and SPE treatment groups (Figure 5B, $p < 0.001$). The forskolin-induced I_{sc} of the distal colon was also lower in the constipated control group (29.65 ± 1.92 μAm/cm^2) than in the normal control ($p < 0.001$), positive control ($p < 0.01$), and SPE treatment ($p < 0.001$) groups (Figure 5C).

Table 1. Transepithelial potential difference (V_{te}), transepithelial resistance (R_{te}), and equivalent short-circuit current (I_{sc}) of distal colonic epithelium membrane of normal control, constipation control, positive control, and SPE-pretreated mice.

Treatment	V_{te} (V)	R_{te} (Ω.cm^2)	I_{sc} (μA/cm^2)
Control	8.33 ± 1.89	71.57 ± 7.28	119.74 ± 23.50
0 mg/kg SPE + Loperamide	8.22 ± 1.63	57.23 ± 7.38	147.51 ± 25.31
100 mg/kg SPE + Loperamide	8.53 ± 1.93	59.47 ± 6.55	136.40 ± 22.98
500 mg/kg SPE + Loperamide	6.51 ± 1.18	58.68 ± 5.45	108.59 ± 14.58
1000 mg/kg SPE + Loperamide	8.58 ± 1.35	72.18 ± 10.24	121.79 ± 12.04
500mg/kg Lactulose + Loperamide	5.37 ± 0.88	57.72 ± 8.19	100.08 ± 21.06

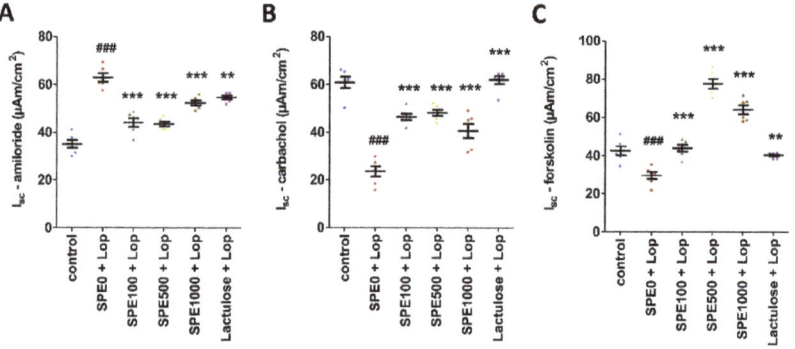

Figure 5. Effects of *Sargassum plagiophyllum* extract (SPE) pretreatment on transport of electrolytes across cell membranes of constipated mice. The charts show short-circuit current (I_{sc}) responses to (**A**) amiloride, (**B**) carbachol, and (**C**) forskolin of distal colon in normal control group (control); constipation control group (SPE0 + Lop); 100, 500, and 1000 mg/kg SPE treatment groups (SPE100 + Lop, SPE500 + Lop, and SPE1000 + Lop, respectively); and positive control group (Lactulose + Lop). Symbols above the bars indicate significant differences from normal control or constipation control (### mean $p < 0.001$, respectively, when compared with the normal control group, and ** and *** mean $p < 0.01$ and 0.001, respectively, when compared with the constipation control group).

3.5. Effect of SPE Pretreatment on Composition of Gut Microbiota in Constipate Mice

Cecal contents were collected and weighed to estimate the numbers of total bacteria, Bifidobacteria, Lactobacilli, Enterobacteriaceae, and Enterococci in the cecum of mice from every control group and all SPE treatment groups. The cecal content weight of the mice in the 1000 mg/kg SPE treatment group (0.1584 ± 0.0117 g) was significantly higher than the cecal content weight of the mice in the constipation control group (0.0960 ± 0.0061 g) (Figure 6A, $p < 0.01$), but the numbers of total bacteria were not significantly different among groups (Figure 6B, $p > 0.05$). The number of Bifidobacteria was not significantly different between the constipation control and the normal control groups

($p > 0.05$), but it was significantly higher in the 500 mg/kg SPE treatment group ($1.33 \pm 0.66 \times 10^9$ cells/g cecal content) than in the constipation control group ($6.78 \pm 3.42 \times 10^7$ cells/g cecal content) (Figure 6C, $p < 0.05$). The numbers of Lactobacilli, Enterobacteriaceae, and Enterococcus were not significantly different among groups (Figure 6D–F, $p > 0.05$). Our results suggest that pretreatment with 500 mg/kg SPE could modulate the composition of bacteria, especially Bifidobacteria, in the cecum of constipated mice.

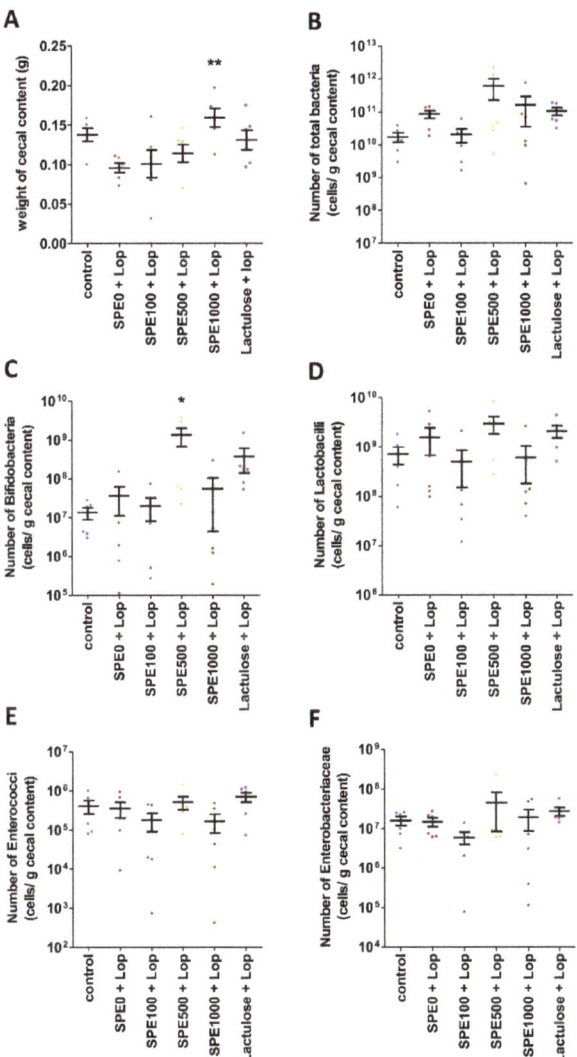

Figure 6. Effects of *Sargassum plagiophyllum* extract (SPE) pretreatment on gut microbiota in constipated mice. (**A**) Weight of cecal contents and number of (**B**) total bacteria, (**C**) Bifidobacteria, (**D**) Lactobacilli, (**E**) Enterococci, and (**F**) Enterobacteriaceae in cecal contents of normal control group (control); constipation control group (SPE0 + Lop); 100, 500, and 1000 mg/kg SPE treatment groups (SPE100 + Lop, SPE500 + Lop, and SPE1000 + Lop, respectively); and positive control group (Lactulose + Lop). Symbols above the bars indicate significant differences from constipation control (* and ** mean $p < 0.05$ and 0.01, respectively, when compared with the constipation control group).

4. Discussion

Our results suggest that SPE pretreatment increased the frequency of contractions in the colonic smooth muscle and effectively increased both the propagation contractions and the total contractions of the colon in constipated mice. Moreover, the frequency of the contractions of the constipation control mice was lower than that of the others; therefore, the total gut transit time of the constipation control mice was longer than that of the normal control and SPE pretreatment groups. This indicates that SPE is capable of preventing constipation by enhancing colonic contraction and reducing the gut transit time and evacuation time. The results of this study are consistent with the results of a previous study of the marine algae *Ulva* (*Enteromorpha*), which indicated that dried *Ulva* enhanced colonic contraction and reduced gut transit time in constipated mice [46].

A recent study found polysaccharides, such as alginates, laminarins, and fucoidans, in *Sargassum* [47]. These polysaccharides have been used as substrates for the fermentation and production of short-chain fatty acids (SCFAs) by gut microbiota [48]. The present study showed that the Bifidobacteria population in the cecal contents of constipated mice was significantly increased in mice pretreated with 500 mg/kg SPE. Bifidobacteria are beneficial microorganisms that stimulate the growth of butyrate-producing bacteria, such as *Faecalibacterium, Eubacterium,* and *Roseburia* [49]. Acetate, propionate, and butyrate have been shown to interact with the free fatty acid receptors 2 and 3 (FFA2 and FFA3) of enterochromaffin cells (ECs) to induce serotonin (5-HT) release and trigger peristalsis [50]. Our results show that the frequency of the total colonic contractions was higher and the total gut transit time was shorter in the SPE treatment groups than in the constipation control group. Pretreatment with SPE was therefore able to prevent constipation by enhancing colonic contractions and reducing the gut transit time and evacuation time. Therefore, SPE pretreatment prevented constipation in the loperamide-induced mice by promoting the beneficial bacteria that might enhance the butyrate production, which leads to increased colonic contractility. In this study, we observed four selected bacteria that were reported to be involved with constipation. For further studies, we suggest that 16S rRNA gene sequence analysis should be performed to observe the changes in the microbiota of SPE-treated mice.

Furthermore, the results of this study also suggest that SPE pretreatment increases fecal water content in constipated mice. Our results are consistent with those of previous studies that revealed a reduction in fecal water content and the secretion of water in the distal colon of constipated rats [51]. The feces of mice supplemented with lactulose and SPE in this study contained more water than the feces of mice in the constipation control group. This result supports the findings of studies of the marine algae *Ulva* and *Chondrus*. These algae induced the secretion of water into the colon and increased fecal water content [46,52,53]. Moreover, lactulose was also found to increase fecal water content by absorption [54].

The study of electrolyte transport across the epithelial cell membrane of the distal colon showed that the basal transepithelial potential difference (V_{te}), transepithelial resistance (R_{te}), and equivalent short-circuit current (I_{sc}) were not significantly different among all groups. This result indicates that pretreatment with SPE did not affect the colonic tissue or the ion channels [39]. However, the functioning of the ion channels in the distal colon of constipated mice treated with SPE changed. Cl^- secretion increased, and Na^+ absorption was inhibited in SPE-pretreated mice. These changes increased the fecal water content in these groups compared with the constipation control group. The increased Cl^- secretion was confirmed by the increased I_{sc} induced by carbachol in the distal colon of SPE-supplemented mice. SPE induced an influx of Ca^{2+} into gut epithelial cells, which activated the CaCC [55]. Moreover, the forskolin-induced I_{sc} was also higher in the SPE pretreatment groups, indicating that cAMP increased in the cell and then activated CFTR and increased Cl^- secretion [56]. *Sargassum* has been shown to contain flavonoids [57], which increase cyclic adenosine monophosphate (cAMP) in gut epithelial cells and then induce the release of Ca^{2+} from the endoplasmic reticulum to the cytosol via protein kinase A (PKA) [54,58]. Recent studies revealed that increased cellular Ca^{2+} levels are not only important for the activation of CaCC but that they also activate CFTR via the PI3K/Akt pathway [56,59].

Therefore, SPE pretreatment might increase fecal water content by increasing cellular Ca^{2+} levels to induce Cl^- secretion in the colonic lumen.

High cellular Ca^{2+} levels also inhibited Na^+ absorption and reduced water absorption in the colon [60]. In the present study, the amiloride-induced I_{sc} of the distal colon of mice treated with SPE decreased. This result indicates that Na^+ absorption in the distal colon reduced, and fecal water content therefore increased. In a recent study, it was found that goblet cell numbers on the villi of ileum increased in constipated mice pretreated with SPE [34]. This finding implied that mucus secretion in the ileum might also have increased, which supports our finding that fecal water content increased in constipated mice supplemented with SPE.

In conclusion, SPE is a natural supplement that enhances colonic contractility and increases the numbers of Bifidobacteria. Pretreatment with SPE reduced the gut transit time and the evacuation time of constipated mice. SPE also increased the secretion of Cl^- and reduced Na^+ absorption in the distal colon, leading to increased fecal water content. Therefore, SPE was able to prevent constipation.

Author Contributions: Conceptualization, S.P., P.K., C.T. and N.H.; methodology and data analysis, S.P., N.H., C.T. and P.K.; investigation, S.P., N.J., S.T., W.P. and S.C.; writing—original draft preparation, S.P.; writing—review and editing, S.P., P.K., C.T. and N.H.; project administration, S.P. and P.K.; funding acquisition, S.P. All authors have read and agreed to the published version of the manuscript.

Funding: This research was supported by the National Science, Research and Innovation Fund (NSRF) and the Prince of Songkla University (Grant No. SCI6405072S).

Institutional Review Board Statement: The study was conducted according to the guidelines of the Declaration of Helsinki and approved by the Animal Ethics Committee of the Prince of Songkla University, Thailand (ethical approval code: MOE 0521.11/1555 Ref.68/2018, date of approval: 28 December 2018).

Informed Consent Statement: Not applicable.

Data Availability Statement: The data supporting the research for this study are available within the manuscript.

Acknowledgments: We are grateful to Supattra Pongparadorn and Jaruwan Mayakun from the Excellence Center for Biodiversity of Peninsular Thailand (Prince of Songkla University, Thailand) for the identification and collection of *Sargassum plagiophyllum*.

Conflicts of Interest: The authors declare no conflict of interest.

References

1. Tamura, A.; Tomita, T.; Oshima, T.; Toyoshima, F.; Yamasaki, T.; Okugawa, T.; Kondo, T.; Kono, T.; Tozawa, K.; Ikehara, H.; et al. Prevalence and self-recognition of chronic constipation: Results of an internet survey. *J. Neurogastroenterol. Motil.* **2016**, *22*, 677–685. [CrossRef] [PubMed]
2. Zhang, Q.; Zhong, D.; Sun, R.; Zhang, Y.; Pegg, R.B.; Zhong, G. Prevention of loperamide induced constipation in mice by KGM and the mechanisms of different gastrointestinal tract microbiota regulation. *Carbohydr. Polym.* **2021**, *256*, 117418. [CrossRef] [PubMed]
3. Boland, J.W.; Boland, E.G. Constipation and malignant bowel obstruction in palliative care. *Medicine* **2020**, *48*, 18–22. [CrossRef]
4. Milosavljevic, T.; Popovic, D.D.; Mijac, D.D.; Milovanovic, T.; Krstic, S.; Krstic, M.N. Chronic constipation, gastroenterohepatologist's approach. *Dig. Dis.* **2021**. [CrossRef] [PubMed]
5. Forootan, M.; Bagheri, N.; Darvishi, M. Chronic constipation. *Medicine* **2018**, *97*, e10631. [CrossRef]
6. Hu, T.G.; Wen, P.; Fu, H.Z.; Lin, G.Y.; Liao, S.T.; Zou, Y.X. Protective effect of mulberry (*Morus atropurpurea*) fruit against diphenoxylate-induced constipation in mice through the modulation of gut microbiota. *Food Funct.* **2019**, *10*, 1513–1528. [CrossRef]
7. Tabbers, M.M.; de Milliano, I.; Roseboom, M.G.; Benninga, M.A. Is *Bifidobacterium* breve effective in the treatment of childhood constipation? Results from a pilot study. *Nutr. J.* **2011**, *10*, 19. [CrossRef] [PubMed]
8. Tsukahara, T.; Bukawa, W.; Kan, T.; Ushida, K. Effect of a cell preparation of *Enterococcus faecalis* strain EC-12 on digesta flow and recovery from constipation in a pig model and human subjects. *Microb. Ecol. Health Dis.* **2005**, *17*, 107–113.
9. Zhao, Y.; Yu, Y.-B. Intestinal microbiota and chronic constipation. *SpringerPlus* **2016**, *5*, 1130. [CrossRef]

10. Chassard, C.; Dapoigny, M.; Scott, K.P.; Crouzet, L.; Del'homme, C.; Marquet, P.; Martin, J.C.; Pickering, G.; Ardid, D.; Eschalier, A.; et al. Functional dysbiosis within the gut microbiota of patients with constipated-irritable bowel syndrome. *Aliment. Pharmacol. Ther.* **2012**, *35*, 828–838. [CrossRef]
11. Parkes, G.C.; Rayment, N.B.; Hudspith, B.N.; Petrovska, L.; Lomer, M.C.; Brostoff, J.; Whelan, K.; Sanderson, J.D. Distinct microbial populations exist in the mucosa-associated microbiota of sub-groups of irritable bowel syndrome. *Neurogastroenterol. Motil.* **2012**, *24*, 31–39. [CrossRef] [PubMed]
12. Durban, A.; Abellan, J.J.; Jimenez-Hernandez, N.; Salgado, P.; Ponce, M.; Ponce, J.; Garrigues, V.; Latorre, A.; Moya, A. Structural alterations of faecal and mucosa-associated bacterial communities in irritable bowel syndrome. *Environ. Microbiol. Rep.* **2012**, *4*, 242–247. [CrossRef] [PubMed]
13. Portalatin, M.; Winstead, N. Medical Management of Constipation. *Clin. Colon Rectal Surg.* **2012**, *25*, 12–19. [CrossRef] [PubMed]
14. Krogh, K.; Chiarioni, G.; Whitehead, W. Management of chronic constipation in adults. *United Eur. Gastroenterol. J.* **2017**, *5*, 465–472. [CrossRef]
15. Tropini, C.; Moss, E.L.; Merrill, B.D.; Ng, K.M.; Higginbottom, S.K.; Casavant, E.P.; Gonzalez, C.G.; Fremin, B.; Bouley, D.M.; Elias, J.E.; et al. Transient osmotic perturbation causes long-term alteration to the gut microbiota. *Cell* **2018**, *173*, 1742–1754. [CrossRef]
16. Vriesman, M.H.; Koppen, I.J.N.; Camilleri, M.; Di Lorenzo, C.; Benninga, M.A. Management of functional constipation in children and adults. *Nat. Rev. Gastroenterol. Hepatol.* **2020**, *17*, 21–39. [CrossRef]
17. Ngatu, R.N.; Ikeda, M.; Watanabe, H.; Tanaka, M.; Inoue, M. Laxative effects of dietary supplementation with sujiaonori algal biomaterial in Japanese adult women with functional constipation: A case study. *J. Funct. Biomater.* **2017**, *8*, 15. [CrossRef]
18. Peñalver, R.; Lorenzo, J.M.; Ros, G.; Amarowicz, R.; Pateiro, M.; Nieto, G. Seaweeds as a functional ingredient for a healthy diet. *Mar. Drugs* **2020**, *18*, 301. [CrossRef]
19. Dewinta, A.F.; Susetya, I.E.; Suriani, M. Nutritional profile of *Sargassum* sp. from Pane Island, Tapanuli Tengah as a component of functional food. *J. Phys. Conf. Ser.* **2020**, *1542*, 012040. [CrossRef]
20. K-da, S.; Peerakietkhajorn, S.; Siringoringo, B.; Muangnil, P.; Wichienchot, S.; Khuituan, P. Oligosaccharides from *Gracilaria fisheri* ameliorate gastrointestinal dysmotility and gut dysbiosis in colitis mice. *J. Funct. Foods* **2020**, *71*, 104021. [CrossRef]
21. Siringoringo, B.; Huipao, N.; Tipbunjong, C.; Nopparat, J.; Wichienchot, S.; Hutapea, A.M.; Khuituan, P. *Gracilaria fisheri* oligosaccharides ameliorate inflammation and colonic epithelial barrier dysfunction in mice with acetic acid-induced colitis. *Asian Pac. J. Trop. Biomed.* **2021**, *11*, 440–449.
22. Chamidah, A. Prebiotic index evaluation of crude laminaran of *Sargassum* sp. using feces of wistar rats. *IOP Conf. Ser. Earth Environ. Sci.* **2018**, *139*, 012043. [CrossRef]
23. Ramnani, P.; Chitarrari, R.; Tuohy, K.; Grant, J.; Hotchkiss, S.; Philp, K.; Campbell, R.; Gill, C.; Rowland, I. In vitro fermentation and prebiotic potential of novel low molecular weight polysaccharides derived from agar and alginate seaweeds. *Anaerobe* **2012**, *18*, 1–6. [CrossRef]
24. Shang, Q.; Shan, X.; Cai, C.; Hao, J.; Li, G. Dietary fucoidan modulates the gut microbiota in mice by increasing the abundance of *Lactobacillus* and Ruminococcaceae. *Food Funct.* **2016**, *7*, 3224–3232. [CrossRef] [PubMed]
25. Yangthong, M.; Hutadilok-Towatana, N.; Thawonsuwan, J.; Wutiporn, P. An aqueous extract from *Sargassum* sp. enhances the immune response and resistance against *Streptococcus iniae* in the Asian sea bass (Lates calcarifer Bloch). *J. Appl. Phycol.* **2016**, *28*, 3587–3598. [CrossRef]
26. Zheng, L.X.; Chen, X.Q.; Cheong, K.L. Current trends in marine algae polysaccharides: The digestive tract, microbial catabolism, and prebiotic potential. *Int. J. Biol. Macromol.* **2020**, *151*, 344–354. [CrossRef]
27. Liu, L.; Heinrich, M.; Myers, S.; Dworjanyn, S.A. Towards a better understanding of medicinal uses of the brown seaweed *Sargassum* in traditional Chinese medicine: A phytochemical and pharmacological review. *J. Ethnopharmacol.* **2012**, *142*, 591–619. [CrossRef]
28. Zhang, Y.; Zuo, J.; Yan, L.; Cheng, Y.; Li, Q.; Wu, S.; Chen, L.; Thring, R.W.; Yang, Y.; Gao, Y.; et al. *Sargassum fusiforme* fucoidan alleviates high-fat diet-induced obesity and insulin resistance associated with the improvement of hepatic oxidative stress and gut microbiota profile. *J. Agric. Food Chem.* **2020**, *68*, 10626–10638. [CrossRef]
29. Edison, E.; Diharmi, A.; Ariani, N.M.; Ilza, M. Komponen bioactive dan aktivitas antioksidan ekstrak kasar *Sargassum plagyophyllum*. *J. Pengolah. Has. Perikan. Indones.* **2020**, *20*, 58–66.
30. Saeton, U.; Nontasak, P.; Palasin, K.; Wonglapsuwan, M.; Mayakun, J.; Pongparadon, S.; Chotigeat, W. Potential health benefits of fucoidan from the brown seaweeds *Sargassum plagiophyllum* and *Sargassum polycystum*. *J. Appl. Phycol.* **2021**, *33*, 3357–3364. [CrossRef]
31. Suresh, V.; Senthilkumar, N.; Thangam, R.; Rajkumar, M.; Anbazhagan, C.; Rengasamy, R.; Gunasekaran, P.; Kannan, S.; Palani, P. Separation, purification and preliminary characterization of sulfated polysaccharides from *Sargassum plagiophyllum* and its in vitro anticancer and antioxidant activity. *Process Biochem.* **2013**, *48*, 364–373. [CrossRef]
32. Kalasariya, H.S.; Yadav, V.K.; Yadav, K.K.; Tirth, V.; Algahtani, A.; Islam, S.; Gupta, N.; Jeon, B.-H. Seaweed-based molecules and their potential biological activities: An eco-sustainable cosmetics. *Molecules* **2021**, *26*, 5313. [CrossRef] [PubMed]
33. Kumar, Y.; Tarafdar, A.; Badgujar, P.C. Seaweed as a source of natural antioxidants: Therapeutic activity and food applications. *Hindawi* **2021**, 5753391. [CrossRef]

34. Sengkhim, R.; Peerakietkhajorn, S.; Jeanmard, N.; Pongparadorn, S.; Khuituan, P.; Thitiphatphuvanon, T.; Surinlert, P.; Tipbunjong, C. Effects of *Sargassum plagiophyllum* extract pretreatment on tissue histology of constipated mice. *Trop. J. Pharm. Res.* **2021**, *20*, 2339–2346. [CrossRef]
35. Zahra, R.; Mehrnaz, M.; Farzaneh, V.; Kohzad, S. Antioxidant activity of extract from a brown alga, *Sargassum boveanum*. *Afr. J. Biotechnol.* **2007**, *6*, 2740–2745.
36. Hayeeawaema, F.; Wichienchot, S.; Khuituan, P. Amelioration of gut dysbiosis and gastrointestinal motility by konjac oligo-glucomannan on loperamide-induced constipation in mice. *Nutrition* **2020**, *73*, 110715. [CrossRef]
37. Khuituan, P.; K-da, S.; Bannob, K.; Hayeeawaema, F.; Peerakietkhajorn, S.; Tipbunjong, C.; Charoenphandhu, N. Prebiotic oligosaccharides from dragon fruits alter gut motility in mice. *Biomed. Pharmacother.* **2019**, *114*, 108821. [CrossRef]
38. Li, H.; Sheppard, D.N.; Hug, M.J. Transepithelial electrical measurements with the Ussing chamber. *J. Cyst. Fibros* **2004**, *3*, 123–126. [CrossRef]
39. Clarke, L.L. A guide to Ussing chamber studies of mouse intestine. *Am. J. Physiol. Gastrointest. Liver Physiol.* **2009**, *296*, G1151–G1166. [CrossRef]
40. Peerakietkhajorn, S.; Jeanmard, N.; Chuenpanitkit, P.; K-da, S.; Bannob, K.; Khuituan, P. Effects of plant oligosaccharides derived from dragon fruit on gut microbiota in proximal and distal colon of mice. *Sains Malays.* **2020**, *49*, 603–611. [CrossRef]
41. Kaufmann, P.; Pfefferkorn, A.; Teuber, M.; Meile, L. Identification and quantification of *Bifidobacterium* species isolated from food with genus-specific 16S rRNA-targeted probes by colony hybridization and PCR. *Appl. Environ. Microbiol.* **1997**, *63*, 1268–1273. [CrossRef] [PubMed]
42. Matsuki, T.; Watanabe, K.; Fujimoto, J.; Kado, Y.; Takada, T.; Matsumoto, K.; Tanaka, R. Quantitative PCR with 16S rRNA-gene-targeted species-specific primers for analysis of human intestinal bifidobacteria. *Appl. Environ. Microbiol.* **2004**, *70*, 167–173. [CrossRef]
43. Fu, C.J.; Carter, J.N.; Li, Y.; Porter, J.H.; Kerley, M.S. Comparison of agar plate and real-time PCR on enumeration of *Lactobacillus*, *Clostridium perfringens* and total anaerobic bacteria in dog faeces. *Lett. Appl. Microbiol.* **2006**, *42*, 490–494. [CrossRef]
44. Leser, T.D.; Amenuvor, J.Z.; Jensen, T.K.; Lindecrona, R.H.; Boye, M.; Møller, K. Culture-independent analysis of gut bacteria: The pig gastrointestinal tract microbiota revisited. *Appl. Environ. Microbiol.* **2002**, *68*, 673–690. [CrossRef] [PubMed]
45. Sghir, A.; Gramet, G.; Suau, A.; Rochet, V.; Pochart, P.; Dore, J. Quantification of bacterial groups within human fecal flora by oligonucleotide probe hybridization. *Appl. Environ. Microbiol.* **2000**, *66*, 2263–2266. [CrossRef] [PubMed]
46. Ren, X.; Liu, L.; Gamallat, Y.; Zhang, B.; Xin, Y. *Enteromorpha* and polysaccharides from enteromorpha ameliorate loperamide-induced constipation in mice. *Biomed. Pharmacother.* **2017**, *96*, 1075–1081. [CrossRef] [PubMed]
47. Cherry, P.; Yadav, S.; Strain, C.R.; Allsopp, P.J.; Mcsorley, E.M.; Ross, R.P.; Stanton, C. Prebiotics from seaweeds: An ocean of opportunity? *Mar. Drugs* **2019**, *17*, 327. [CrossRef] [PubMed]
48. Binn, N. Role of the GI tract microbiota in health and disease. In *Probiotics, Prebiotics and the Gut Microbiota*; Gibson, G.R., Ed.; International Life Science Institute Europe: Brussels, Belgium, 2013; pp. 4–10.
49. Rivière, A.; Selak, M.; Lantin, D.; Leroy, F.; De Vuyst, L. Bifidobacteria and butyrate-producing colon bacteria: Importance and strategies for their stimulation in the human gut. *Front. Microbiol.* **2016**, *7*, 979. [CrossRef]
50. Hurst, N.R.; Kendig, D.M.; Murthy, K.S.; Grider, J.R. The Short chain fatty acids, butyrate and propionate, have differential effects on the motility of the guinea pig colon. *Neurogastroenterol. Motil.* **2014**, *26*, 1586–1596. [CrossRef]
51. Shimotoyodome, A.; Meguro, S.; Hase, T.; Tokimitsu, I.; Sakata, T. Decreased colonic mucus in rats with loperamide-induced constipation. *Comp. Biochem. Physiol. Part A Mol. Integr. Physiol.* **2000**, *126*, 203–212. [CrossRef]
52. Barcelo, A.; Claustre, J.; Moro, F.; Chayvialle, J.A.; Cuber, J.C.; Plaisancié, P. Mucin secretion is modulated by luminal factors in the isolated vascularly perfused rat colon. *Gut* **2000**, *46*, 218–224. [CrossRef] [PubMed]
53. Liu, J.; Kandasamy, S.; Zhang, J.; Kirby, C.W.; Karakach, T.; Hafting, J.; Critchley, A.T.; Evans, F.; Prithiviraj, B. Prebiotic effects of diet supplemented with the cultivated red seaweed *Chondrus crispus* or with fructo-oligo-saccharide on host immunity, colonic microbiota and gut microbial metabolites. *BMC Complement. Altern. Med.* **2015**, *15*, 279. [CrossRef] [PubMed]
54. Jabeen, A.; Baig, M.T.; Shaikh, S.; Sarosh, N.A.; Kashif, S.S.; Shahnaz, S.; Vengus, P.; Soomro, H.; Shahid, U. In vivo study on laxative effect of *Prunus amygdalus* oil. *Int. J. Med. Res. Health Sci.* **2019**, *8*, 121–125.
55. Yu, B.; Jiang, Y.; Jin, L.; Ma, T.; Yang, H. Role of quercetin in modulating chloride transport in the intestine. *Front. Physiol.* **2016**, *7*, 549. [CrossRef]
56. Billet, A.; Hanrahan, J.W. The secret life of CFTR as a calcium-activated chloride channel. *J. Physiol.* **2013**, *591*, 5273–5278. [CrossRef] [PubMed]
57. Ranjani, D.M.; Longanathan, P.; Arputharaj, P.; Kalaiarasi, J. Pharmacognostical and phytochemical analysis of *Sargassum cinereum* (Turner) C. Agardh. *J. Pharmacogn. Phytochem.* **2018**, *7*, 2233–2238.
58. Yue, G.G.L.; Yip, T.W.N.; Huang, Y.; Ko, W.H. Cellular mechanism for potentiation of Ca^{2+}-mediated Cl^- secretion by the flavonoid baicalein in intestinal epithelia. *J. Biol. Chem.* **2004**, *279*, 39310–39316. [CrossRef]
59. Yang, X.; Wen, G.; Tuo, B.; Zhang, F.; Wan, H.; He, J.; Yang, S.; Dong, H. Molecular mechanisms of calcium signaling in the modulation of small intestinal ion transports and bicarbonate secretion. *Oncotarget* **2018**, *9*, 3727–3740. [CrossRef]
60. Alli, A.A.; Bao, H.F.; Liu, B.C.; Yu, L.; Aldrugh, S.; Montgomery, D.S.; Ma, H.P.; Eaton, D.C. Calmodulin and CaMKII modulate ENaC activity by regulating the association of MARCKS and the cytoskeleton with the apical membrane. *Am. J. Physiol.-Ren. Physiol.* **2015**, *309*, 456–463. [CrossRef]

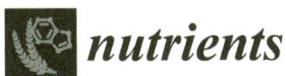

Review

Treatment of Glaucoma with Natural Products and Their Mechanism of Action: An Update

Ru Hui Sim [1], Srinivasa Rao Sirasanagandla [2], Srijit Das [2,*] and Seong Lin Teoh [3,*]

[1] Tanglin Health Clinic, Kuala Lumpur 50480, Malaysia; simruhui@gmail.com
[2] Department of Human & Clinical Anatomy, College of Medicine & Health Sciences, Sultan Qaboos University, Al-Khoud, Muscat 123, Oman; srinivasa@squ.edu.om
[3] Department of Anatomy, Faculty of Medicine, Universiti Kebangsaan Malaysia Medical Centre, Cheras, Kuala Lumpur 56000, Malaysia
* Correspondence: s.das@squ.edu.om (S.D.); teohseonglin@ppukm.ukm.edu.my (S.L.T.)

Abstract: Glaucoma is one of the leading causes of irreversible blindness. It is generally caused by increased intraocular pressure, which results in damage of the optic nerve and retinal ganglion cells, ultimately leading to visual field dysfunction. However, even with the use of intraocular pressure-lowering eye drops, the disease still progresses in some patients. In addition to mechanical and vascular dysfunctions of the eye, oxidative stress, neuroinflammation and excitotoxicity have also been implicated in the pathogenesis of glaucoma. Hence, the use of natural products with antioxidant and anti-inflammatory properties may represent an alternative approach for glaucoma treatment. The present review highlights recent preclinical and clinical studies on various natural products shown to possess neuroprotective properties for retinal ganglion cells, which thereby may be effective in the treatment of glaucoma. Intraocular pressure can be reduced by baicalein, forskolin, marijuana, ginsenoside, resveratrol and hesperidin. Alternatively, *Ginkgo biloba*, *Lycium barbarum*, *Diospyros kaki*, *Tripterygium wilfordii*, saffron, curcumin, caffeine, anthocyanin, coenzyme Q10 and vitamins B3 and D have shown neuroprotective effects on retinal ganglion cells via various mechanisms, especially antioxidant, anti-inflammatory and anti-apoptosis mechanisms. Extensive studies are still required in the future to ensure natural products' efficacy and safety to serve as an alternative therapy for glaucoma.

Keywords: glaucoma; herbs; traditional medicine; retinal ganglion cells; intraocular pressure

1. Introduction

Glaucoma is one of the leading causes of irreversible blindness, causing 6.6% of all blindness in 2010 [1]. According to the World Health Organization's (WHO) World Report on Vision, of the estimated 2.2 billion people having a vision impairment around the world, glaucoma affects an estimated 6.9 million people [2]. It has been further estimated that by 2040, approximately 111.8 million people worldwide aged between 40 and 80 years old will be affected by glaucoma [3]. Glaucoma is generally caused by intraocular pressure (IOP, >21 mmHg) build-up, resulting from blockage of intraocular fluid and aqueous humor drainage [4]. The elevated IOP progressively damages the retinal ganglion cells (RGCs) and optic nerve, causing visual field constriction that affects the peripheral field initially and the central vision field gradually [5]. Glaucoma patients require lifelong treatment and follow-up, and the disease has a significant negative impact on patients' quality of life in terms of anxiety, psychological well-being, daily life, driving and confidence in healthcare [6]. The main risk factors for glaucoma prevalence include age, family history with glaucoma, African American race, thinner central corneal thickness, pseudoexfoliation, pigment dispersion and myopia [7]. Additionally, an association between diabetes, hypertension, triglyceride levels and glaucoma were also identified [7,8]. Furthermore, genetic factors are also known to be risk factors for glaucoma, in which single-nucleotide polymorphisms in numerous genes (e.g., myocilin, apolipoprotein E, X-ray repair cross-complementing group 1, zona pellucida glycoprotein 4) have been shown to be associated with an increased risk of glaucoma [9,10].

Glaucoma can be classified into two major types, i.e., open-angle (OAG) and angle-closure glaucoma (ACG), according to the physical obstruction of the aqueous humor drainage system, and the appearance of the iridocorneal angle and trabecular meshwork (TM) [11]. Alternatively, it can also be categorized as primary (idiopathic, not associated with other diseases or conditions) or secondary (attributed to underlying diseases or conditions, such as trauma, long-term medication, ophthalmic surgery, uveitis, necrotic tumors, diabetes or syndromic conditions) [11,12].

In primary OAG (POAG), aqueous humor drainage is obstructed or inadequate as there is an internal blockage within the TM [13]. In contrast, primary ACG (PACG) is characterized by the presence of a physical obstacle to the aqueous drainage as the iris is adhered to the cornea, obstructing the flow of aqueous humor to the TM and the uveoscleral drainage [12,14]. Symptoms appear more drastically in PACG, which results in a rapid reduction in the vision field, leading to total blindness. Other symptoms include ocular pain, headache, nausea, vomiting, multicolored halos and blurred vision [12]. Additionally, PACG is an ophthalmic emergency that requires immediate treatment to prevent the progression of irreversible ocular damage [12].

2. Pathogenesis of Glaucoma

The exact pathogenesis of glaucoma is complex and has not yet been fully elucidated. The potential mechanism involved in the neurodegeneration of glaucoma has been postulated to involve an amalgamation of mechanical, vascular, genetic and immunological factors.

2.1. Mechanical Hypothesis

The mechanical hypothesis explains the relationship between the IOP and RGC pathophysiology. The perforated lamina cribrosa (LC) is the weakest part of the sclera, and it is where the RGC axons pierce through the minute perforations to form the optic nerve, while the central retinal artery and vein pass through the LC via a larger central aperture [15]. Elevated IOP resulted from the imbalance between the production and drainage of aqueous humor, which led to the irreversible backwards bowing of the LC, in the process known as 'cupping' [16]. Optic nerve cupping is characterized by the remodeling of the extracellular matrix (ECM) and fibrosis in the LC [17]. Glaucomatous LC cells showed increased ECM gene expression and elevated intracellular calcium, which is known to promote proliferation, activation and contractility in fibroblasts via the nuclear factor of activated T cells/calcium signaling pathway [17]. This deformation damages the optic nerve and capillaries passing through the LC, disturbing the anterograde axonal transportation of RGCs, which then ultimately triggers visual field defects in glaucoma [16]. Furthermore, elevated IOP also resulted in activated pro-fibrotic pathway-induced ECM accumulation in the TM, leading to less efficient aqueous humor outflow, thereby causing further damage to the LC [18].

Ivers et al. [19] demonstrated that in experimental glaucoma monkeys, the first structural abnormality induced by elevated IOP was an increased anterior LC surface depth, followed by a decreased minimum rim width, and, lastly, a reduced retinal nerve fiber layer (RNFL) thickness. Different levels of increased IOP showed a remarkable effect on the visual field, best-corrected visual acuity and LC parameters (cup depth, LC depth, LC curvature index and prelaminar tissue thickness) [20]. Additionally, greater posterior displacement of the LC was significantly associated with a faster rate of loss of the RNFL [21]. RGC axonal degeneration and anterograde axonal transport deficits at the optic nerve head (ONH, the location where RGC axons converge to form the optic nerve and traverse the LC) precede the structural and functional loss of RGCs [22]. Disturbance of the RGC anterograde axonal transport leads to the accumulation of metabolic waste in the cells and deprives the metabolic needs of the RGCs, subsequently causing their apoptosis [23].

In normal-tension glaucoma (NTG), patients also present with glaucomatous optic disc excavation, despite a normal IOP [24]. This suggests other risk factors are involved in the optic neurodegeneration of glaucoma. The LC serves as a barrier between the IOP within the eye, and the intracranial pressure within the cerebrospinal fluid-filled subarachnoid space surrounding the optic nerve; the pressure gradient between the LC is known as the translaminar pressure gradient (TLPG) [25,26]. The TLPG is higher in glaucoma patients, including NTG patients, and is associated with mechanical damage to the optic nerve fibers, anterograde axonal transportation disruption and altered blood flow, leading to glaucomatous damage [26–28].

2.2. Vascular Hypothesis

The blood flow of the ONH was significantly reduced in the eyes of pre-perimetric glaucoma patients, where there are characteristic glaucomatous changes in the optic disc, but without the presence of visual field defects [29,30]. POAG and PACG patients possess a lower capillary density, but with greater tortuosity and more dilated capillaries, compared to healthy individuals [31]. Similarly, both NTG and POAG patients showed lower retrobulbar velocities, and higher retinal venous saturation and choroidal thickness asymmetries, when compared to control subjects [32]. Decreased ocular blood flow was also shown to be correlated with structural glaucomatous progression, as indicated by retinal and optic nerve changes [33]. A recent retrospective longitudinal study revealed that reduced blood flow in the ONH precedes glaucomatous neurodegeneration in POAG patients [34]. The vascular hypothesis is thus based on the reduced perfusion pressure, faulty vascular autoregulation or loss of neurovascular coupling, which leads to optic nerve degeneration in glaucoma [35]. Due to the reduced ocular blood flow, this hypothesis proposes that the RGC axons suffer from oxygen and nutrient insufficiency, ultimately causing their degeneration. In a glaucoma rat model, ocular hypertension (OHT) led to selective hypoxia in the LC, which was associated with injured RGC axons, and axonal transport disruption [36]. This study also demonstrated upregulation of hypoxia-inducible enzyme heme oxygenase-1 (HO-1) and the anaerobic glycolytic enzyme lactate dehydrogenase, and increased generation of superoxide radicals in the retina and ONH, as well as the active subunit of the superoxide-generating enzyme NADPH oxidase, suggesting the involvement of oxidative stress [36]. Similarly, hypoxic RGCs were observed in young and aged glaucoma model DBA/2J (D2) mouse retinas, with a significant increase in the hypoxia-inducible factor-1α (HIF-1α) protein and reactive oxygen species (ROS), followed by a significant decrease in the antioxidant capacity and mitochondrial mass in the aged retinas [37].

2.3. Oxidative Stress and Neuroinflammation in Glaucoma

In accordance with animal studies, numerous studies have provided evidence of increased oxidative stress in glaucoma patients. In addition, blood and aqueous humor levels of oxidative stress-related molecular biomarkers, i.e., protein carbonyls and advanced glycation end products, significantly increased in glaucomatous samples compared with healthy controls [38]. Similarly, PACG patients presented with decreased serum levels of total antioxidant status (TAS) and superoxide dismutase (SOD), as well as increased levels of malondialdehyde (MDA), compared to healthy controls [39]. A meta-analysis further indicated that POAG patients had lower TAS in the blood and higher levels of SOD, glutathione peroxidase (GPX) and catalase (CAT) in the aqueous humor [40]. Oxidative stress is known to induce or dysregulate inflammation in the event of optic neurodegeneration from glaucoma.

Studies have shown that inflammation contributes to the disease progression of glaucoma. In glaucomatous human optic nerves, the number of CD163+ cells (a commonly used marker for anti-inflammatory macrophages involved in tissue repair and remodeling) was significantly increased [41]. Systemic inflammatory status markers, i.e., the neutrophil-to-lymphocyte ratio, platelet-to-lymphocyte ratio and systemic immune inflammation index, were significantly increased in POAG patients compared with the control group [42]. POAG patients exhibited a significant increase in various cytokines, i.e., serum interleukin (IL)-4, -6 and -12p70 and tumor necrosis factor-alpha (TNF-α), compared with the controls [43]. Similarly, elevated plasma TNF-α levels in patients with POAG and pseudoexfoliation glaucoma were detected [44,45]. Additionally, aqueous humor samples collected from chronic PACG patients showed significantly increased levels of eotaxin, macrophage inflammatory protein-1-alpha and interferon gamma (IFN-γ)-induced protein-10, and lower levels of TNF-α, IL-5, -9 and -17 and granulocyte-macrophage colony-stimulating factor, compared to the control group [46].

Glial cells in the retina, i.e., astrocytes, Müller cells and microglial cells having an important role in mediating inflammatory responses, have been shown to become reactive, leading to the production of inflammatory cytokines, causing further neuronal damage in glaucoma patients and experimental glaucoma models [47,48]. In general, cytokine signaling is linked to the inflammatory transducer nuclear factor-kappa B (NF-κB). In D2 mice, low energy-induced 5′ adenosine monophosphate-activated protein kinase (AMPK) phosphorylation in the retina and optic nerve triggered NF-κB p65 signaling, leading to increased pro-inflammatory TNF-α, IL-6 and nitric oxide synthase (NOS)-2 expression [49]. Injection administration of TGF-β2 increased IOP and ECM deposition in the TM of wild-type mice. In contrast, mice harboring a mutation in NF-κB blocked the effect, suggesting NF-κB is necessary for TGF-β2-induced ECM production and OHT [50]. Additionally, transgenic inhibition of astroglial NF-κB restrained the neuroinflammatory (reduced pro-inflammatory cytokine expressions, i.e., IL-1A, -1B, -2, -6, -10, -12 and -13, TNF-α and IFN-γ) and neurodegenerative outcomes (attenuated loss of RGCs and axons) of the eyes of an experimental OHT mouse model [51].

The current evidence indeed supports the contribution of neuroinflammation in the pathogenesis of glaucoma, but it is still not clear as to when neuroinflammation takes part in the sequence of pathological events in glaucoma. Neuroinflammation has been suggested to be secondary to the initial pathology (i.e., optic nerve crush injury) [52]. Optic nerve crush injury induced glial activation in the retina, which was significantly muted if RGC death was blocked by deletion of the Bax gene [52]. On the other hand, the inhibition of monocyte infiltration and microglial activation by X-ray treatment prevented neuronal damage and dysfunction in the ONH [53]. Nevertheless, immunomodulation has been shown to be beneficial in the progression of glaucomatous changes.

2.4. Excitotoxicity of Glutamate

In addition to the inflammatory response, glial cells in the retina also play a vital role in the function of the retina by providing homeostatic and metabolic support to the photoreceptors and retinal neurons [54]. Müller cells and astrocytes possess uptake and exchange systems for various neurotransmitters, including glutamate, via the glutamate/aspartate transporter (GLAST) in rodents, also known as the Na^+-dependent high-affinity glutamate transporter-1 (EAAT-1) in humans [54,55]. Glaucomatous eyes have been shown to have decreased levels of EAAT-1, and the glutamate receptor subunit *N*-methyl-d-aspartate (NMDA)-R1 [56]. Furthermore, mice deficient in GLAST demonstrate spontaneous RGC loss and optic nerve degeneration without elevated IOP, suggesting the decrease in GLAST expression leads to glutamate excitotoxicity in the retina, as a possible pathogenesis of glaucoma [57].

As reviewed by others, perhaps the most accepted hypothesis involved in glaucoma pathogenesis currently may include the mechanical damage to the ONH induced by increased IOP, followed by vascular dysregulation (reduced ocular blood flow) and neuroinflammation (glial activation), which then disrupt axonal transport due to axonal mitochondrial function loss in the RGCs, ultimately leading to RGC axonal degeneration and

RGC cell death (Figure 1) [58–60]. However, the combination of mechanisms described earlier may vary greatly among different glaucoma patients [60].

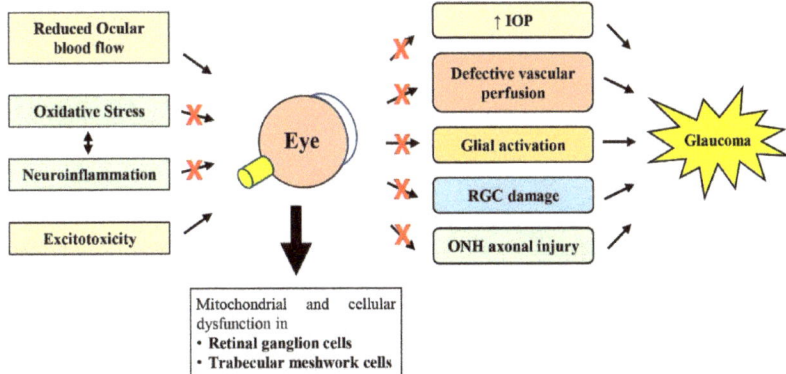

Figure 1. Schematic diagram showing how oxidative stress, neuroinflammation, reduced ocular blood flow and excitotoxicity lead to subsequent pathological changes observed in glaucoma. The therapeutic potential of natural products against glaucomatous changes at various steps is shown with the symbol ×. RGC, retinal ganglion cell; IOP, intraocular pressure; ONH, optic nerve head.

3. Glaucoma Research Models

Numerous research models have been used to gain a considerable understanding of the pathogenesis of glaucoma, and to assess therapeutic approaches for glaucoma treatments [61–64]. In this section, we provide a brief overview of some of these models used by the studies presented in this review (summarized in Table 1); this helps to provide a better understanding of the discussions in the following sections.

There are several genetic glaucomatous animal models that present with an elevated or normal IOP. For instance, the D2 mouse presents a late-onset, chronic pigmentary glaucoma due to the high IOP that progresses with age, resulting from tyrosinase-related protein 1 (*Tyrp1*) mutation and a premature stop codon in glycoprotein non-metastatic melanoma protein B (*Gpnmb*), which collectively lead to anterior segment anomalies, iris atrophy, peripheral anterior synechiae and pigment dispersion [64,65]. In contrast, D2-*Gpnmb*⁺ mice are the wild types for the *Gpnmb* mutation that do not develop increased IOP and glaucoma [66]. Alternatively, the *Vav2/Vav3*-deficient and connective tissue growth factor (βB1-CTGF) mouse models are other murine models of spontaneous glaucoma that present with elevated IOP, which leads to subsequent RGC loss [67,68]. Transgenic mice with a low overexpression of E50K mutant optineurin (E50K-OPTN) have been reported to present with enhanced axonal degeneration and decreased RGC survival, under normal IOP [69].

Glaucoma can also be induced in wild-type animal models by elevating the IOP experimentally. A high IOP can be achieved by blocking aqueous humor drainage with the injection of various substances (e.g., microbeads, hydroxypropyl methylcellulose and hyaluronic acid) into the anterior chamber [70–72]. Alternatively, injection of hypertonic saline into the episcleral vein [73], and cauterization [74] or laser photocoagulation [75–77] of the episcleral or limbal veins lead to TM scarring, which increases the resistance to aqueous humor drainage, resulting in an elevation in IOP. The elevated IOP in these models leads to varying degrees of RGC loss, glial activation and visual defects [75–78].

To investigate the role of excitotoxicity in glaucoma, RGC loss can be induced with the injection of NMDA intravitreally [79]. The optic nerve crush (performed by applying a crush injury to the optic nerve with a pair of cross-action forceps) or the complete optic nerve transection model causes all RGC axons to be damaged simultaneously, which results in the gradual loss of RGCs [80,81]. This non-IOP-related axonal degeneration research model is commonly used to assess the RGC neuroprotection properties of various substances [82]. The partial optic nerve transection model causes damage to only a portion of the RGC axons; thus, this model can study both primary (the death of RGCs whose axons have been cut off) and delayed secondary neurodegeneration (the death of RGCs whose axons are intact) [83]. Retinal ischemia/reperfusion (I/R) injury is known to be associated with glaucoma, and other eye diseases, and has been widely used as an animal model for OAG. I/R injury reduces retinal blood flow, which creates a state of retinal hypersensitivity to oxygen and other nutrients, precipitating severe oxidative and inflammatory damage when the circulation is subsequently reinstated (reperfusion) [84,85].

Table 1. Overview of glaucoma research models.

Research Models			Genes Involved	Mechanisms	References
Genetic in vivo model	D2 mice		Tyrosinase-related protein 1 (*Tyrp1*) Glycoprotein non-metastatic melanoma protein B (*Gpnmb*)	Blockage of aqueous humor drainage, leading to progressive elevated IOP	[65]
	Methods		Surgery involved	Mechanisms	References
Experimental in vivo model	Injection		Injection of microbeads into the anterior chamber	Blockage of aqueous humor drainage, leading to elevated IOP	[70]
			Injection of hydroxypropyl methylcellulose into the anterior chamber	Blockage of aqueous humor drainage, leading to elevated IOP	[71]
			Injection of hyaluronic acid into the anterior chamber	Blockage of aqueous humor drainage, leading to elevated IOP	[72]
			Injection of hypertonic saline into the episcleral vein	Produced scarring in the TM, increasing resistance to aqueous humor drainage, leading to elevated IOP	[73]
			Intravitreal injection of NMDA	NMDA induced excitotoxicity, leading to RGC death	[79]
	Cauterization/laser photocoagulation		Episcleral vein cauterization	Produced scarring in the TM, increasing resistance to aqueous humor drainage, leading to elevated IOP	[74]
			Argon laser photocoagulation of the episcleral/limbal vein	Produced scarring in the TM, increasing resistance to aqueous humor drainage, leading to elevated IOP	
	Nerve injury		Optic nerve crush	Optic nerve injury leading to axonal degeneration and gradual RGC loss	[80]
			Complete optic nerve transection	Optic nerve injury leading to axonal degeneration and gradual RGC loss	[81]
			Partial optic nerve transection	Optic nerve injury leading to axonal degeneration and gradual RGC loss	[83]
	Retinal I/R injury		Reduced retinal blood flow by induction of elevated IOP (ischemia), followed by reinstation of blood flow (reperfusion)	Extreme acute OHT-induced ischemic injury to RGC, followed by severe oxidative and inflammatory damage to RGCs after reperfusion	[84,85]

D2, DBA/2J; I/R, ischemia/reperfusion; IOP, intraocular pressure; NMDA, *N*-methyl-d-aspartate; RGC, retinal ganglion cell.

Numerous in vitro studies have utilized the RGC-5 cell line in glaucoma research to evaluate the neuroprotective properties of various supplements, including the studies reviewed here. However, it has now become clear that RGC-5 cells that were originally identified as immortalized rat RGCs were contaminated early in their development by the immortalized photoreceptor 661W cell line (RGC precursor-like cells) in the laboratory they originated from [86,87]. Therefore, the RGC-5 cells used by many of the studies described in the following section may not reflect the true phenotype of a mature RGC. Perhaps the use of primary RGCs from animal models would be better to investigate glaucomatous RGC responses to therapies in vitro [88].

In general, the various research models described represent only some aspects of glaucoma, thus each having different advantages over other models. It is important to use a suitable model based on the objective of the study.

4. Natural Products Used for Glaucoma Treatment and Their Mechanism of Action

In view of the role played by oxidative stress and neuroinflammation in glaucoma, the use of antioxidants may represent an alternative approach for glaucoma treatment. Currently, the mainstay of glaucoma treatment is the reduction in IOP, using IOP-lowering eye drops [89]. Other glaucoma treatments include laser trabeculoplasty and cyclodestruction, or surgical trabeculectomy, trabeculotomy, deep sclerectomy and viscocanalostomy, based on the European Glaucoma Society guidelines [90]. However, even when the IOP normalizes, the disease still progresses and affects visual function in some patients.

There has been significant research interest in complementary and alternative medicine (CAM), and it has been widely used in the treatment of glaucoma. In a survey involving a total of 1516 glaucoma patients in Canada, 10% of patients used CAM therapy specifically for glaucoma, and half of them believed that the treatments were beneficial [91]. Other recent surveys reported the prevalence of CAM usage to be 22% in Saudi Arabia and 67% in Palestine among eye patients [92,93]. The present review highlights recent studies on various CAMs used for the treatment of glaucoma.

4.1. Gingko biloba L.

Ginkgo biloba L. (GB) belongs to the Ginkgoceae family, and its leaves and seeds have been used for medicinal purposes for centuries [94]. With more than 70 different flavonoids having been identified in GB, it has been suggested to have broad-spectrum free radical scavenging activities [95]. Indeed, treatment with GB extract was able to increase the survival of a rat RGC line, following exposure to oxidative stress induced by hydrogen peroxide (H_2O_2) [96]. Furthermore, POAG patients treated with 120 mg of GB extract daily for at least 6 months demonstrated a lower rate of single-stranded DNA breaks in circulating leukocytes, indicating reduced oxidative stress [97].

Numerous clinical trials have also demonstrated that GB extract supplementation slows the progression of visual field damage and improves visual function in NTG patients [98,99]. However, Shim et al. [99] demonstrated that supplementation with 40 mg of GB extract, three times per day, showed no effect on the mean defect or contrast sensitivity in NTG patients, compared to those receiving placebo. Based on the vascular hypothesis of glaucoma pathogenesis, NTG patients receiving 80 mg GB extract tablets, twice a day for four weeks, showed a significant increase in ocular blood flow, volume and velocity, in comparison to the placebo group [100]. Furthermore, GB supplementation increased the radial peripapillary capillary vascular density in healthy subjects who received a 120 mg GB extract capsule daily for 4 weeks [101]. Table 2 summarizes clinical trials of natural products used for glaucoma treatment.

In animal studies, intraperitoneal injections of GB extract administered after optic nerve injury in rats were associated with a higher survival rate of RGCs [96,102]. This could be due to the anti-apoptosis property of GB, as demonstrated by the inhibition of apoptosis of RGCs via the modulation of mitogen-activated protein kinase (MAPK) signaling pathways, in the adult rat optic nerve injury model, following the retrobulbar injection of diterpene ginkgolides meglumine injection (DGMI, made from GB extracts, including ginkgolides A, B and K) [103]. Mechanistically, DGMI could inhibit cell apoptosis by inhibiting p38, JNK and Erk1/2 activation [103]. Additionally, GB extract-derived procyanidin B2 and rutin were shown to be able to protect human retinal pigment epithelial cells subjected to tert-butyl hydroperoxide-induced oxidative stress by modulating nuclear factor erythroid 2-related factor (Nrf)-2 and Erk1/2 signaling [104]. Another study proposed that P53, Bax, Bcl-2 and caspase-3/-9 could be considered as the core targets for GB extract against apoptosis in H$_2$O$_2$-treated RGCs [105]. A summary of preclinical studies of natural products used for glaucoma treatment is provided in Table 3.

4.2. Scutellaria baicalensis Georgi—Baicalin, Baicalein and Wogonin

Scutellaria baicalensis Georgi, commonly known as Baikal skullcap or Chinese skullcap, is a widely used Chinese medicinal herb [106]. *S. baicalensis* extract and its three major active flavonoids, namely, baicalin, baicalein and wogonin showed low cytotoxicity and possessed neuroprotective, antioxidant, anti-inflammatory and anti-cancer properties [106–108].

Intragastric administration of 200 mg/kg of baicalein for 28 days significantly reduced IOP in a rat model of chronic OHT [109]. The decreased thickness of the RGC complex and the reduced nucleus of the RGC layer mediated by OHT were significantly ameliorated by baicalein treatment and associated with reduced apoptosis of RGCs by upregulating the expression of the anti-apoptotic protein Bcl-2 [109]. Additionally, baicalein protects RGCs against retinal ischemia via the downregulation of HIF-1α, matrix metalloproteinase (MMP)-9 and vascular endothelial growth factor (VEGF), and upregulation of HO-1 [110].

The intraperitoneal administration of wogonin, 10 min after the establishment of the optic nerve crush rat model, reduced the loss of RGCs and inhibited RGC apoptosis [111]. The study also demonstrated the anti-inflammatory property of wogonin in preventing TLR4-NF-κB-mediated neuroinflammation, as indicated by the reduced gliosis response, microglial activation and pro-inflammatory cytokine (TNF-α, monocyte chemoattractant protein-1 (MCP-1), iNOS, IL-6 and -1β and cyclooxygenase (COX-2)) expressions in the retina following optic nerve crush [111].

Intraperitoneal administration of baicalin increased the number of RGCs and attenuated pathological changes (indistinct layer of retinas, decrease in the thickness of the RGC layer (GCL, a retinal layer where RGCs and displaced amacrine cells reside) and RGC density) in a model of episcleral venous occlusion with cauterization to establish a mouse model of glaucoma with chronic elevated IOP [112]. Baicalin treatment also inhibited autophagy and activated PI3K/AKT signaling in glaucoma mice, as PI3K/AKT signaling was shown to restrain the apoptosis and inflammatory response of RGCs in glaucoma development [112]. Additionally, treatment with baicalin significantly increased cell survival, reduced ROS production and inhibited pro-inflammatory factor IL-1α and endothelial leucocyte adhesion molecule-1 (ELAM-1) production in cultured human TM cells exposed to H$_2$O$_2$ [113].

4.3. Coleus forskohlii (willd.) Briq.—Forskolin

Coleus forskohlii (willd.) Briq. is a medicinal plant indigenous to India and Southeast Asia [114]. The leaves, roots and tubers of *C. forskohlii* are a rich source of a diterpenoid called forskolin, which acts as a second messenger cyclic adenosine 3′,5′-monophosphate (cAMP) booster, via the direct stimulation of adenylate cyclase [114]. Studies have revealed that cAMP is important in regulating aqueous humor dynamics in the ciliary body and TM [115]. Indeed, a previous study has shown that forskolin perfused arterially at 30, 100 and 1000 nM caused a significant reduction in the rate of aqueous humor formation in an isolated bovine eye preparation [116]. This may explain the hypotensive effect of forskolin administration, as shown in a double-blind, randomized controlled trial where POAG patients treated with forskolin 1% w/v aqueous solution eye drops, at two drops thrice a day, for 4 weeks, showed a significant decrease in IOP [117,118].

In animal studies, a dietary combination of forskolin, homotaurine, spearmint and vitamins B1, B6 and B12 was able to protect against RGC loss in a rodent model of optic nerve injury [119] and hypertensive glaucoma [120]. Both studies demonstrated that the forskolin supplement mixture may counteract the inflammatory processes via the reduction in cytokine (iNOS, IL-6 and TNF-α) secretion, thereby leading to decreased apoptotic markers (Bax/Bcl-2 ratio and active caspase-3), finally sparing RGC death and the preservation of visual function [119,120]. However, in contrast to the clinical studies, the forskolin supplement mixture did not affect IOP elevation in glaucomatous rodents [120].

4.4. Erigeron breviscapus (vant.) Hand. Mazz.—Scutellarin

Erigeron breviscapus (vant.) Hand. Mazz. (DengZhanHua in Chinese) is a dicotyledonous plant in the Compositae chrysanthemum family found primarily in southwest China, especially in Yunnan [121]. It has been used in traditional Chinese medicine, for the prevention and treatment of cardiovascular diseases [121]. *E. breviscapus* supplements administered for 6 months showed no obvious adverse effects, with a significant decrease in the mean defect and an increase in the mean sensitivity, in POAG patients with a controlled IOP, demonstrating its partial protective effect on the visual field in glaucoma [122]. In chronic elevated IOP animal models, *E. breviscapus* oral supplements were shown to reduce IOP, improve impaired visual function, increase the RGC density and reduce RGC axonal degeneration caused by elevated IOP [123,124]. In RGCs, *E. breviscapus* extract was shown to suppress the outward potassium channel currents, which was suggested to be one of the key mechanisms behind *E. breviscapus*'s beneficial effects against glaucoma-induced RGC damage and visual impairment [125].

The flavonoid scutellarin is one of the major constituents of *E. breviscapus*. A 3-week oral scutellarin treatment ameliorated retinal thinning and visual deficits in an induced chronic OHT glaucoma model [126]. Scutellarin protected RGCs and reduced impaired retinal microglial cells by inhibiting NLRP3 inflammasome-mediated inflammatory reactions, which was associated with a reduced upregulation of apoptosis-associated speck-like protein (a caspase recruitment domain), cleaved caspase-1 and IL-18 and -1β following acute OHT [127].

4.5. Lycium barbarum L.

Lycium barbarum L., commonly known as goji berry or wolfberry, has been widely used in China to treat various diseases, i.e., blurry vision, abdominal pain, infertility, dry cough, fatigue, dizziness and headaches, and has been used as a potent anti-aging agent [128]. The most abundant component in goji berries is represented by carbohydrates, and isolated *L. barbarum* polysaccharides (LBPs) have been found to exert various pharmacological properties, i.e., neuroprotective, hypoglycemic, anti-cancer, immunomodulatory and antioxidant properties [129,130]. LBP supplementation has been shown to protect RGC survival and preserve retinal function in various glaucoma models, i.e., acute OHT [131,132], chronic OHT [133,134] and partial optic nerve transection [135]. In the partial optic nerve transection model, LBP pre-treatment for 7 days prior to the injury was shown to delay secondary degeneration of RGCs [136]. The study also reported LBP exerting its neuroprotective effects by inhibiting oxidative stress and the JNK/c-jun pathway, and by transiently increasing the expression of insulin-like growth factor-1, which is a known neurotrophic factor determining the survival of RGCs during the early stages of optic nerve injury [136].

LBP has been shown to protect RGCs against oxidative stress injury by inhibiting the generation of ROS and reducing the mitochondrial membrane potential following cobalt chloride ($CoCl_2$)-induced hypoxia [137]. Additionally, LBP significantly promoted cell viability, reduced apoptosis and decreased cleaved caspase-3/-9 and ROS levels in human TM cells after H_2O_2 administration [138]. Alternatively, LBP treatment has been shown to promote M2 polarization of microglia and downregulate autophagy after partial optic nerve resection, which contributes to the delayed secondary degeneration of RGCs [139]. Other studies have also suggested that LBP provides neuroprotection to the RGCs and retina by inhibiting vascular damage, probably via the regulation of endothelin-1 (ET-1)-mediated biological effects [131,133]. In a recent study, LBP treatment also promoted blood–retinal barrier maintenance and survival of RGCs in acute OHT mice, which were mediated through the regulation of amyloid-β production and advanced glycosylation end product receptor expression [140]. Furthermore, *L. barbarum* ethanolic extracts reduced angiopoietin-like 7 protein (ANGPTL7) expression while increasing that of caveolin-1 in PC12 neuronal cells exposed to hydrostatic pressures, which was associated with decreased gene expressions of ECM proteins, i.e., MMP-2, MMP-9, collagen I and TGF-β [141]. Previous studies have indeed indicated that ANGPTL7 modulates the TM's ECM [142] and

MMP-mediated ECM turnover in the TM, which leads to a reduction in outflow resistance in the conventional outflow pathway, and to maintenance of IOP homeostasis [143].

LBP treatment significantly reduced neuronal death and glial activation in the retina following I/R injury [144,145]. Furthermore, LBP treatment was able to alleviate ischemia-induced retinal dysfunction (exhibiting greater b-wave and oscillatory potential responses) [144,146]. The antioxidant levels (glutathione, SOD and CAT) in the retina were significantly higher, while the MDA level was lower, in the submicron and blended *L. barbarum* extract-treated groups, compared to the control [146]. Further studies demonstrated that LBP exerted its neuroprotective effects via the activation of Nrf2 and an increase in HO-1 protein expression in the retina after I/R injury [145].

4.6. Diospyros kaki L.

Persimmon (*Diospyros kaki* L.), belonging to the family Ebenaceae, is a well-known fruit rich in carbohydrates, dietary fibers, vitamins, minerals, carotenoids, phenolic compounds and other bioactive phytochemicals [147]. In addition to its fruit, persimmon's leaves are also rich in flavonoids that exhibit antioxidant properties [148]. Pre-treatment of RGCs exposed to excessive oxidative stress and excitotoxicity with an ethanolic extract of persimmon leaves (EEDK) increased cell viability in a concentration-dependent manner [149]. Further studies revealed that the neuroprotective effect of EEDK was associated with decreased levels of apoptotic markers, i.e., poly (ADP-ribose) polymerase, p53 and cleaved caspase-3, and increased expression levels of antioxidant enzymes, i.e., SOD, GPX and glutathione S-transferase [149]. The same study demonstrated that EEDK treatment protects the retina and RGCs in a partial optic nerve crush mouse model [149]. Additionally, EEDK was also shown to reduce elevated IOP in a glaucoma mouse model, by regulating the soluble guanylate cyclase α-1 (sGCα-1, a primary regulator of vascular hypertension) signal [150].

4.7. Tripterygium wilfordii Hook F.—Triptolide and Celastrol

Tripterygium wilfordii Hook F., commonly known as thunder god vine, is a traditional Chinese medicine widely used to treat autoimmune and inflammatory diseases including rheumatoid arthritis, systemic lupus erythematosus and dermatomyositis [151]. Triptolide and celastrol are the predominant active phytochemicals isolated from this plant, which exhibit similar pharmacological activities, i.e., anti-cancer, anti-inflammatory, immunosuppressive, anti-obesity and anti-diabetic activities [152]. Triptolide treatment improved RGC survival via the inhibition of microglial activation in glaucoma models [153–155]. Additionally, triptolide treatment inhibited the expression of TNF-α and the nuclear translocation of NF-κB in an optic nerve crush model, suggesting that the neuroprotective effect of triptolide was attributed, partly, to its anti-inflammatory property [155]. Similarly, celastrol treatment also improved RGC survival in glaucoma models [156,157].

4.8. Crocus sativus L.—Crocetin and Crocin

Saffron (the dried stigma of *Crocus sativus* L.) is a spice that is widely used in food preparation, as a flavoring and coloring agent [158]. Referred to as the 'golden spice', saffron is the highest-priced aromatic medicinal plant in the world, with numerous pharmacological properties such as anti-cancer, anti-diabetic, anti-inflammatory, antioxidant, immunomodulatory, antifungal and antimicrobial properties [158]. Oral administration of saffron extract was shown to decrease microglial numbers and their activation following increased IOP, and this led to the prevention of RGC death [159]. A randomized interventional pilot study revealed that 30 mg/day saffron supplementation significantly reduced IOP in POAG patients, after 3 weeks of treatment [160].

More than 150 chemical compounds have been extracted from saffron, with crocin and crocetin being the two major active ingredients [161]. Intraperitoneal treatment with crocin can inhibit I/R-induced RGC death, and the effect of crocin may be mediated, partly, by its antioxidant action through the ERK pathway [162], or activation of the PI3K/AKT signaling pathway [163]. Additionally, crocin protects RGCs against H_2O_2-induced damage by reducing ROS production and activating NF-κB [164]. Similarly, crocetin, an aglycone of crocin, prevented cell loss and apoptosis in the GCL in mice following NMDA- [165] and I/R-induced retinal damage [166].

4.9. Curcuma longa L.—Curcumin

Curcumin is a yellow pigment and an active component of the rhizome of *Curcuma longa* L., or turmeric [167]. It is known to possess antioxidant, anti-inflammatory, anti-cancer, anti-arthritis, anti-asthmatic, antimicrobial, antiviral and antifungal properties [167,168]. Considering that curcumin is a powerful antioxidant natural compound, it may represent another potential treatment to alleviate oxidative stress in glaucoma. Using an elevated IOP rodent model, curcumin treatment decreased the intracellular level of ROS and alleviated RGC apoptosis induced by oxidative stress [169]. In the same study, it was also observed that curcumin inhibited pro-apoptotic factors, such as caspase-3 and Bax, and upregulated the anti-apoptotic factor Bcl-2 [169]. In an ex vivo optic nerve injury model, thinning of retinal layers, especially the GCL, and strong RGC apoptosis were observed after 24 h post-injury, which correlated with a time-dependent increase in caspase-3 and -9 and pro-apoptotic marker levels, and a powerful activation of the JNK, c-Jun and ERK signaling (MAPK) pathways [170]. Curcumin prevented alterations in the apoptotic cascade and MAPK pathways, preserving RGC survival and retinal thickness [170]. In another experimental study in a rat retinal I/R injury model, curcumin supplementation in the diet for 2 days before I/R was able to protect the retina from ischemic injury [171]. Additionally, curcumin pre-treatment inhibited I/R-induced degeneration of retinal capillaries, which may occur through its inhibitory effects on injury-induced activation of NF-κB and signal transducer and activator of transcription 3 (STAT3), and on overexpression of MCP-1, a chemokine involved in the inflammatory response via recruitment of monocytes to injury sites [172].

Studies using TM cells exposed to H_2O_2-induced oxidative stress as an in vitro model observed that pre-treatment with curcumin reduced the production of intracellular ROS in a dose-dependent manner [173,174]. Curcumin alleviated oxidative stress-induced pro-inflammatory factors such as IL-1a, -6 and -8 and ELAM-1 and inhibited the apoptosis of TM cells [173]. Curcumin has also been shown to protect TM cells against oxidative stress and apoptosis via the Nrf2-keap1 pathway [174].

4.10. Camellia sinensis (L.) Kuntze—Epigallocatechin-3-Gallate

Camellia sinensis (L.) Kuntze, commonly known as green tea, is consumed as a beverage and is popular in China and Japan [175]. Green tea extract treatment administered orally to retinal I/R injury rats showed a higher number of surviving RGCs, and less apoptotic RGCs were observed [176]. Green tea extract treatment also reduced the increased protein expression (i.e., of apoptotic markers (activated caspase-3 and -8) and inflammation-related proteins (Toll-like receptor 4 (TLR4), IL-1β and TNF-α)) and p38 phosphorylation caused by the ischemic injury [176]. Additionally, green tea extract treatment led to suppression of activated microglia, astrocytes and Müller cells following lipopolysaccharide (LPS)-induced retinal inflammation in rats [177]. The green tea anti-inflammatory effects were associated with a reduction in the phosphorylation of STAT3 and NF-κB in the retina [177].

The major polyphenolic compounds contained in green tea are catechins, which include epigallocatechin-3-gallate (EGCG), which is also a powerful antioxidant, anti-angiogenic and anticarcinogenic agent [175,178]. EGCG treatment was shown to preserve the RGC density in acute [179] and chronic elevated IOP rats [180], an optic nerve crush rat model [181], a retinal I/R injury rabbit model [182] and NMDA-induced excitotoxicity in rats [183]. Zhang et al. [179] reported that EGCG treatment significantly decreased inflammation-associated cytokine levels (IL-4, -6, -1β and -13, TNF-α and IFN-γ), and the proliferation rate of T lymphocytes. Furthermore, EGCG treatment inhibited the increase in the phosphorylation of nuclear factor of kappa light polypeptide gene enhancer in B cells inhibitor, alpha (IκBα) and p65, leading to the suppression of NF-κB signaling pathway activation [179].

4.11. Panax ginseng—Ginsenoside

Panax ginseng, in the family Araliaceae, is considered as one of the most frequently employed medicinal herbs and functional foods [184,185]. In a randomized, placebo-controlled, crossover study, daily consumption of 3 g of Korean red ginseng (KRG) for 4 weeks was shown to improve daytime contrast sensitivity and ocular pain in glaucoma patients [186]. Following 8 weeks of KRG supplementation, glaucoma patients showed significant improvement in their tear film stability and total Ocular Surface Disease Index score, suggesting KRG improved dry eye syndrome in glaucoma patients [187]. Additionally, OAG patients receiving 1.5 g of KRG, orally 3 times daily for 12 weeks, showed significant improvement in the retinal peripapillary blood flow in the temporal peripapillary region [188].

Ginseng contains numerous phytochemicals such as ginsenoside (triterpenoid saponin), phenols and acidic polysaccharides [189]. These phytochemicals have been shown to protect RGCs. Total *Panax notoginseng* saponin treatment increased RGC survival and inhibited the cell apoptosis pathway induced by an optic nerve crush rat model [190]. Similarly, ginsenoside Rg1 treatment was able to reduce RGC damage in an ultrasound-targeted microbubble optic nerve damage rabbit model [191]. Furthermore, ginsenoside Rb1 protects RGCs against apoptosis caused by $CoCl_2$-induced hypoxia and H_2O_2-induced oxidative stress [192].

4.12. Cannabis sativa—Cannabinoids

Cannabis sativa, commonly known as marijuana, is one of the most used psychoactive substances in the world [193]. The *C. sativa* plant contains more than 60 lipid-based cannabinoids, which are the signaling molecules of the endocannabinoid system; these include Δ^9-tetrahydrocannabinol (Δ^9-THC), Δ^8-tetrahydrocannabinol (Δ^8-THC), cannabidiol and cannabinol [194]. A reduction in IOP was observed in glaucoma patients associated with tachycardia, within the first 30 min after marijuana inhalation, with the duration of action limited to 4 h [195]. Similarly, Δ^9-THC inhalation reduced IOP significantly from baseline in healthy adult subjects, detected from 40 min post-treatment and lasting up to 4 h [196].

In animal studies, a topically applied 2% Δ^9-THC ophthalmic solution was shown to reduce IOP in clinically normal dogs [197]. To prolong the IOP reduction duration, the use of Δ^9-THC-valine-hemisuccinate nanoemulsions, which help to increase absorption, produced a greater drop in IOP, compared to latanoprost and timolol in normal rabbits [198]. Similarly, a submicron emulsion of Δ^8-THC treatment to normal and OHT rabbits also demonstrated a reduced IOP [199]. The IOP-lowering and RGC neuroprotective effects of cannabinoids have been shown to be mediated by CB1 cannabinoid receptors [200,201].

4.13. Anthocyanins

Anthocyanins, considered as flavonoids, are blue, red or purple pigments commonly found in the flowers, fruits and tubers of many plants [202]. Hence, the primary sources of anthocyanins are found in berries, currants, grapes and some tropical fruits [202]. Studies have demonstrated that anthocyanins provide numerous health benefits such as antioxidative and neuroprotective properties, prevention of cardiovascular diseases, anti-angiogenesis, anti-cancer, anti-diabetic, anti-obesity and antimicrobial activities and improved visual health [202,203].

OAG patients receiving supplementation of 50 mg of black currant anthocyanins daily for 24 months also showed a reduced IOP and improved visual field damage progression [204]. Black currant anthocyanin supplementation also enhanced blood flow to the ONH and its surrounding retina in OAG patients, with no changes in systemic conditions such as blood pressure and pulse rates observed [204,205]. Black currant anthocyanin supplementation also normalized the abnormal serum concentration levels of ET-1 in OAG patients, suggesting that anthocyanins possibly affect the ET-1 receptor functions such as pharmacological reactivity and hypersensitivity [206].

The natural anthocyanins delphinidin, luteolinidin and peonidin were shown to be non-toxic to human retinal pigment epithelial (ARPE19) and RGC-5 cells, with luteolinidin and peonidin increasing the survival rates of the RGC-5 cells following exposure to H_2O_2 [207]. Administration of oral bilberry extracts rich in anthocyanins was shown to suppress RGC death following an optic nerve injury mouse model [208]. Bilberry extract administration increased chaperone molecule (Grp78 and Grp94) protein levels, an effect which may underlie the neuroprotective effect of bilberry extract after optic nerve crush [208]. In a model of light-induced retinal damage in pigmented rabbits, administration of bilberry anthocyanin extract at dosages of 250 and 500 mg/kg/day for 7 days significantly inhibited retinal dysfunction, as evidenced by the increased retinal outer nuclear layer thicknesses and lengths of the outer segments of the photoreceptor cells, compared to untreated rabbits with retinal degeneration [209]. Additionally, anthocyanin treatment attenuated the changes caused by light to the apoptotic proteins Bax, Bcl-2 and caspase-3 and increased the antioxidant enzyme levels (SOD, GPX and CAT), but it decreased the MDA level in the retinal cells [209].

4.14. Resveratrol

Resveratrol (trans-3,4′,5-trihydroxystilbene) is a polyphenol found in berries, grapes, pomegranates and red wine [210]. It has been reported to possess a wide range of pharmacological effects, including cardioprotection, neuroprotection and anti-diabetic activity, due to its potent antioxidant and anti-inflammatory properties [210]. Resveratrol has been reported to increase oxidative stress markers, and the nitric oxide level in human glaucomatous TM cells, possibly by increasing endothelial nitric oxide synthase (eNOS) expression and reducing inducible NOS expressions [211]. In experimental glaucoma models, resveratrol treatment was shown to reduce RGC death [212,213]. Cao et al. [213] further demonstrated that intravitreal administration of resveratrol rescued RGCs by the decreased ROS generation in RGCs of a microbead-induced high-IOP mouse model. These studies support the antioxidant properties of resveratrol, which could be beneficial in glaucoma treatment.

Resveratrol protects RGC-5 cells against H_2O_2-induced apoptosis, by reversing H_2O_2-induced increased expressions of cleaved caspase-3/-9, production of ROS and the expressions of p-p38, p-ERK and p-JNK, proposing that resveratrol suppresses MAPK cascades to exert its neuroprotective effects in RGCs [214]. Additionally, resveratrol also mitigates retinal I/R injury-induced RGC loss, glial activation and retinal function impairment by inhibiting the HIF-1a/VEGF and p38/p53 pathways while activating the PI3K/AKT pathway [215–217].

In both the chronic OHT rat model and RGC-5 cells incubated under elevated pressure, RGCs showed apoptosis and mitochondrial dysfunction [218]. Resveratrol treatment improved the expression of proteins involved in mitochondrial biogenesis and dynamics, i.e., AMPK, Nrf-1, mitochondrial transcription factor A (Tfam), mitofusin 2 (mfn-2) and optic atrophy 1 (OPA1), which led to a decrease in RGC apoptosis, mitochondrial membrane potential depolarization and ROS generation [218,219]. Another recent study identified a potential mechanism involving the protective role of resveratrol in preventing ONH astrocyte dysfunction and degeneration, which would enable the astrocytes to continue providing structural and nutrient support to the optic nerve [220].

4.15. Hesperidin

Hesperidin is a flavanone commonly found in citrus fruits such as oranges, tangerines, lemons and grapefruits, known for its anti-inflammatory, antioxidant and anticarcinogenic properties [221]. The antioxidant profile of a novel supplement containing hesperidin, and two other food-derived antioxidants, i.e., crocetin and *Tamarindus indica* (tamarind), was assessed in a prospective, single-arm design trial involving 30 NTG patients receiving the supplements for 8 weeks [222]. In patients with relatively high oxidative stress, the supplement significantly reduced the urinary 8-hydroxy-2′-deoxyguanosine (8-OHdG; a marker of oxidative DNA damage) level, and the biological antioxidant potential was also significantly elevated [222].

In an animal study, a single dose of oral hesperidin pre-treatment (25, 50 and 100 mg/kg) significantly reduced the increased IOP level in dextrose- and prednisolone acetate-induced OHT rats [223]. Additionally, hesperidin treatment increased the glutathione level in the aqueous humor and reduced morphological alteration in the ciliary bodies caused by elevated IOP [223]. Furthermore, hesperidin treatment ameliorated NMDA-induced retinal injury by suppressing oxidative stress [224] and excessive calpain activation [225] while also alleviating hypobaric hypoxia-induced retinal impairment through the activation of the Nrf2/HO-1 pathway [226].

4.16. Caffeine

Caffeine (1, 3, 7-trimethylxanthine) is a natural alkaloid commonly consumed through coffee, tea, carbonated soft drinks, energy drinks, chocolate and other cocoa-containing foods [227]. Caffeine acts as a central nervous system stimulant through its A_1 and A_{2a} adenosine receptor antagonist properties [227]. The effect of caffeine consumption on IOP was found to be controversial in the literature. Tran et al. [228] demonstrated a reduced IOP following 45 and 60 min consumption of caffeine in POAG patients, when compared to the water-drinking group. However, another study reported that 1% caffeine eye drops administered daily for a week showed no effect on IOP in POAG patients [229]. In contrast, healthy individuals receiving a single dose of a 4 mg/kg caffeine capsule showed an increase in IOP, with low-caffeine consumers reporting a more abrupt IOP increase compared to the high-caffeine consumers [230]. Further studies suggested the increase in IOP was associated with a reduction in the anterior chamber angle, which led to resistance to aqueous humor outflow [231]. Recent cross-sectional studies showed caffeine consumption was weakly associated with a lower IOP but was not associated with a decreased risk of developing glaucoma [232,233]. An in vivo study demonstrated a reduced IOP and prevention of loss of RGCs in the caffeine-drinking animals following laser-induced OHT in experimental rats [234]. However, the same study also reported that caffeine treatment did not ameliorate OHT-induced impairment in the RGC retrograde transport, although caffeine treatment appeared to partially attenuate axonal degeneration of the optic nerve induced by OHT [234]. Interestingly, caffeine drinking led to increased microglia reactivity, inflammatory response (IL-1β and TNF mRNA levels) and cell death following 24 h post-I/R injury in a mouse model, which were then reduced at day 7 post-injury [235]. Additionally, caffeine was shown to preserve the integrity of the blood–retinal barrier in LPS-treated ARPE19 cells, which can be considered as a new strategy to treat retinal degenerative diseases [236].

4.17. Coenzyme Q10

Coenzyme Q10 (CoQ10), or ubiquinone-10, is a natural lipophilic vitamin-like molecule with antioxidant and anti-inflammatory properties and is involved in the production and control of cellular bioenergy, pyrimidine synthesis, physicochemical properties of cellular membranes and gene expression [237,238]. It is predominantly found in animal organs (kidney, liver and heart) and is also present in meat, fish, soy oil and peanuts [238].

Treatment with CoQ10, either topically applied or supplemented in the diet, was shown to promote RGC survival by inhibition of RGC apoptosis in glaucoma models [239–241]. CoQ10 treatment has also been shown to inhibit glaucomatous mitochondrial alteration by the preservation of the mtDNA content and Tfam/oxidative phosphorylation (OXPHOS) complex IV protein expressions [239,240]. Furthermore, CoQ10 treatment inhibited the activation of astrocytes and microglial cells in the retina [239,240]. In a clinical study, CoQ10 and vitamin E eye drop administration in POAG patients for 12 months showed a beneficial effect on the inner retinal function (PERG improvement), with a consequent enhancement of the visual cortical responses (VEP improvement) [242]. Additionally, CoQ10 and vitamin E topical treatment increased RGC numbers, inhibited apoptosis and activated astrocytes and microglial cells in a mechanical optic nerve injury rat model [243].

4.18. Vitamins

A cross-sectional study involving a total of 2912 participants in the United States 2005–2006 National Health and Nutrition Examination Survey reported that supplementary consumption and serum levels of vitamins A and E were not associated with glaucoma prevalence [244]. A meta-analysis did not find an association between serum vitamin B_6, vitamin B_{12} and vitamin D levels and different types of glaucoma [245]. Another recent systematic review concluded that blood levels of vitamins (A, B complex, C, D and E) did not demonstrate an association with OAG as well [246]. However, the same study reported that dietary intake of vitamins A and C showed a beneficial association with OAG [246].

The nicotinamide adenine dinucleotide (NAD^+, an important metabolite for mitochondrial metabolism and oxidative stress protection) level in the retina of D2-$Gpnmb^+$ mice decreased with age [247]. Oral administration of vitamin B_3 (nicotinamide, precursor of NAD^+) was protective as both prophylaxis and an intervention of glaucoma, as shown by the reduced incidence of optic nerve degeneration, prevention of RGC soma and axonal loss and retinal nerve fiber layer thinning and preserved visual function [247,248]. In a crossover, randomized clinical trial involving 57 glaucoma patients, oral vitamin B_3 supplementation for 6 weeks at 1.5 g/day, then for 6 weeks at 3.0 g/day, improved RGC function, but without affecting the IOP and RNFL thickness [249].

Table 2. Clinical trials evaluating natural products for glaucoma treatment.

Natural Products	Subjects	Treatment Regime	Clinical Findings	References
Ginkgo biloba	POAG patients	120 mg GB extract, 1 tablet daily, 6 months	Lower rate of single-stranded DNA breaks in circulating leukocytes (vs. untreated patients, $p < 0.001$)	[97]
	NTG patients	80 mg GB extract, 2 tablets daily, 4 years	No effect on IOP (vs. pre-treatment, $p = 0.509$) Slowed visual field damage progression ($p < 0.001$)	[98]
	NTG patients	80 mg GB extract, 2 tablets daily, 2 years	Improved HVF deviation (vs. untreated patients, $p = 0.002$)	[99]
	NTG patients	80 mg GB extract, 2 tablets daily, 4 weeks	Increased ocular blood flow, volume and velocity (vs. placebo-treated patients, $p < 0.03$)	[100]
	Healthy subjects	120 mg GB extract, 1 tablet daily, 4 weeks	Increased radial peripapillary capillary vascular density (vs. pre-treatment, $p < 0.021$)	[101]
Forskolin	POAG patients	Forskolin 1% w/v aqueous solution eye drops, 2 drops thrice a day, 4 weeks	Reduced IOP (vs. timolol-treated patients, $p < 0.05$) No adverse events	[117]
Erigeron breviscapus	POAG patients	E. breviscapus extract, 2 tablets, 3 times daily, 6 months	No obvious adverse effects Decreased mean defect (vs. pre-treatment, $p < 0.01$) Increased mean sensitivity ($p < 0.01$)	[122]
Saffron	POAG patients	Aqueous saffron extract, 30 mg daily, 4 weeks	Reduced IOP (vs. pre-treatment, $p = 0.0046$) No obvious adverse effects	[160]

Table 2. Cont.

Natural Products	Subjects	Treatment Regime	Clinical Findings	References
Ginseng	Glaucoma patients	Korean red ginseng, 3 g daily, 4 weeks	Improved daytime contrast sensitivity (vs. pre-treatment, $p = 0.004$) and ocular pain ($p < 0.001$)	[186]
	Glaucoma patients	Korean red ginseng, 3 g daily, 8 weeks	Improved tear film stability and total OSDI score (vs. placebo-treated patients, $p < 0.01$)	[187]
	OAG patients	Korean red ginseng, 1.5 g, 3 times daily, 12 weeks	Improved retinal peripapillary blood flow in the temporal peripapillary region (vs. pre-treatment, $p = 0.005$) No changes in blood pressure, heart rate, IOP and visual field indices	[188]
Marijuana	Glaucoma patients	Marijuana smoking, single dose	Reduced IOP (vs. placebo-treated patients, p value not defined) Increased heart rate	[195]
	Healthy subjects	Marijuana smoking, single dose	Reduced IOP (vs. pre-treatment, $p < 0.01$) No effect on systemic blood pressure	[196]
Anthocyanins	NTG patients	60 mg, 2 tablets daily, 2 years	Improved best-corrected visual acuity (vs. untreated patients, $p = 0.008$), and HVF deviation ($p = 0.001$)	[99]
	OAG patients	50 mg black currant anthocyanins daily, 2 years	Increased ocular blood flows (vs. placebo-treated patients, $p = 0.01$) Improved visual field damage progression ($p = 0.039$)	[204]
	OAG patients	50 mg black currant anthocyanins daily, 24 months	Reduced IOP (vs. pre-treatment, $p = 0.027$) Improved HVF deviation ($p = 0.017$) No changes in systemic blood pressure or pulse rates	[205]
	OAG patients	50 mg black currant anthocyanins daily, 24 months	Normalized serum ET-1 concentrations (vs. healthy subjects, $p < 0.05$) No changes in advanced oxidation protein products, and antioxidative activities	[206]
Hesperidin, crocetin and *Tamarindus indica*	NTG patients	Food supplement containing hesperidin (50 mg), crocetin (7.5 mg) and *T. indica* (25 mg), 4 tablets twice a day, 8 weeks	Reduced 8-OHdG level in high-oxidative stress patients (vs. pre-treatment, $p < 0.01$) Elevated BAP in high-oxidative stress patients ($p = 0.03$)	[222]
Caffeine	POAG patients	Coffee containing 1.3% caffeine (104 mg caffeine), single dose	Reduced IOP (vs. water-drinking patients, $p = 0.012$) Reduced IOP fluctuation ($p = 0.013$)	[228]
	POAG patients	1% caffeine eye drop, thrice a day, 1 week	No effect on IOP (vs. pre-treatment, $p > 0.05$)	[229]
	Healthy subjects	Caffeine capsule, 4 mg/kg, single dose	Increased IOP (vs. pre-treatment, $p < 0.05$)	[230]
	Healthy subjects	Caffeine capsule, 4 mg/kg, single dose	Increased IOP (vs. placebo-treated subjects, $p < 0.05$) Reduced anterior chamber angle ($p < 0.05$)	[231]

Table 2. Cont.

Natural Products	Subjects	Treatment Regime	Clinical Findings	References
Coenzyme Q10	POAG patients	CoQ10 and vitamin E eye drop, 2 drops daily, 12 months	Decreased ERG P50 and VEP P100 implicit times (vs. pre-treatment, $p < 0.01$) Increased PERG P50-N95 and VEP N75-P100 amplitudes ($p < 0.01$)	[242]
Vitamin B_3	Glaucoma patients	Vitamin B_3 tablet, 1.5 g/day 6 weeks, followed by 3.0 g/day for 6 weeks	Improved RGC functions—PhNR Vmax (vs. placebo-treated patients, $p = 0.03$), Vmax ratio ($p = 0.02$) and visual field mean deviation ($p = 0.02$) No effect on IOP ($p = 0.59$) and RNFL thickness ($p = 0.11$)	[249]

8-OhdG, 8-hydroxydeoxyguanosine; BAP, biological antioxidant potential; ET-1, endothelin-1; HVF, Humphrey visual field; IOP, intraocular pressure; NTG, normal-tension glaucoma; OAG, open-angle glaucoma; OSDI, Ocular Surface Disease Index; PhNR, photopic negative; POAG, primary open-angle glaucoma; PERG, pattern electroretinogram; RGC, retinal ganglion cell; RNFL, retinal nerve fiber layer.

Previous studies have reported that serum vitamin D levels are significantly lower in glaucoma patients as compared to healthy subjects [250,251]. Additionally, the presence of polymorphisms in vitamin D receptors, e.g., the BsmI 'B' allele and TaqI 't' allele, was shown to be a relevant risk factor in the development of POAG [251]. Vitamin D deficiency subjects were reported to have higher, although not significant, IOP values compared to healthy individuals [252]. Treatment with 1α,25-dihydroxyvitamin D_3 and its analog 2-methylene-19-nor-(20S)-1α,25-dihydroxyvitamin D_3 through eye drops reduced the IOP in normal monkeys [253]. D2 mice treated with 1 µg/kg of 1α,25-dihydroxyvitamin D_3, intraperitoneally for 5 weeks, showed improved RGC function (increased PERG and FERG amplitudes) and reduced RGC death, compared to vehicle-treated controls [254]. Additionally, the same study also reported decreased microglial and astrocyte activation, reduced inflammatory cytokines (IL-1β and -6, IFN-γ and CCL-3) and increased expression of neuroprotective factors (BDNF, VEGF-A and PlGF) in the 1α,25-dihydroxyvitamin D_3 treatment group [254].

Induced OHT rats fed with a vitamin E-supplemented diet showed no difference in RGC cell death, compared to normal diet-treated rats [255]. However, the same study demonstrated that dietary vitamin E deficiency aggravated RGC apoptosis following induced OHT, which was found to be related to the increased level of lipid peroxidation [255]. In contrast, both topical and systemic α-tocopherol administration preserved the RGC numbers and retinal morphology in an optic nerve crush rat model [256].

Table 3. Preclinical studies on natural products used for glaucoma treatment and their mechanism of action.

Natural Products	Model	RGC	IOP	Ocular Vasculation	Other Findings	References
Ginkgo biloba	Rat RGC cells exposed to H_2O_2	Increased survival rate	-	-	-	[96]
	Rat optic nerve crush model	Increased RGC density	-	-	-	[96]
	Rat optic nerve crush model	Increased survival rate	-	-	-	[102]
	Mouse RGC-5 cells exposed to H_2O_2	Reduced cell apoptosis	-	-	Increased antioxidant capacity (reduced T-AOC, SOD and CAT depletion)	[105]
Diterpene ginkgolides meglumine injection	Rat optic nerve injury model	Reduced cell apoptosis	-	-	Decreased conduction time of F-VEP	[103]
Scutellaria baicalensis—Baicalein	Rat episcleral vein cauterization-induced chronic OHT model	-	Reduced IOP	-	-	[109]
	Rat ischemic model	Reduced cell apoptosis	-	-	Upregulation of HO-1 Downregulation of HIF-1α, VEGF and MMP-9	[110]
S. baicalensis—Wogonin	Rat optic nerve crush model	Reduced cell apoptosis	-	-	Decreased caspase-3 activation Decreased gliosis response and microglial activation Decreased pro-inflammatory cytokine (TNF-α, MCP-1, iNOS, IL-6 and-1β and COX-2) expression	[111]
S. baicalensis—Baicalin	NMDA-stimulated RGC	Reduced cell apoptosis	-	-	Alleviated NMDA-induced oxidative stress (reduced ROS and MDA levels) Inhibited NMDA-induced autophagy	[112]
	Mouse episcleral venous occlusion-induced chronic OHT model	Increased RGC density Increased GCL thickness	-	-	Inhibited OHT-induced autophagy Activated PI3K/AKT signaling	[112]
Forskolin	Isolated bovine eye	-	Reduced IOP	-	Reduced peak calcium response to ATP	[116]
Forskolin, homotaurine, spearmint extract and vitamins B1, B2 and B12 mixture	Mouse optic nerve crush model	Increased RGC numbers	-	-	Reduced cytokine (iNOS and IL-6) secretion Decreased apoptotic marker (Bax/Bcl-2 ratio and active caspase-3) levels	[119]
	Rat methylcellulose-induced OHT model	Increased RGC numbers	No effect	-	Prevented the reduction in retinal function (increased PhNR amplitude, PERG amplitude and implicit time) Prevented microglial and Müller cell activation Decreased inflammatory markers (NF-κB, TNF-α and IL-6) Decreased apoptotic marker (Bax/Bcl-2 ratio and active caspase-3) levels	[120]

Table 3. Cont.

Natural Products	Model	RGC	IOP	Ocular Vasculation	Other Findings	References
Sodium alginate poly (vinyl alcohol) electrospun nanofibers of forskolin	Normal rabbit	-	Reduced IOP	-	-	[257]
Erigeron breviscapus	Rat episcleral vein cauterization-induced OHT model	-	Reduced IOP	-	Improved visual function	[123]
	Rabbit methylcellulose-induced OHT model	Increased RGC density Increased RNFL thickness Reduced RGC axonal degeneration	-	-	-	[124]
Scutellarin	Mouse clear hydrogel-induced OHT model	-	-	-	Reduced retinal thinning Reduced visual behavioral deficits	[126]
	BV-2 cells exposed to low oxygen level	-	-	-	Increased cell viability Inhibited expression of NLRP3 Reduced the upregulation of ASC, cleaved caspase-1 and IL-18 and -1β	[127]
	Rat saline-induced acute OHT model	Increased survival rate	-	-	Reduced impaired microglial cells Inhibited NLRP3 expression Reduced upregulation of ASC, cleaved caspase-1 and IL-18 and -1β	[127]
Lycium barbarum	Rat argon laser photocoagulation-induced OHT model	Reduced ET-1 expression in RGCs	-	-	-	[131]
	Mouse acute OHT model	Increased RGC numbers Increased IRL thickness	-	Recovered blood vessel density in retina	Protected retinal vasculature stability (reduced IgG leakage, more continued structure of tight junctions associated with increased occludin protein level) Downregulation of RAGE, ET-1, Aβ and AGE	[131]
	Rat acute OHT model	Normalized GCL density Preserved IRL thickness Preserved RGCs	-	-	Preserved positive scotopic threshold response functions	[132]
	Rat suture implantation-induced chronic OHT model	-	-	-	-	[134]
	Rat partial optic nerve transection model	-	-	-	Preserved visual function	[135]
	Rat complete and partial optic nerve transection	Delayed RGC degeneration	-	-	Increased MnSOD and IGF-1 expressions	[136]
	RGC-5 cells exposed to CoCl$_2$-induced hypoxia	Reduced cell apoptosis	-	-	Inhibited ROS generation Inhibited reduction in mitochondrial membrane potential	[137]

Table 3. Cont.

Natural Products	Model	RGC	IOP	Ocular Vasculation	Other Findings	References
	Human TM cells exposed to H_2O_2	-	-	-	Promoted cell viability Reduced apoptosis Reduced cleaved caspase-3/-9 and ROS levels	[138]
	Rat partial optic nerve transection model	Delayed secondary degeneration of RGCs	-	-	Promoted M2 polarization of microglia/macrophages Downregulated autophagy level	[139]
	PC12 cells exposed to hydrostatic pressures	-	-	-	Reduced ANGPTL7, MMP-2 and -9, collagen I and TGF-β expressions	[141]
	Mouse retinal I/R injury model	Retinal cellular organization remained normal Fewer pyknotic nuclei in GCL and INL	-	-	Reduced glial activation	[144]
	Rat retinal I/R injury model	Reduced apoptosis in GCL and INL	-	-	Increased Nrf2 nuclear accumulation Increased HO-1 expression	[145]
	Rat saline-induced acute OHT model	Downregulation of APP and RAGE expressions	-	Reverse loss of function of astrocyte endfeet around blood vessels	Reduced numbers of astrocytes and microglia Decreased glutamine toxicity in astrocytes (downregulation of glutamine synthetase)	[146]
	Rat retinal I/R injury model	-	-	-	Preserved retinal thickness Increased antioxidant levels (GSSH + GSH, SOD and CAT) Reduced MDA level	[146]
Diospyros kaki	Mouse microbead-induced OHT model, and D2 mouse	Reduced RGC loss	Reduced IOP	-	Increased sGCα-1 expression	[149]
	RGC-5 cells exposed to glutamate	Increased cell viability	-	-	Decreased apoptotic protein levels (poly (ADP-ribose) polymerase, p53 and cleaved caspase-3) Increased antioxidant-associated protein expression levels (SOD, GST and GPX)	[150]
	Mouse partial optic nerve crush model	Reduced RGC death	-	-	-	[150]
T. wilfordii—Triptolide	D2 mouse	Improved RGC survival	No effect	-	Suppressed microglia activation Reduced microglia count	[153]
	Angle photocoagulation-induced chronic glaucoma rat model	Improved RGC survival	-	-	Reduced TNF-α expression	[154]
	Mouse optic nerve crush model	Improved RGC survival	-	-	Reduced TNF-α expression Inhibited nuclear translocation of NF-κB	[155]
T. wilfordii—celastrol	Mouse optic nerve crush model	Improved RGC survival	-	-	Reduced TNF-α expression	[156]
	Rat trabecular laser photocoagulation model	Improved RGC survival	-	-		[157]

Table 3. Cont.

Natural Products	Model	RGC	IOP	Ocular Vasculation	Other Findings	References
Crocus sativus L.	Mouse laser-induced OHT model	Prevented RGC death	-	-	Decreased microglial numbers and their activation Partially reversed downregulation of P2RY12	[159]
C. sativus—Crocin	Rat retinal I/R injury model	Increased RGC survival	-	-	Inhibited retinal thinning Decreased cleaved caspase-3 and p-ERK protein expressions Increased GSH and T-SOD activities Decreased ROS and MDA levels	[162]
	Rat retinal I/R injury model	Increased RGC survival Reduced RGC apoptosis	-	-	Upregulation of Bcl-2/Bax level Enhanced p-AKT levels	[163]
	RGC-5 cells exposed to H_2O_2	Protected RGCs from apoptosis Enhanced cell viability	-	-	Decreased LDH release Decreased ROS levels Increased ΔΨm Downregulated Bax and cytochrome c protein expressions Promoted Bcl-2 protein expression Activated NF-κB	[164]
C. sativus—Crocetin	Mouse NMDA-induced retinal injury model	Increased GCL density	-	-	Reduced TUNEL-positive cells Inhibited activated caspase-3/-7 Increased cleaved caspase-3 expression	[165]
	Rat retinal I/R injury model	Increased GCL density Reduced INL thinning	-	-	Decreased TUNEL-positive cells and 8-OHdG-positive cells Decreased phosphorylation levels of p38, JNK, NF-κB and c-Jun	[166]
Curcumin	BV-2 cells exposed to H_2O_2	-	-	-	Increased cell viability Decreased ROS and apoptosis Downregulated caspase-3, cytochrome c and Bax Upregulated Bcl-2	[169]
	Rat episcleral vein cauterization	Prevented RGC loss	-	-	Downregulated caspase-3, cytochrome c and Bax Upregulated Bcl-2	[169]
	Ex vivo optic nerve cut model	Increased RGC survival Preserved retinal thickness	-	-	Prevented alterations in apoptotic cascades and MAPK and SUMO-1 pathways	[170]
	Rat retinal I/R injury model	-	-	-	Prevented retinal damage	[171]
	Rat retinal I/R injury model	Inhibited GCL cell loss Reduced cell apoptosis	-	-	Inhibited retinal capillary degeneration Inhibited upregulation of MCP-1, IKKα, p-IκBα and p-STAT3 (Tyr), and downregulation of β-tubulin II	[172]

Table 3. *Cont.*

Natural Products	Model	RGC	IOP	Ocular Vasculation	Other Findings	References
	Primary porcine TM cells exposed to H_2O_2	-		-	Prevented cell death Reduced ROS production Inhibited pro-inflammatory factors (IL-6, -1α and -8 and ELAM-1) Decreased SA-β-gal activity Reduced carbonylated proteins and apoptotic cell numbers	[173]
	Primary porcine TM cells exposed to H_2O_2	-		-	Reduced ROS level Reduced apoptosis Upregulated Bcl-2 Downregulated Bax and activated caspase-3 levels Reduced Nrf2, HO-1 and NQO1 expressions Increased Keap1 expression	[174]
	Rat partial optic nerve transection model	Improved RGC density ratio	No effect	-		[258]
	Human TM cells exposed to H_2O_2	-		-	Reduced TNF and IL-1α and -6 expression Reduced mitochondrial ROS production Reduced cleaved caspase-3 proteins Reduced TUNEL-positive cells	[259]
Green tea	Rat retinal I/R injury model	Increased RGC numbers Reduced apoptotic RGCs	-	-	Reduced activated caspase-3 and -8, SOD2 and inflammation-related proteins expressions Reduced p38 phosphorylation Enhanced JAK phosphorylation	[176]
	Rat LPS-induced retinal inflammation model	-	-	-	Suppressed activated microglia, astrocytes and Müller glia Reduced pro-inflammatory cytokine expressions (IL-1β and -6 and TNF-α in retina and vitreous humor)	[177]
Green tea—EGCG	Rat saline-induced acute OHT model	-	-	-	Decreased inflammation-associated cytokine levels Decreased the proliferation rate of T lymphocyte cells Reduced IκBα and p65 phosphorylation	[179]
	Mouse microbead-induced OHT model	Increased RGC numbers	No effect	-		[180]
	Rat optic nerve crush model	Increase RGC density	-	-	Increased NF-L protein expression Reduced retinal gliosis Reduced MDA level	[181]
	Rabbit retinal I/R injury model	Preserved organization of GCL, IPL and INL	-	-		[182]

Table 3. Cont.

Natural Products	Model	RGC	IOP	Ocular Vasculation	Other Findings	References
	Rat NMDA-induced excitotoxicity model	Increased GCL cell density	-	-	-	[183]
Ginseng	Rat optic nerve crush injury model	Increased cell survival Reduced cell apoptosis	-	-	Increased Bcl-2/Bax protein ratio Decreased c-Jun, P-c-Jun and P-JNK protein expressions	[190]
	Rabbit ultrasound-targeted microbubble optic nerve injury model	Reduced RGC damage	Reduced IOP	-	Reduced oxidative stress level Reduced MDA and NO levels Increased SOD level	[191]
	RGC-5 cells exposed to $CoCl_2$ or H_2O_2	Reduced cell apoptosis	-	-	Reduced cleaved caspase-3 and -9 expressions	[192]
Marijuana—Δ^9-THC	Normal dogs	-	Reduced IOP	-	No effect on aqueous humor flow rate	[197]
	Normal rabbit	-	Reduced IOP	-	-	[198]
Marijuana—Δ^8-THC	Rabbit chymotrypsin-induced OHT model	-	Reduced IOP	-	-	[199]
Marijuana	Rat retinal I/R injury model	Reduced RGC damage	-	-	-	[201]
Anthocyanins	RGC-5 cells exposed to H_2O_2	Increased survival rate	-	-	-	[207]
	Mouse optic nerve crush model	Increased survival rate	-	-	Increased Grp78 and Grp94 levels	[208]
Resveratrol	Glaucomatous human TM cells	-	-	-	Increased eNOS and NO levels Decreased iNOS expressions Increased IL-1α level with low dose Decreased IL-1α level with high dose	[211]
	Rat hyaluronic acid-induced chronic OHT model	Preserved RGC numbers	No effect	-	-	[212]
	Mouse microbead-induced OHT model	Preserved RGC numbers	-	-	Decreased ROS generation and acetyl-p53 expression Upregulated BDNF and TrkB expressions	[213]
	RGC-5 cells exposed to H_2O_2	Increased cell viability	-	-	Reduced expressions of cleaved caspase-3 and -9 Reduced ROS production Reduced loss of mitochondrial membrane potential and p-p38, p-ERK and p-JNK expressions	[214]
	Mouse retinal I/R injury model	Ameliorated retinal thickness damage Increased RGC numbers	-	-	Promoted SOD, CAT and GSH activities Downregulated mitochondrial apoptosis-related proteins (Bax and cleaved caspase-3) Increased Bcl-2 expression	[215]
	Mouse retinal I/R injury model	Reduced RGC loss Reduced retinal damage	-	-	Reduced TUNEL staining Reduced Bax and cleaved caspase-3 levels	[216]

Table 3. Cont.

Natural Products	Model	RGC	IOP	Ocular Vasculation	Other Findings	References
	Mouse retinal I/R injury model	Reduced RGC loss	-	-	Reduced Bcl-2, Bax, caspase-3, GFAP, COX-2 and iNOS expressions	[217]
	Rat superparamagnetic iron oxide-induced chronic OHT model	No effect on GCL density Decreased cell apoptosis	No effect	-	Improved retinal morphology Improved expressions of proteins involved in mitochondrial biogenesis and dynamics	[218]
	RGC-5 cells exposed to elevated pressure	Decreased cell apoptosis	-	-	Decreased mitochondrial membrane potential depolarization Decreased ROS production Upregulated expressions of proteins involved in mitochondrial biogenesis and dynamics	[218]
	Mouse retinal I/R injury model	Decreased cell apoptosis Restored retina thickness	-	-	Increased Opa1 expression, and long Opa1 isoform-to-short Opa1 isoform ratios	[219]
	Normal rabbit	-	Reduced IOP	-	-	[260]
Hesperidin	Rat dextrose- or prednisolone acetate-induced OHT model	-	Reduced IOP	-	Increased glutathione Reduced morphological alteration in ciliary bodies	[223]
	Mouse NMDA-induced retinal injury model	-	-	-	Reduced inflammatory cytokine (TNF-α, IL-1b and -6 and MCP-1) expressions	[224]
	Mouse NMDA-induced retinal injury model	Prevented reductions in RGC markers Prevented RGC death	-	-	Reduced calpain activation, ROS generation and TNF-α gene expression Improved electrophysiological function and visual function	[225]
	Rat hypobaric hypoxia-induced retinal injury model	-	-	-	Enhanced Nrf2 and HO-1 activation Attenuated apoptotic caspase levels Reduced Bax and preserved Bcl-2 expressions Downregulated PARP1 expression Upregulated CNTF expression	[226]
Caffeine	Rat laser-induced OHT model	Increased survival rate	Reduced IOP	-	Downregulated TNF and IL-1β mRNA and protein levels Suppressed microglia activation (downregulated MHC-II, TSPO, CD11b and TREM2 expressions)	[234]
	Rat retinal I/R injury model	-	-	-	Reduced microglial activation at 7 days post-injury (reduced Iba1 and MHC-II cells; reduced TSPO and MHC-II mRNA levels) Reduced TUNEL-positive cells	[235]

Table 3. Cont.

Natural Products	Model	RGC	IOP	Ocular Vasculation	Other Findings	References
	Human retinal pigment epithelial cells exposed to LPS	-	-	-	Reduced LPS-induced inflammatory cytokines (TNF-α, IL-1β and -6) Restored BDNF expression Reduced p-NF-κB p65 nuclear translocation Restored blood–retinal barrier (increased transepithelial electrical resistance value and ZO-1 tight junction expression)	[236]
	Mouse retinal I/R injury model	-	-	-	Increased PERG amplitude Reduced IL-6 mRNA expression Increased BDNF mRNA expression	[236]
Coenzyme Q10	Mouse retinal ischemia model	Promoted RGC survival	-	-	Prevented upregulation of SOD2 and HO-1 protein expression Blocked activation of astrocytes and microglial cells Blocked apoptosis by decreasing caspase-3 protein expression Decreased Bax protein expression Preserved Tfam protein expression	[239]
	D2-Gpnmb+ mice	Promoted RGC survival	-	-	Preserved axons in the ONH Inhibited astrocytes activation Blocked the upregulation of NR1, NR2A, SOD2 and HO1 protein expressions Decreased Bax protein expression Preserved mtDNA content and Tfam/OXPHOS complex IV protein expressions	[240]
	Rat chronic OHT model	Prevented RGC apoptosis and RGC loss	No effect	-	-	[241]
	Rat mechanic optic nerve injury model	Increased RGC numbers	-	-	Reduced activation of astroglia and microglial cells Increased Bcl-xL protein expression	[243]
Vitamin B$_3$	D2-Gpnmb+ mouse	Prevented RGC loss Prevented RNFL thinning	Reduced IOP at high dose	-	Prevented the decline in NAD levels Reduced incidence of optic nerve degeneration Improved PERG amplitude Inhibited formation of dysfunctional mitochondria Decreased PARP activation Reduced DNA damage	[247]
	D2 mouse	Increased RGC density	-	-	Reduced HIF-1α transcriptional induction Increased F-PERG adaptation	[248]

Table 3. Cont.

Natural Products	Model	RGC	IOP	Ocular Vasculation	Other Findings	References
Vitamin D	Normal monkeys	-	Reduced IOP	-	-	[253]
	D2 mouse	Reduced RGC death	-	-	Improved PERG and FERG amplitudes Increased neuroprotective factor (BDNF, VEGF-A and PlGF) mRNA levels Decreased microglial and astrocyte activation Decreased inflammatory cytokine (IL-1β, -6, IFN-γ and CCL-3) expressions Decreased NF-κB activation	[254]
Vitamin E	Rat episcleral vein cauterization	No effect	No effect	-	Increased serum vitamin E level	[255]
	Rat optic nerve crush model	Preserved RGC numbers	-	-	-	[256]

Δ9-THC, Δ-9-tetrahydrocannabinol; Aβ, amyloid beta; AGE, advanced glycation end products; ANGPTL7, angiopoietin-like protein 7; APP, amyloid precursor protein; ASC, caspase recruitment domain; Bax, Bcl-2-like protein 4; Bcl-2, B cell lymphoma 2; CAT, catalase; CNTF, ciliary neurotrophic factor; COX-2, cyclooxygenase; D2, DBA/2J; ELAM-1, endothelial leucocyte adhesion molecule-1; eNOS endothelial nitric oxide synthase; ET-1, endothelin-1; F-VEP, flash visual evoked potentials; GCL, ganglion cell layer; GPX, glutathione peroxidase; GSH, glutathione; HIF-1α, hypoxia–inducible factor-1α; HO-1, heme oxygenase-1; IGF-1, insulin-like growth factor 1; IL, interleukin; iNOS, inducible nitric oxide synthase; IRL, insulin receptor-like; LDH, lactate de ydrogenase; LPS, lipopolysaccharide; MCP-1, monocyte chemoattractant protein-1; MDA, malondialdehyde; MHC-II, major histocompatibility complex class II; MMP, metalloproteinase; NF-κB, nuclear factor-kappa B; NF-L, neurofilament light chain; NLRP3, NOD-, LRR- and pyrin domain-containing protein 3; NMDA, N-methyl-d-aspartate; Nrf, nuclear factor erythroid 2-related factor; NQO1, NAD(P)H:quinone oxidoreductase; OHT, ocular hypertension; ONH, optic nerve head; OPA1, optic atrophy 1; OXPHOS, oxidative phosphorylation; PARP1, poly [ADP-ribose] polymerase 1; PERG, pattern electroretinogram; PhNR, photopic negative response; PlGF, placental growth factor; ROS, reactive oxygen species; RAGE receptor for advanced glycation end products; RGC, retinal ganglion cell; RNFL, retinal nerve fiber layer; sGCα-1, soluble guanylate cyclase α1; SOD, superoxide dismutase; T-AOC, total antioxidant capacity colorimetric; TNF-α, tumor necrosis factor-alpha; TGF-β, transforming growth factor-beta; Tfam, mitochondrial transcription factor A; TREM2, trigge"ing receptor expressed on myeloid cells 2; TSPO, translocator protein (18 kDa); VEGF, vascular endothelial growth factor.

5. Challenges for Natural Product Application in Glaucoma Treatment

The WHO has defined guidelines for evaluating the safety and efficacy of natural products, which is important to further supporting the use of CAM in the healthcare system [261]. This guideline provides general principles for both preclinical and clinical studies on evaluating herbal medicines, i.e., quality and preparation of plant materials, and general pharmacological, pharmacodynamic and toxicological analyses. Although the use of crude extracts from whole plants or a particular part of any herbal plant proves to be useful in the treatment of glaucoma, as described in this review, the identification and isolation of an active phytochemical may also be important, especially in the drug development process. Crude extracts contain a wide range of phytochemicals that may work synergistically or individually to provide a polypharmacy effect in the treatment of glaucoma [262]. Similarly, several studies have reported the use of a mixture of molecules to be effective in reducing IOP in POAG patients. Researchers may have difficulty in identifying the exact mechanism or compound responsible for such findings. For instance, oral administration of two tablets per day of a food supplement containing 150 mg of *C. forskohlii* extract (containing 15 mg forskolin), 200 mg of rutin, 0.7 mg of vitamin B1 and 0.8 mg of vitamin B2 for 30 days contributed to reducing IOP in POAG patients [263]. The same supplementation has also been shown to reduce ocular discomfort in POAG patients due to chronic use of multi-dose eye drops containing preservatives [264], and to prevent IOP spikes after neodymium:YAG laser iridotomy in patients at risk of POAG [265]. Additionally, supplementation with tablets containing *C. forskohlii* extract, homotaurine, carnosine, folic acid, vitamins of the B group and magnesium in POAG patients compensated by IOP-lowering drugs during a period of 12 months showed a significant further decrease in IOP and an improvement in the pattern electroretinogram amplitude at 6, 9 and 12 months, and foveal sensitivity at 12 months [266]. In another study, daily intake of a similar supplement for 4 months showed a decrease in IOP, improved light sensitivity and contrast sensitivity and a better quality of life in POAG patients [267]. Additionally, supplementation with French maritime pine bark/bilberry fruit extracts rich in anthocyanins to POAG patients for 4 weeks showed a reduced IOP [268].

Numerous eye drops of various classes, such as prostaglandin analogs, beta blockers, carbonic anhydrase inhibitors, adrenergic agonists, miotics and hyperosmotic agents, are often preferred over surgeries for the treatment of glaucoma [269]. One of the major issues in glaucoma treatment is patients' noncompliance, due to improper techniques of administering eye drops [270]. Another major issue is poor drug bioavailability across the blood–retinal barrier, limited retention capacity of the cul-de-sac (usually 7–10 μL, maximum 50 μL), rapid drainage of the medication caused by gravity and washout by tearing or through the nasolacrimal duct [271]. The use of various nanoformulations such as nanoparticles, nanoemulsions and nano lipid vesicles to transport phytochemicals may be able to increase the bioavailability of the drugs to the eye. For instance, baicalein loaded in trimethyl chitosan nanoparticles showed a longer pre-ocular retention time and improved baicalein bioavailability, compared to baicalein solution [272]. Davis et al. [258] reported the use of a curcumin-loaded nanocarrier formulation using D-α-tocopherol polyethene glycol 1000 succinate nanoparticles, with each particle measuring <20 nm in diameter. In an OHT rat model, topical application of curcumin nanocarriers administered twice daily for three weeks was shown to significantly reduce RGC loss, but not in the free curcumin treatment group [258]. Additionally, the same study showed that curcumin nanocarriers protected retinal cells against $CoCl_2$-induced hypoxia and glutamate-induced toxicity in vitro, by significantly increasing cell viability [258]. Similarly, a chitosan–gelatin-based hydrogel containing curcumin-loaded nanoparticles decreased the inflammation (reduced expression of TNF and IL-1α and -6, associated with downregulated mitochondrial ROS production) and apoptosis levels (reduced TUNEL-positive cells and cleaved caspase-3 protein level) of human TM cells exposed to H_2O_2-induced oxidative stress [259]. Apart from curcumin, co-encapsulated resveratrol and quercetin in chitosan nanoparticles, and sodium alginate-poly (vinyl alcohol) electrospun nanofibers of forskolin showed an efficient IOP reduction in adult normotensive rabbits [257,260]. These studies demonstrated that phytochemical nanoformulations hold promising results, promoting their use as an alternative to existing glaucoma eye drops in clinical practice.

Lastly, it is important to use a suitable methodology to address the objectives of a study. Numerous studies used the Bcl-2/Bax ratio to imply that the therapeutic substance influences the activation of the intrinsic apoptotic pathway in RGCs, as shown by the numerous studies which have been reviewed here. However, the concept that both Bcl-2 and Bax expressions are in a stoichiometric 1:1 balance in cells reflects the old 'rheostat' model of the Bcl-2 family's protein function, a hypothetical model that was debunked over two decades ago when it was shown that a 1:1 interaction of these proteins was a laboratory artifact [273,274]. Additionally, the predominant anti-apoptotic protein expressed in the retinal cells, including the GCL, is the long form of Bcl-X (Bcl-X_L), which was found to be 16 times more abundant than Bcl-2 [275]. Furthermore, it is even questionable whether Bcl-2 is expressed in adult RGCs and may, in fact, be limited to Müller cells in the retina [276]. Therefore, the reporting of the Bcl-2/Bax ratio may not be a suitable marker to imply apoptosis in RGCs, and instead, the changes in Bcl-X_L expression may correlate better with RGC apoptosis.

6. Conclusions

One of the most common causes of vision loss is glaucoma. Recent data have gained insight into glaucoma pathogenesis, which involves a complex interaction of LC cupping, insufficient ocular blood supply, oxidative stress and neuroinflammation. The use of natural products with antioxidant, anti-inflammatory and anti-apoptotic properties may prove to be beneficial in the treatment of glaucoma. Furthermore, natural products are easily available and are cost effective. Natural products have been shown to protect against RGC loss in in vitro and in vivo preclinical studies, as well as in clinical trials. The present review highlighted various natural products such as GBE, *L. barbarum*, *D. kaki*, *T. wilfordii*, saffron, curcumin, anthocyanin, caffeine, coenzyme Q10 and vitamins B_3, D and E that confer neuroprotective effects on RGCs. Additionally, IOP has been shown to be reduced by treatment with marijuana, baicalein, forskolin, ginsenoside, resveratrol and hesperidin. GB, ginseng, anthocyanins and *L. barbarum* were reported to increase ocular blood flow in glaucoma. Additionally, caffeine administration has been shown to reduce IOP through its adenosine receptor antagonist properties. Although these may serve as alternative targets for glaucoma treatment other than IOP-lowering drugs, more evidence is required to warrant the recommendation of these novel targets. Admittedly, a few of these natural products have had no or limited clinical testing, restricting their potential use in the treatment of glaucoma. Nevertheless, it is important to ensure that the bioavailability and safety of these natural products are checked in well-designed randomized clinical trials to further determine their therapeutic potential in glaucoma.

Author Contributions: Conceptualization, R.H.S. and S.D.; writing—original draft preparation, R.H.S. and S.R.S.; writing—review and editing, S.L.T. and S.D. All authors have read and agreed to the published version of the manuscript.

Funding: This research received no external funding.

Institutional Review Board Statement: Not applicable.

Informed Consent Statement: Not applicable.

Conflicts of Interest: The authors declare no conflict of interest.

References

1. Bourne, R.R.; Taylor, H.R.; Flaxman, S.R.; Keeffe, J.; Leasher, J.; Naidoo, K.; Pesudovs, K.; White, R.A.; Wong, T.Y.; Resnikoff, S.; et al. Number of people blind or visually impaired by glaucoma worldwide and in world regions 1990–2010: A meta-analysis. *PLoS ONE* **2016**, *11*, e0162229. [CrossRef]
2. World Health Organization. *World Report on Vision*; World Health Organization: Geneva, Switzerland, 2019; pp. 1–160.

3. Tham, Y.C.; Li, X.; Wong, T.Y.; Quigley, H.A.; Aung, T.; Cheng, C.Y. Global prevalence of glaucoma and projections of glaucoma burden through 2040: A systematic review and meta-analysis. *Ophthalmology* **2014**, *121*, 2081–2090. [CrossRef]
4. Bajwa, M.N.; Malik, M.I.; Siddiqui, S.A.; Dengel, A.; Shafait, F.; Neumeier, W.; Ahmed, S. Two-stage framework for optic disc localization and glaucoma classification in retinal fundus images using deep learning. *BMC Med. Inform. Decis. Mak.* **2019**, *19*, 136. [CrossRef]
5. Tharmathurai, S.; Muhammad-Ikmal, M.K.; Razak, A.A.; Che-Hamzah, J.; Azhany, Y.; Fazilawati, Q.; Liza-Sharmini, A.T. Depression and severity of glaucoma among older adults in urban and suburban areas. *J. Glaucoma* **2021**, *30*, e205–e212. [CrossRef] [PubMed]
6. Chandramohan, H.; Wan Abdul Halim, W.H.; Azizi, H.A.; Hing, S.T.; Zainal Rain, S.L.; Abdul Rahman, G.Y.; Mohd Khialdin, S. Quality of life and severity of glaucoma: A study using Glaucol-36 Questionnaire at Universiti Kebangsaan Malaysia Medical Centre (UKMMC). *Int. Med. J.* **2017**, *24*, 61–64.
7. Ko, F.; Boland, M.V.; Gupta, P.; Gadkaree, S.K.; Vitale, S.; Guallar, E.; Zhao, D.; Friedman, D.S. Diabetes, triglyceride levels, and other risk factors for glaucoma in the National Health and Nutrition Examination Survey 2005–2008. *Investig. Ophthalmol. Vis. Sci.* **2016**, *57*, 2152–2157. [CrossRef] [PubMed]
8. Kreft, D.; Doblhammer, G.; Guthoff, R.F.; Frech, S. Prevalence, incidence, and risk factors of primary open-angle glaucoma—A cohort study based on longitudinal data from a German public health insurance. *BMC Public Health* **2019**, *19*, 851. [CrossRef]
9. Chen, M.; Yu, X.; Xu, J.; Ma, J.; Chen, X.; Chen, B.; Gu, Y.; Wang, K. Association of gene polymorphisms with primary open angle glaucoma: A systematic review and meta-analysis. *Investig. Ophthalmol. Vis. Sci.* **2019**, *60*, 1105–1121. [CrossRef]
10. Han, X.; Souzeau, E.; Ong, J.S.; An, J.; Siggs, O.M.; Burdon, K.P.; Best, S.; Goldberg, I.; Healey, P.R.; Graham, S.L.; et al. Myocilin gene Gln368Ter variant penetrance and association with glaucoma in population-based and registry-based studies. *JAMA Ophthalmol.* **2019**, *137*, 28–35. [CrossRef] [PubMed]
11. Choplin, N.T. Classification of glaucoma. In *Atlas of Glaucoma*; Choplin, N.T., Traverso, C.E., Eds.; CRC Press: Boca Raton, FL, USA, 2014; pp. 7–12.
12. Khaled Alsirhani, E.; Sahli Abdulaziz Ali, Y.; Mutlaq Ayidh Alosaimi, S.; Ahmed Ali Alkhawajah, S.; Khalifah Alsaqer, S.; Alanazi, M.S.H.; Alanzi, H.O.H.; Alghamdi, L.S.A.; Salman Alfaifi, A.; Almutairi, J.A. An overview of glaucoma diagnosis & management: A literature review. *Arch. Pharm. Pract.* **2020**, *11*, 66–69.
13. Weinreb, R.N.; Leung, C.K.; Crowston, J.G.; Medeiros, F.A.; Friedman, D.S.; Wiggs, J.L.; Martin, K.R. Primary open-angle glaucoma. *Nat. Rev. Dis. Primers* **2016**, *2*, 16067. [CrossRef] [PubMed]
14. Wright, C.; Tawfik, M.A.; Waisbourd, M.; Katz, L.J. Primary angle-closure glaucoma: An update. *Acta Ophthalmol.* **2016**, *94*, 217–225. [CrossRef] [PubMed]
15. Standring, S. *Gray's Anatomy: The Anatomical Basis of Clinical Practice*, 42nd ed.; Standring, S., Ed.; Elsevier Limited: New York, NY, USA, 2020; pp. 1–1606.
16. Li, L.; Song, F. Biomechanical research into lamina cribrosa in glaucoma. *Natl. Sci. Rev.* **2020**, *7*, 1277–1279. [CrossRef]
17. Irnaten, M.; Zhdanov, A.; Brennan, D.; Crotty, T.; Clark, A.; Papkovsky, D.; O'Brien, C. Activation of the NFAT-calcium signaling pathway in human lamina cribrosa cells in glaucoma. *Investig. Ophthalmol. Vis. Sci.* **2018**, *59*, 831–842. [CrossRef] [PubMed]
18. Zhavoronkov, A.; Izumchenko, E.; Kanherkar, R.R.; Teka, M.; Cantor, C.; Manaye, K.; Sidransky, D.; West, M.D.; Makarev, E.; Csoka, A.B. Pro-fibrotic pathway activation in trabecular meshwork and lamina cribrosa is the main driving force of glaucoma. *Cell Cycle* **2016**, *15*, 1643–1652. [CrossRef]
19. Ivers, K.M.; Sredar, N.; Patel, N.B.; Rajagopalan, L.; Queener, H.M.; Twa, M.D.; Harwerth, R.S.; Porter, J. In Vivo changes in lamina cribrosa microarchitecture and optic nerve head structure in early experimental glaucoma. *PLoS ONE* **2015**, *10*, e0134223. [CrossRef]
20. Wu, J.; Du, Y.; Li, J.; Fan, X.; Lin, C.; Wang, N. The influence of different intraocular pressure on lamina cribrosa parameters in glaucoma and the relation clinical implication. *Sci. Rep.* **2021**, *11*, 9755. [CrossRef]
21. Kim, J.A.; Kim, T.W.; Weinreb, R.N.; Lee, E.J.; Girard, M.J.A.; Mari, J.M. Lamina cribrosa morphology predicts progressive retinal nerve fiber layer loss in eyes with suspected glaucoma. *Sci. Rep.* **2018**, *8*, 738. [CrossRef]
22. Maddineni, P.; Kasetti, R.B.; Patel, P.D.; Millar, J.C.; Kiehlbauch, C.; Clark, A.F.; Zode, G.S. CNS axonal degeneration and transport deficits at the optic nerve head precede structural and functional loss of retinal ganglion cells in a mouse model of glaucoma. *Mol. Neurodegener.* **2020**, *15*, 48. [CrossRef]
23. Berdahl, J.P.; Ferguson, T.J.; Samuelson, T.W. Periodic normalization of the translaminar pressure gradient prevents glaucomatous damage. *Med. Hypotheses* **2020**, *144*, 110258. [CrossRef]
24. Li, L.; Bian, A.; Cheng, G.; Zhou, Q. Posterior displacement of the lamina cribrosa in normal-tension and high-tension glaucoma. *Acta Ophthalmol.* **2016**, *94*, e492–e500. [CrossRef]
25. Pircher, A.; Remonda, L.; Weinreb, R.N.; Killer, H.E. Translaminar pressure in Caucasian normal tension glaucoma patients. *Acta Ophthalmol.* **2017**, *95*, e524–e531. [CrossRef]
26. Siaudvytyte, L.; Januleviciene, I.; Ragauskas, A.; Bartusis, L.; Meiliuniene, I.; Siesky, B.; Harris, A. The difference in translaminar pressure gradient and neuroretinal rim area in glaucoma and healthy subjects. *J. Ophthalmol.* **2014**, *2014*, 937360. [CrossRef]
27. Trivli, A.; Koliarakis, I.; Terzidou, C.; Goulielmos, G.N.; Siganos, C.S.; Spandidos, D.A.; Dalianis, G.; Detorakis, E.T. Normal-tension glaucoma: Pathogenesis and genetics. *Exp. Ther. Med.* **2019**, *17*, 563–574. [CrossRef]

28. Burgoyne, C.F. A biomechanical paradigm for axonal insult within the optic nerve head in aging and glaucoma. *Exp. Eye Res.* **2011**, *93*, 120–132. [CrossRef]
29. Shiga, Y.; Kunikata, H.; Aizawa, N.; Kiyota, N.; Maiya, Y.; Yokoyama, Y.; Omodaka, K.; Takahashi, H.; Yasui, T.; Kato, K.; et al. Optic nerve head blood flow, as measured by laser speckle flowgraphy, is significantly reduced in preperimetric glaucoma. *Curr. Eye Res.* **2016**, *41*, 1447–1453. [CrossRef]
30. Shiga, Y.; Aizawa, N.; Tsuda, S.; Yokoyama, Y.; Omodaka, K.; Kunikata, H.; Yasui, T.; Kato, K.; Kurashima, H.; Miyamoto, E.; et al. Preperimetric glaucoma prospective study (PPGPS): Predicting visual field progression with basal optic nerve head blood flow in normotensive PPG eyes. *Transl. Vis. Sci. Technol.* **2018**, *7*, 11. [CrossRef] [PubMed]
31. Rong, X.; Cai, Y.; Li, M.; Chen, X.; Kang, L.; Yang, L. Relationship between nailfold capillary morphology and retinal thickness and retinal vessel density in primary open-angle and angle-closure glaucoma. *Acta Ophthalmol.* **2020**, *98*, e882–e887. [CrossRef] [PubMed]
32. Abegao Pinto, L.; Willekens, K.; Van Keer, K.; Shibesh, A.; Molenberghs, G.; Vandewalle, E.; Stalmans, I. Ocular blood flow in glaucoma—The Leuven Eye Study. *Acta Ophthalmol.* **2016**, *94*, 592–598. [CrossRef] [PubMed]
33. Tobe, L.A.; Harris, A.; Hussain, R.M.; Eckert, G.; Huck, A.; Park, J.; Egan, P.; Kim, N.J.; Siesky, B. The role of retrobulbar and retinal circulation on optic nerve head and retinal nerve fibre layer structure in patients with open-angle glaucoma over an 18-month period. *Br. J. Ophthalmol.* **2015**, *99*, 609–612. [CrossRef]
34. Kiyota, N.; Shiga, Y.; Omodaka, K.; Pak, K.; Nakazawa, T. Time-course changes in optic nerve head blood flow and retinal nerve fiber layer thickness in eyes with open-angle glaucoma. *Ophthalmology* **2021**, *128*, 663–671. [CrossRef] [PubMed]
35. Ahmad, S.S. Controversies in the vascular theory of glaucomatous optic nerve degeneration. *Taiwan J. Ophthalmol.* **2016**, *6*, 182–186. [CrossRef]
36. Chidlow, G.; Wood, J.P.M.; Casson, R.J. Investigations into hypoxia and oxidative stress at the optic nerve head in a rat model of glaucoma. *Front. Neurosci.* **2017**, *11*, 478. [CrossRef] [PubMed]
37. Jassim, A.H.; Fan, Y.; Pappenhagen, N.; Nsiah, N.Y.; Inman, D.M. Oxidative stress and hypoxia modify mitochondrial homeostasis during glaucoma. *Antioxid. Redox Signal.* **2021**, *35*, 1341–1357. [CrossRef]
38. Hondur, G.; Goktas, E.; Yang, X.; Al-Aswad, L.; Auran, J.D.; Blumberg, D.M.; Cioffi, G.A.; Liebmann, J.M.; Suh, L.H.; Trief, D.; et al. Oxidative stress-related molecular biomarker candidates for glaucoma. *Investig. Ophthalmol. Vis. Sci.* **2017**, *58*, 4078–4088. [CrossRef]
39. Li, S.; Shao, M.; Li, Y.; Li, X.; Wan, Y.; Sun, X.; Cao, W. Relationship between oxidative stress biomarkers and visual field progression in patients with primary angle closure glaucoma. *Oxidative Med. Cell. Longev.* **2020**, *2020*, 2701539. [CrossRef] [PubMed]
40. Tang, B.; Li, S.; Cao, W.; Sun, X. The association of oxidative stress status with open-angle glaucoma and exfoliation glaucoma: A systematic review and meta-analysis. *J. Ophthalmol.* **2019**, *2019*, 1803619. [CrossRef]
41. Margeta, M.A.; Lad, E.M.; Proia, A.D. CD163+ macrophages infiltrate axon bundles of postmortem optic nerves with glaucoma. *Graefes Arch. Clin. Exp. Ophthalmol.* **2018**, *256*, 2449–2456. [CrossRef]
42. Tang, B.; Li, S.; Han, J.; Cao, W.; Sun, X. Associations between blood cell profiles and primary open-angle glaucoma: A retrospective case-control study. *Ophthalmic Res.* **2020**, *63*, 413–422. [CrossRef]
43. Huang, P.; Qi, Y.; Xu, Y.S.; Liu, J.; Liao, D.; Zhang, S.S.; Zhang, C. Serum cytokine alteration is associated with optic neuropathy in human primary open angle glaucoma. *J. Glaucoma* **2010**, *19*, 324–330. [CrossRef] [PubMed]
44. Kondkar, A.A.; Azad, T.A.; Almobarak, F.A.; Kalantan, H.; Al-Obeidan, S.A.; Abu-Amero, K.K. Elevated levels of plasma tumor necrosis factor alpha in patients with pseudoexfoliation glaucoma. *Clin. Ophthalmol.* **2018**, *12*, 153–159. [CrossRef]
45. Kondkar, A.A.; Sultan, T.; Almobarak, F.A.; Kalantan, H.; Al-Obeidan, S.A.; Abu-Amero, K.K. Association of increased levels of plasma tumor necrosis factor alpha with primary open-angle glaucoma. *Clin. Ophthalmol.* **2018**, *12*, 701–706. [CrossRef]
46. Duvesh, R.; Puthuran, G.; Srinivasan, K.; Rengaraj, V.; Krishnadas, S.R.; Rajendrababu, S.; Balakrishnan, V.; Ramulu, P.; Sundaresan, P. Multiplex cytokine analysis of aqueous humor from the patients with chronic primary angle closure glaucoma. *Curr. Eye Res.* **2017**, *42*, 1608–1613. [CrossRef]
47. Wang, L.; Cioffi, G.A.; Cull, G.; Dong, J.; Fortune, B. Immunohistologic evidence for retinal glial cell changes in human glaucoma. *Investig. Ophthalmol. Vis. Sci.* **2002**, *43*, 1088–1094.
48. Wang, X.; Tay, S.S.; Ng, Y.K. An immunohistochemical study of neuronal and glial cell reactions in retinae of rats with experimental glaucoma. *Exp. Brain Res.* **2000**, *132*, 476–484. [CrossRef] [PubMed]
49. Harun-Or-Rashid, M.; Inman, D.M. Reduced AMPK activation and increased HCAR activation drive anti-inflammatory response and neuroprotection in glaucoma. *J. Neuroinflamm.* **2018**, *15*, 313. [CrossRef]
50. Hernandez, H.; Roberts, A.L.; McDowell, C.M. Nuclear factor-kappa beta signaling is required for transforming growth factor Beta-2 induced ocular hypertension. *Exp. Eye Res.* **2020**, *191*, 107920. [CrossRef]
51. Yang, X.; Zeng, Q.; Baris, M.; Tezel, G. Transgenic inhibition of astroglial NF-κB restrains the neuroinflammatory and neurodegenerative outcomes of experimental mouse glaucoma. *J. Neuroinflamm.* **2020**, *17*, 252. [CrossRef] [PubMed]
52. Mac Nair, C.E.; Schlamp, C.L.; Montgomery, A.D.; Shestopalov, V.I.; Nickells, R.W. Retinal glial responses to optic nerve crush are attenuated in Bax-deficient mice and modulated by purinergic signaling pathways. *J. Neuroinflamm.* **2016**, *13*, 93. [CrossRef] [PubMed]

53. Howell, G.R.; Soto, I.; Zhu, X.; Ryan, M.; Macalinao, D.G.; Sousa, G.L.; Caddle, L.B.; MacNicoll, K.H.; Barbay, J.M.; Porciatti, V.; et al. Radiation treatment inhibits monocyte entry into the optic nerve head and prevents neuronal damage in a mouse model of glaucoma. *J. Clin. Investig.* **2012**, *122*, 1246–1261. [CrossRef]
54. Reichenbach, A.; Bringmann, A. Glia of the human retina. *Glia* **2020**, *68*, 768–796. [CrossRef]
55. Magi, S.; Piccirillo, S.; Amoroso, S.; Lariccia, V. Excitatory amino acid transporters (EAATs): Glutamate transport and beyond. *Int. J. Mol. Sci.* **2019**, *20*, 5674. [CrossRef] [PubMed]
56. Naskar, R.; Vorwerk, C.K.; Dreyer, E.B. Concurrent downregulation of a glutamate transporter and receptor in glaucoma. *Investig. Ophthalmol. Vis. Sci.* **2000**, *41*, 1940–1944.
57. Harada, T.; Harada, C.; Nakamura, K.; Quah, H.M.; Okumura, A.; Namekata, K.; Saeki, T.; Aihara, M.; Yoshida, H.; Mitani, A.; et al. The potential role of glutamate transporters in the pathogenesis of normal tension glaucoma. *J. Clin. Investig.* **2007**, *117*, 1763–1770. [CrossRef]
58. Osborne, N.N.; Nunez-Alvarez, C.; Joglar, B.; Del Olmo-Aguado, S. Glaucoma: Focus on mitochondria in relation to pathogenesis and neuroprotection. *Eur. J. Pharmacol.* **2016**, *787*, 127–133. [CrossRef]
59. Muench, N.A.; Patel, S.; Maes, M.E.; Donahue, R.J.; Ikeda, A.; Nickells, R.W. The influence of mitochondrial dynamics and function on retinal ganglion cell susceptibility in optic nerve disease. *Cells* **2021**, *10*, 1593. [CrossRef]
60. Evangelho, K.; Mogilevskaya, M.; Losada-Barragan, M.; Vargas-Sanchez, J.K. Pathophysiology of primary open-angle glaucoma from a neuroinflammatory and neurotoxicity perspective: A review of the literature. *Int. Ophthalmol.* **2019**, *39*, 259–271. [CrossRef] [PubMed]
61. Almasieh, M.; Levin, L.A. Neuroprotection in glaucoma: Animal models and clinical trials. *Annu. Rev. Vis. Sci.* **2017**, *3*, 91–120. [CrossRef] [PubMed]
62. Kimura, A.; Noro, T.; Harada, T. Role of animal models in glaucoma research. *Neural Regen. Res.* **2020**, *15*, 1257–1258. [CrossRef]
63. Evangelho, K.; Mastronardi, C.A.; de-la-Torre, A. Experimental models of glaucoma: A powerful translational tool for the future development of new therapies for glaucoma in humans-a review of the literature. *Medicina* **2019**, *55*, 280. [CrossRef] [PubMed]
64. Harada, C.; Kimura, A.; Guo, X.; Namekata, K.; Harada, T. Recent advances in genetically modified animal models of glaucoma and their roles in drug repositioning. *Acta Br. J. Ophthalmol.* **2019**, *103*, 161–166. [CrossRef] [PubMed]
65. Yang, X.L.; van der Merwe, Y.; Sims, J.; Parra, C.; Ho, L.C.; Schuman, J.S.; Wollstein, G.; Lathrop, K.L.; Chan, K.C. Age-related Changes in eye, brain and visuomotor behavior in the DBA/2J mouse model of chronic glaucoma. *Sci. Rep.* **2018**, *8*, 4643. [CrossRef]
66. Porciatti, V.; Chou, T.H.; Feuer, W.J. C57BL/6J, DBA/2J, and DBA/2J. Gpnmb+ mice have different visual signal processing in the inner retina. *Mol. Vis.* **2010**, *16*, 2939–2947.
67. Fujikawa, K.; Iwata, T.; Inoue, K.; Akahori, M.; Kadotani, H.; Fukaya, M.; Watanabe, M.; Chang, Q.; Barnett, E.M.; Swat, W. *VAV2* and *VAV3* as candidate disease genes for spontaneous glaucoma in mice and humans. *PLoS ONE* **2010**, *5*, e9050. [CrossRef]
68. Reinehr, S.; Koch, D.; Weiss, M.; Froemel, F.; Voss, C.; Dick, H.B.; Fuchshofer, R.; Joachim, S.C. Loss of retinal ganglion cells in a new genetic mouse model for primary open-angle glaucoma. *J. Cell. Mol. Med.* **2019**, *23*, 5497–5507. [CrossRef]
69. Tseng, H.C.; Riday, T.T.; McKee, C.; Braine, C.E.; Bomze, H.; Barak, I.; Marean-Reardon, C.; John, S.W.; Philpot, B.D.; Ehlers, M.D. Visual impairment in an optineurin mouse model of primary open-angle glaucoma. *Neurobiol. Aging* **2015**, *36*, 2201–2212. [CrossRef]
70. Sappington, R.M.; Carlson, B.J.; Crish, S.D.; Calkins, D.J. The microbead occlusion model: A paradigm for induced ocular hypertension in rats and mice. *Investig. Ophthalmol. Vis. Sci.* **2010**, *51*, 207–216. [CrossRef]
71. Vaghela, J.J.; Barvaliya, M.J.; Parmar, S.J.; Tripathi, C.R. Evaluation of efficacy of *Aloe vera* (L.) Burm. f. gel solution in methylcellulose-induced ocular hypertension in New Zealand white rabbits. *J. Basic Clin. Physiol. Pharmacol.* **2020**, *32*, 20190158. [CrossRef] [PubMed]
72. Moreno, M.C.; Marcos, H.J.; Oscar Croxatto, J.; Sande, P.H.; Campanelli, J.; Jaliffa, C.O.; Benozzi, J.; Rosenstein, R.E. A new experimental model of glaucoma in rats through intracameral injections of hyaluronic acid. *Exp. Eye Res.* **2005**, *81*, 71–80. [CrossRef] [PubMed]
73. Morrison, J.C.; Johnson, E.C.; Cepurna, W.O. Hypertonic saline injection model of experimental glaucoma in rats. In *Glaucoma. Methods in Molecular Biology*; Jakobs, T., Ed.; Humana Press: New York, NY, USA, 2018; Volume 1695, pp. 11–21.
74. Bai, Y.; Zhu, Y.; Chen, Q.; Xu, J.; Sarunic, M.V.; Saragovi, U.H.; Zhuo, Y. Validation of glaucoma-like features in the rat episcleral vein cauterization model. *Chin. Med. J.* **2014**, *127*, 359–364. [CrossRef]
75. Feng, L.; Chen, H.; Suyeoka, G.; Liu, X. A laser-induced mouse model of chronic ocular hypertension to characterize visual defects. *J. Vis. Exp.* **2013**, *10*, 50440. [CrossRef]
76. Yun, H.; Lathrop, K.L.; Yang, E.; Sun, M.; Kagemann, L.; Fu, V.; Stolz, D.B.; Schuman, J.S.; Du, Y. A laser-induced mouse model with long-term intraocular pressure elevation. *PLoS ONE* **2014**, *9*, e107446. [CrossRef]
77. Biermann, J.; van Oterendorp, C.; Stoykow, C.; Volz, C.; Jehle, T.; Boehringer, D.; Lagreze, W.A. Evaluation of intraocular pressure elevation in a modified laser-induced glaucoma rat model. *Exp. Eye Res.* **2012**, *104*, 7–14. [CrossRef] [PubMed]
78. Biswas, S.; Wan, K.H. Review of rodent hypertensive glaucoma models. *Acta Ophthalmol.* **2019**, *97*, e331–e340. [CrossRef] [PubMed]

79. Honda, S.; Namekata, K.; Kimura, A.; Guo, X.; Harada, C.; Murakami, A.; Matsuda, A.; Harada, T. Survival of alpha and intrinsically photosensitive retinal ganglion cells in NMDA-induced neurotoxicity and a mouse model of normal tension glaucoma. *Investig. Ophthalmol. Vis. Sci.* **2019**, *60*, 3696–3707. [CrossRef]
80. Tang, Z.; Zhang, S.; Lee, C.; Kumar, A.; Arjunan, P.; Li, Y.; Zhang, F.; Li, X. An optic nerve crush injury murine model to study retinal ganglion cell survival. *J. Vis. Exp.* **2011**, *10*, e2685. [CrossRef]
81. Rovere, G.; Nadal-Nicolas, F.M.; Agudo-Barriuso, M.; Sobrado-Calvo, P.; Nieto-Lopez, L.; Nucci, C.; Villegas-Perez, M.P.; Vidal-Sanz, M. Comparison of retinal nerve fiber layer thinning and retinal ganglion cell loss after optic nerve transection in adult albino rats. *Investig. Ophthalmol. Vis. Sci.* **2015**, *56*, 4487–4498. [CrossRef] [PubMed]
82. Ing, E.; Ivers, K.M.; Yang, H.; Gardiner, S.K.; Reynaud, J.; Cull, G.; Wang, L.; Burgoyne, C.F. Cupping in the monkey optic nerve transection model consists of prelaminar tissue thinning in the absence of posterior laminar deformation. *Investig. Ophthalmol. Vis. Sci.* **2016**, *57*, 2914–2927. [CrossRef]
83. Yan, F.; Guo, S.; Chai, Y.; Zhang, L.; Liu, K.; Lu, Q.; Wang, N.; Li, S. Partial optic nerve transection in rats: A model established with a new operative approach to assess secondary degeneration of retinal ganglion cells. *J. Vis. Exp.* **2017**, *10*, e56272. [CrossRef]
84. Minhas, G.; Sharma, J.; Khan, N. Cellular stress response and immune signaling in retinal ischemia-reperfusion injury. *Front. Immunol.* **2016**, *7*, 444. [CrossRef]
85. Hartsock, M.J.; Cho, H.; Wu, L.; Chen, W.J.; Gong, J.; Duh, E.J. A Mouse Model of Retinal Ischemia-Reperfusion Injury through Elevation of Intraocular Pressure. *J. Vis. Exp.* **2016**, *10*, e54065. [CrossRef]
86. Van Bergen, N.J.; Wood, J.P.; Chidlow, G.; Trounce, I.A.; Casson, R.J.; Ju, W.K.; Weinreb, R.N.; Crowston, J.G. Recharacterization of the RGC-5 retinal ganglion cell line. *Investig. Ophthalmol. Vis. Sci.* **2009**, *50*, 4267–4272. [CrossRef]
87. Krishnamoorthy, R.R.; Clark, A.F.; Daudt, D.; Vishwanatha, J.K.; Yorio, T. A forensic path to RGC-5 cell line identification: Lessons learned. *Investig. Ophthalmol. Vis. Sci.* **2013**, *54*, 5712–5719. [CrossRef]
88. Chintalapudi, S.R.; Djenderedjian, L.; Stiemke, A.B.; Steinle, J.J.; Jablonski, M.M.; Morales-Tirado, V.M. Isolation and molecular profiling of primary mouse retinal ganglion cells: Comparison of phenotypes from healthy and glaucomatous retinas. *Front. Aging Neurosci.* **2016**, *8*, 93. [CrossRef]
89. Lusthaus, J.; Goldberg, I. Current management of glaucoma. *Med. J. Aust.* **2019**, *210*, 180–187. [CrossRef] [PubMed]
90. European Glaucoma Society Terminology and Guidelines for Glaucoma, 4th Edition—Chapter 3: Treatment principles and options Supported by the EGS Foundation: Part 1: Foreword; Introduction; Glossary; Chapter 3 Treatment principles and options. *Acta Br. J. Ophthalmol.* **2017**, *101*, 130–195. [CrossRef] [PubMed]
91. Wan, M.J.; Daniel, S.; Kassam, F.; Mutti, G.; Butty, Z.; Kasner, O.; Trope, G.E.; Buys, Y.M. Survey of complementary and alternative medicine use in glaucoma patients. *J. Glaucoma* **2012**, *21*, 79–82. [CrossRef]
92. AlSalman, S.; AlHussaini, M.A.; Khandekar, R.B.; Edward, D.P. The proportion of complementary and alternative medicine utilization among Saudi population for eye care: Cross-sectional study. *Cureus* **2021**, *13*, e13109. [CrossRef] [PubMed]
93. Jaber, D.; Ghannam, R.A.; Rashed, W.; Shehadeh, M.; Zyoud, S.H. Use of complementary and alternative therapies by patients with eye diseases: A hospital-based cross-sectional study from Palestine. *BMC Complementary Med. Ther.* **2021**, *21*, 3. [CrossRef]
94. Achete de Souza, G.; de Marqui, S.V.; Matias, J.N.; Guiguer, E.L.; Barbalho, S.M. Effects of *Ginkgo biloba* on diseases related to oxidative stress. *Planta Med.* **2020**, *86*, 376–386. [CrossRef]
95. Liu, X.G.; Wu, S.Q.; Li, P.; Yang, H. Advancement in the chemical analysis and quality control of flavonoid in *Ginkgo biloba*. *J. Pharm. Biomed. Anal.* **2015**, *113*, 212–225. [CrossRef]
96. Cho, H.K.; Kim, S.; Lee, E.J.; Kee, C. Neuroprotective effect of Ginkgo biloba extract against hypoxic retinal ganglion cell degeneration in vitro and in vivo. *J. Med. Food* **2019**, *22*, 771–778. [CrossRef] [PubMed]
97. Fang, L.; Neutzner, A.; Turtschi, S.; Flammer, J.; Mozaffarieh, M. The effect of Ginkgo biloba and Nifedipine on DNA breaks in circulating leukocytes of glaucoma patients. *Expert Rev. Ophthalmol.* **2015**, *10*, 313–318. [CrossRef]
98. Lee, J.; Sohn, S.W.; Kee, C. Effect of *Ginkgo biloba* extract on visual field progression in normal tension glaucoma. *J. Glaucoma* **2013**, *22*, 780–784. [CrossRef] [PubMed]
99. Shim, S.H.; Kim, J.M.; Choi, C.Y.; Kim, C.Y.; Park, K.H. Ginkgo biloba extract and bilberry anthocyanins improve visual function in patients with normal tension glaucoma. *J. Med. Food* **2012**, *15*, 818–823. [CrossRef]
100. Park, J.W.; Kwon, H.J.; Chung, W.S.; Kim, C.Y.; Seong, G.J. Short-term effects of *Ginkgo biloba* extract on peripapillary retinal blood flow in normal tension glaucoma. *Korean J. Ophthalmol.* **2011**, *25*, 323–328. [CrossRef] [PubMed]
101. Sabaner, M.C.; Dogan, M.; Altin, S.S.; Balaman, C.; Yilmaz, C.; Omur, A.; Zeybek, I.; Palaz, M. *Ginkgo Biloba* affects microvascular morphology: A prospective optical coherence tomography angiography pilot study. *Int. Ophthalmol.* **2021**, *41*, 1053–1061. [CrossRef]
102. Ma, K.; Xu, L.; Zhang, H.; Zhang, S.; Pu, M.; Jonas, J.B. The effect of ginkgo biloba on the rat retinal ganglion cell survival in the optic nerve crush model. *Acta Ophthalmol.* **2010**, *88*, 553–557. [CrossRef]
103. Fan, X.X.; Cao, Z.Y.; Liu, M.X.; Liu, W.J.; Xu, Z.L.; Tu, P.F.; Wang, Z.Z.; Cao, L.; Xiao, W. Diterpene Ginkgolides Meglumine Injection inhibits apoptosis induced by optic nerve crush injury via modulating MAPKs signaling pathways in retinal ganglion cells. *J. Ethnopharmacol.* **2021**, *279*, 114371. [CrossRef]
104. Li, Y.; Cheng, Z.; Wang, K.; Zhu, X.; Ali, Y.; Shu, W.; Bao, X.; Zhu, L.; Fan, X.; Murray, M.; et al. Procyanidin B2 and rutin in *Ginkgo biloba* extracts protect human retinal pigment epithelial (RPE) cells from oxidative stress by modulating Nrf2 and Erk1/2 signalling. *Exp. Eye Res.* **2021**, *207*, 108586. [CrossRef]

105. Yu, H.; Dong, H.; Zhang, Y.; Liu, Q. A network pharmacology-based strategy for predicting the protective mechanism of *Ginkgo biloba* on damaged retinal ganglion cells. *Chin. J. Nat. Med.* **2021**, *19*, 1–13. [CrossRef]
106. Xiao, J.R.; Do, C.W.; To, C.H. Potential therapeutic effects of baicalein, baicalin, and wogonin in ocular disorders. *J. Ocul. Pharmacol. Ther.* **2014**, *30*, 605–614. [CrossRef]
107. Pan, L.; Cho, K.S.; Yi, I.; To, C.H.; Chen, D.F.; Do, C.W. Baicalein, baicalin, and wogonin: Protective effects against ischemia-induced neurodegeneration in the brain and retina. *Oxidative Med. Cell. Longev.* **2021**, *2021*, 8377362. [CrossRef]
108. Song, J.; Kim, Y.S.; Lee, D.; Kim, H. Safety evaluation of root extract of *Pueraria lobata* and *Scutellaria baicalensis* in rats. *BMC Complementary Med. Ther. Vol.* **2020**, *20*, 226. [CrossRef] [PubMed]
109. Yang, J.; Zhang, M.; Song, Q.; Li, S.; Zhao, X.; Kan, L.; Zhu, S. Integrating network pharmacological and experimental models to investigate the therapeutic effects of baicalein in glaucoma. *Chin. Med.* **2021**, *16*, 124. [CrossRef]
110. Chao, H.M.; Chuang, M.J.; Liu, J.H.; Liu, X.Q.; Ho, L.K.; Pan, W.H.; Zhang, X.M.; Liu, C.M.; Tsai, S.K.; Kong, C.W.; et al. Baicalein protects against retinal ischemia by antioxidation, antiapoptosis, downregulation of HIF-1alpha, VEGF, and MMP-9 and upregulation of HO-1. *J. Ocul. Pharmacol. Ther.* **2013**, *29*, 539–549. [CrossRef]
111. Xu, Y.; Yang, B.; Hu, Y.; Lu, L.; Lu, X.; Wang, J.; Xu, F.; Yu, S.; Huang, J.; Liang, X. Wogonin prevents TLR4-NF-κB-medicated neuro-inflammation and improves retinal ganglion cells survival in retina after optic nerve crush. *Oncotarget* **2016**, *7*, 72503–72517. [CrossRef] [PubMed]
112. Zhao, N.; Shi, J.; Xu, H.; Luo, Q.; Li, Q.; Liu, M. Baicalin suppresses glaucoma pathogenesis by regulating the PI3K/AKT signaling in vitro and in vivo. *Bioengineered* **2021**, *12*, 10187–10198. [CrossRef]
113. Gong, L.; Zhu, J. Baicalin alleviates oxidative stress damage in trabecular meshwork cells in vitro. *Naunyn-Schmiedeberg's Arch. Pharmacol.* **2018**, *391*, 51–58. [CrossRef]
114. Srivastava, S.; Misra, A.; Mishra, P.; Shukla, P.; Kumar, M.; Sundaresan, V.; Negi, K.S.; Agrawal, P.K.; Rawat, A.K.S. Molecular and chemotypic variability of forskolin in *Coleus forskohlii* Briq., a high value industrial crop collected from Western Himalayas (India). *RSC Adv.* **2017**, *7*, 8843–8851. [CrossRef]
115. Shim, M.S.; Kim, K.Y.; Ju, W.K. Role of cyclic AMP in the eye with glaucoma. *BMB Rep.* **2017**, *50*, 60–70. [CrossRef] [PubMed]
116. Shahidullah, M.; Wilson, W.S.; Rafiq, K.; Sikder, M.H.; Ferdous, J.; Delamere, N.A. Terbutaline, forskolin and cAMP reduce secretion of aqueous humour in the isolated bovine eye. *PLoS ONE* **2020**, *15*, e0244253. [CrossRef]
117. Majeed, M.; Nagabhushanam, K.; Natarajan, S.; Vaidyanathan, P.; Kumar, S.K. A double-blind, randomized clinical trial to evaluate the efficacy and safety of forskolin eye drops 1% in the treatment of open angle glaucoma—A comparative study. *J. Clin. Trials* **2014**, *4*, 1000184. [CrossRef]
118. Majeed, M.; Nagabhushanam, K.; Natarajan, S.; Vaidyanathan, P.; Karri, S.K.; Jose, J.A. Efficacy and safety of 1% forskolin eye drops in open angle glaucoma—An open label study. *Saudi J. Ophthalmol.* **2015**, *29*, 197–200. [CrossRef]
119. Locri, F.; Cammalleri, M.; Dal Monte, M.; Rusciano, D.; Bagnoli, P. Protective efficacy of a dietary supplement based on forskolin, homotaurine, spearmint extract, and group B vitamins in a mouse model of optic nerve injury. *Nutrients* **2019**, *11*, 2931. [CrossRef] [PubMed]
120. Cammalleri, M.; Dal Monte, M.; Amato, R.; Bagnoli, P.; Rusciano, D. A dietary combination of forskolin with homotaurine, spearmint and B vitamins protects injured retinal ganglion cells in a rodent model of hypertensive glaucoma. *Nutrients* **2020**, *12*, 1189. [CrossRef]
121. Fan, H.; Lin, P.; Kang, Q.; Zhao, Z.L.; Wang, J.; Cheng, J.Y. Metabolism and pharmacological mechanisms of active ingredients in *Erigeron breviscapus*. *Curr. Drug Metab.* **2021**, *22*, 24–39. [CrossRef]
122. Zhong, Y.; Xiang, M.; Ye, W.; Cheng, Y.; Jiang, Y. Visual field protective effect of *Erigeron breviscapus* (vant.) Hand. Mazz. extract on glaucoma with controlled intraocular pressure: A randomized, double-blind, clinical trial. *Drugs R D* **2010**, *10*, 75–82. [CrossRef]
123. Lu, X.J.; Zhang, F.W.; Cheng, L.; Liu, A.Q.; Duan, J.G. Effect on multifocal electroretinogram in persistently elevated intraocular pressure by erigeron breviscapus extract. *J. Ophthalmol.* **2011**, *4*, 349–352. [CrossRef]
124. Zhong, Y.; Xiang, M.; Ye, W.; Huang, P.; Cheng, Y.; Jiang, Y. Neuroprotective effect of *Erigeron Breviscapus (vant) Hand-mazz* extract on retinal ganglion cells in rabbits with chronic elevated intraocular pressure. *Asian Biomed.* **2011**, *5*, 195–203. [CrossRef]
125. Yin, S.; Wang, Z.F.; Duan, J.G.; Ji, L.; Lu, X.J. Extraction (DSX) from *Erigeron breviscapus* modulates outward potassium currents in rat retinal ganglion cells. *Int. J. Ophthalmol.* **2015**, *8*, 1101–1106. [CrossRef]
126. Zhu, J.; Sainulabdeen, A.; Akers, K.; Adi, V.; Sims, J.R.; Yarsky, E.; Yan, Y.; Yu, Y.; Ishikawa, H.; Leung, C.K.; et al. Oral scutellarin treatment ameliorates retinal thinning and visual deficits in experimental glaucoma. *Front. Med.* **2021**, *8*, 681169. [CrossRef] [PubMed]
127. Zhu, J.; Chen, L.; Qi, Y.; Feng, J.; Zhu, L.; Bai, Y.; Wu, H. Protective effects of *Erigeron breviscapus* Hand.- Mazz. (EBHM) extract in retinal neurodegeneration models. *Mol. Vis.* **2018**, *24*, 315–325.
128. Gao, Y.; Wei, Y.; Wang, Y.; Gao, F.; Chen, Z. *Lycium barbarum*: A traditional chinese herb and a promising anti-aging agent. *Aging Dis.* **2017**, *8*, 778–791. [CrossRef]
129. Masci, A.; Carradori, S.; Casadei, M.A.; Paolicelli, P.; Petralito, S.; Ragno, R.; Cesa, S. *Lycium barbarum* polysaccharides: Extraction, purification, structural characterisation and evidence about hypoglycaemic and hypolipidaemic effects. A review. *Food Chem.* **2018**, *254*, 377–389. [CrossRef]

130. Mocan, A.; Vlase, L.; Vodnar, D.C.; Bischin, C.; Hanganu, D.; Gheldiu, A.M.; Oprean, R.; Silaghi-Dumitrescu, R.; Crisan, G. Polyphenolic content, antioxidant and antimicrobial activities of *Lycium barbarum* L. and *Lycium chinense* Mill. leaves. *Molecules* **2014**, *19*, 10056–10073. [CrossRef] [PubMed]
131. Mi, X.S.; Feng, Q.; Lo, A.C.; Chang, R.C.; Lin, B.; Chung, S.K.; So, K.F. Protection of retinal ganglion cells and retinal vasculature by *Lycium barbarum* polysaccharides in a mouse model of acute ocular hypertension. *PLoS ONE* **2012**, *7*, e45469. [CrossRef]
132. Lakshmanan, Y.; Wong, F.S.; Yu, W.Y.; Li, S.Z.; Choi, K.Y.; So, K.F.; Chan, H.H. *Lycium barbarum* polysaccharides rescue neurodegeneration in an acute ocular hypertension rat model under pre- and posttreatment conditions. *Investig. Ophthalmol. Vis. Sci.* **2019**, *60*, 2023–2033. [CrossRef] [PubMed]
133. Mi, X.S.; Chiu, K.; Van, G.; Leung, J.W.; Lo, A.C.; Chung, S.K.; Chang, R.C.; So, K.F. Effect of *Lycium barbarum* polysaccharides on the expression of endothelin-1 and its receptors in an ocular hypertension model of rat glaucoma. *Neural Regen. Res.* **2012**, *7*, 645–651. [CrossRef]
134. Lakshmanan, Y.; Wong, F.S.Y.; Zuo, B.; So, K.F.; Bui, B.V.; Chan, H.H. Posttreatment intervention with *Lycium barbarum* polysaccharides is neuroprotective in a rat model of chronic ocular hypertension. *Investig. Ophthalmol. Vis. Sci.* **2019**, *60*, 4606–4618. [CrossRef]
135. Chu, P.H.; Li, H.Y.; Chin, M.P.; So, K.F.; Chan, H.H. Effect of *Lycium barbarum* (wolfberry) polysaccharides on preserving retinal function after partial optic nerve transection. *PLoS ONE* **2013**, *8*, e81339. [CrossRef] [PubMed]
136. Li, H.; Liang, Y.; Chiu, K.; Yuan, Q.; Lin, B.; Chang, R.C.; So, K.F. *Lycium barbarum* (wolfberry) reduces secondary degeneration and oxidative stress, and inhibits JNK pathway in retina after partial optic nerve transection. *PLoS ONE* **2013**, *8*, e68881. [CrossRef]
137. Liu, L.; Sha, X.Y.; Wu, Y.N.; Chen, M.T.; Zhong, J.X. *Lycium barbarum* polysaccharides protects retinal ganglion cells against oxidative stress injury. *Neural Regen. Res.* **2020**, *15*, 1526–1531. [CrossRef]
138. Liu, Y.; Zhang, Y. *Lycium barbarum* polysaccharides alleviate hydrogen peroxide-induced injury by up-regulation of miR-4295 in human trabecular meshwork cells. *Exp. Mol. Pathol.* **2019**, *106*, 109–115. [CrossRef] [PubMed]
139. Li, H.Y.; Huang, M.; Luo, Q.Y.; Hong, X.; Ramakrishna, S.; So, K.F. *Lycium barbarum* (Wolfberry) increases retinal ganglion cell survival and affects both microglia/macrophage polarization and autophagy after rat partial optic nerve transection. *Cell Transpl.* **2019**, *28*, 607–618. [CrossRef] [PubMed]
140. Mi, X.S.; Feng, Q.; Lo, A.C.Y.; Chang, R.C.; Chung, S.K.; So, K.F. *Lycium barbarum* polysaccharides related RAGE and Abeta levels in the retina of mice with acute ocular hypertension and promote maintenance of blood retinal barrier. *Neural Regen. Res.* **2020**, *15*, 2344–2352. [CrossRef]
141. Xu, S.; Liu, S.; Yan, G. *Lycium barbarum* exerts protection against glaucoma-like injury via inhibition of MMP-9 signaling in vitro. *Med. Sci. Monit.* **2019**, *25*, 9794–9800. [CrossRef] [PubMed]
142. Comes, N.; Buie, L.K.; Borras, T. Evidence for a role of angiopoietin-like 7 (ANGPTL7) in extracellular matrix formation of the human trabecular meshwork: Implications for glaucoma. *Genes Cells* **2011**, *16*, 243–259. [CrossRef]
143. Weinreb, R.N.; Robinson, M.R.; Dibas, M.; Stamer, W.D. Matrix metalloproteinases and glaucoma treatment. *J. Ocul. Pharmacol. Ther.* **2020**, *36*, 208–228. [CrossRef]
144. Yang, D.; So, K.F.; Lo, A.C. *Lycium barbarum* polysaccharide extracts preserve retinal function and attenuate inner retinal neuronal damage in a mouse model of transient retinal ischaemia. *Clin. Exp. Ophthalmol.* **2017**, *45*, 717–729. [CrossRef]
145. He, M.; Pan, H.; Chang, R.C.; So, K.F.; Brecha, N.C.; Pu, M. Activation of the Nrf2/HO-1 antioxidant pathway contributes to the protective effects of Lycium barbarum polysaccharides in the rodent retina after ischemia-reperfusion-induced damage. *PLoS ONE* **2014**, *9*, e84800. [CrossRef] [PubMed]
146. Wu, I.H.; Chan, S.M.; Lin, C.T. The neuroprotective effect of submicron and blended *Lycium barbarum* for experiment retinal ischemia and reperfusion injury in rats. *J. Vet. Med. Sci.* **2020**, *82*, 1719–1728. [CrossRef]
147. Matheus, J.R.V.; Andrade, C.J.d.; Miyahira, R.F.; Fai, A.E.C. Persimmon (Diospyros Kaki L.): Chemical Properties, Bioactive Compounds and Potential Use in the Development of New Products—A Review. *Food Rev. Int.* **2020**, *10*, 1–18. [CrossRef]
148. Hossain, A.; Moon, H.K.; Kim, J.K. Antioxidant properties of Korean major persimmon (*Diospyros kaki*) leaves. *Food Sci. Biotechnol.* **2018**, *27*, 177–184. [CrossRef]
149. Ryul Ahn, H.; Kim, K.A.; Kang, S.W.; Lee, J.Y.; Kim, T.J.; Jung, S.H. Persimmon leaves (*Diospyros kaki*) extract protects optic nerve crush-induced retinal degeneration. *Sci. Rep.* **2017**, *7*, 46449. [CrossRef]
150. Ahn, H.R.; Yang, J.W.; Kim, J.Y.; Lee, C.Y.; Kim, T.J.; Jung, S.H. The intraocular pressure-lowering effect of persimmon leaves (*Diospyros kaki*) in a mouse model of glaucoma. *Int. J. Mol. Sci.* **2019**, *20*, 5268. [CrossRef] [PubMed]
151. Li, J.; Hao, J. Treatment of neurodegenerative diseases with bioactive components of *Tripterygium wilfordii*. *Am. J. Chin. Med.* **2019**, *47*, 769–785. [CrossRef]
152. Chen, S.R.; Dai, Y.; Zhao, J.; Lin, L.; Wang, Y.; Wang, Y. A mechanistic overview of triptolide and celastrol, natural products from *Tripterygium wilfordii* Hook F. *Front. Pharmacol.* **2018**, *9*, 104. [CrossRef] [PubMed]
153. Yang, F.; Wu, L.; Guo, X.; Wang, D.; Li, Y. Improved retinal ganglion cell survival through retinal microglia suppression by a chinese herb extract, triptolide, in the DBA/2J mouse model of glaucoma. *Ocul. Immunol. Inflamm.* **2013**, *21*, 378–389. [CrossRef]
154. Yang, F.; Wang, D.; Wu, L.; Li, Y. Protective effects of triptolide on retinal ganglion cells in a rat model of chronic glaucoma. *Drug Des. Dev. Ther.* **2015**, *9*, 6095–6107. [CrossRef] [PubMed]
155. Li, Y.F.; Zou, Y.F.; Chen, X.F.; Zhang, W. Effect of triptolide on retinal ganglion cell survival in an optic nerve crush model. *Cell Mol. Biol.* **2017**, *63*, 102–107. [CrossRef]

156. Kyung, H.; Kwong, J.M.; Bekerman, V.; Gu, L.; Yadegari, D.; Caprioli, J.; Piri, N. Celastrol supports survival of retinal ganglion cells injured by optic nerve crush. *Brain Res.* **2015**, *1609*, 21–30. [CrossRef] [PubMed]
157. Gu, L.; Kwong, J.M.K.; Yadegari, D.; Yu, F.; Caprioli, J.; Piri, N. The effect of celastrol on the ocular hypertension-induced degeneration of retinal ganglion cells. *Neurosci. Lett.* **2018**, *670*, 89–93. [CrossRef]
158. Rasool, A.; Imran Mir, M.; Zulfajri, M.; Hanafiah, M.M.; Azeem Unnisa, S.; Mahboob, M. Plant growth promoting and antifungal asset of indigenous rhizobacteria secluded from saffron (*Crocus sativus* L.) rhizosphere. *Microb. Pathog.* **2021**, *150*, 104734. [CrossRef] [PubMed]
159. Fernandez-Albarral, J.A.; Ramirez, A.I.; de Hoz, R.; Lopez-Villarin, N.; Salobrar-Garcia, E.; Lopez-Cuenca, I.; Licastro, E.; Inarejos-Garcia, A.M.; Almodovar, P.; Pinazo-Duran, M.D.; et al. Neuroprotective and anti-inflammatory effects of a hydrophilic saffron extract in a model of glaucoma. *Int. J. Mol. Sci.* **2019**, *20*, 4110. [CrossRef]
160. Jabbarpoor Bonyadi, M.H.; Yazdani, S.; Saadat, S. The ocular hypotensive effect of saffron extract in primary open angle glaucoma: A pilot study. *BMC Complement. Altern. Med.* **2014**, *14*, 399. [CrossRef]
161. Maggi, M.A.; Bisti, S.; Picco, C. Saffron: Chemical composition and neuroprotective activity. *Molecules* **2020**, *25*, 5618. [CrossRef]
162. Chen, L.; Qi, Y.; Yang, X. Neuroprotective effects of crocin against oxidative stress induced by ischemia/reperfusion injury in rat retina. *Ophthalmic Res.* **2015**, *54*, 157–168. [CrossRef]
163. Qi, Y.; Chen, L.; Zhang, L.; Liu, W.B.; Chen, X.Y.; Yang, X.G. Crocin prevents retinal ischaemia/reperfusion injury-induced apoptosis in retinal ganglion cells through the PI3K/AKT signalling pathway. *Exp. Eye Res.* **2013**, *107*, 44–51. [CrossRef] [PubMed]
164. Lv, B.; Chen, T.; Xu, Z.; Huo, F.; Wei, Y.; Yang, X. Crocin protects retinal ganglion cells against H_2O_2-induced damage through the mitochondrial pathway and activation of NF-κB. *Int. J. Mol. Med.* **2016**, *37*, 225–232. [CrossRef]
165. Ohno, Y.; Nakanishi, T.; Umigai, N.; Tsuruma, K.; Shimazawa, M.; Hara, H. Oral administration of crocetin prevents inner retinal damage induced by N-methyl-D-aspartate in mice. *Eur. J. Pharmacol.* **2012**, *690*, 84–89. [CrossRef]
166. Ishizuka, F.; Shimazawa, M.; Umigai, N.; Ogishima, H.; Nakamura, S.; Tsuruma, K.; Hara, H. Crocetin, a carotenoid derivative, inhibits retinal ischemic damage in mice. *Eur. J. Pharmacol.* **2013**, *703*, 1–10. [CrossRef]
167. Kevin, T.T.M.; Nur Idanis, A.S.; Anastasha, B.; Mohd Faris, M.R.; Faizah, O.; Taty Anna, K. Curcumin minimises histopathological and immunological progression in the ankle joints of collagen-induced arthritis rats. *Med. Health* **2020**, *15*, 26–36. [CrossRef]
168. Kamal, D.A.M.; Salamt, N.; Yusuf, A.N.M.; Kashim, M.; Mokhtar, M.H. Potential health benefits of curcumin on female reproductive disorders: A review. *Nutrients* **2021**, *13*, 3126. [CrossRef]
169. Yue, Y.K.; Mo, B.; Zhao, J.; Yu, Y.J.; Liu, L.; Yue, C.L.; Liu, W. Neuroprotective effect of curcumin against oxidative damage in BV-2 microglia and high intraocular pressure animal model. *J. Ocul. Pharmacol. Ther.* **2014**, *30*, 657–664. [CrossRef]
170. Buccarello, L.; Dragotto, J.; Hassanzadeh, K.; Maccarone, R.; Corbo, M.; Feligioni, M. Retinal ganglion cell loss in an ex vivo mouse model of optic nerve cut is prevented by curcumin treatment. *Cell Death Discov.* **2021**, *7*, 394. [CrossRef]
171. Esfandiari, A.; Hashemi, F. Protective effects of curcumin on ischemic reperfusion of rat retina. *Comp. Clin. Pathol.* **2019**, *28*, 89–95. [CrossRef]
172. Wang, L.; Li, C.; Guo, H.; Kern, T.S.; Huang, K.; Zheng, L. Curcumin inhibits neuronal and vascular degeneration in retina after ischemia and reperfusion injury. *PLoS ONE* **2011**, *6*, e23194. [CrossRef] [PubMed]
173. Lin, C.; Wu, X. Curcumin protects trabecular meshwork cells from oxidative stress. *Investig. Ophthalmol. Vis. Sci.* **2016**, *57*, 4327–4332. [CrossRef] [PubMed]
174. Luo, Y.; Ding, H.; Li, D.; Luo, J. Curcumin protects trabecular meshwork cells against hydrogen peroxide-induced oxidative stress and apoptosis via Nrf2-keap1 pathway. *Trop. J. Pharm. Res.* **2018**, *17*, 2169–2176. [CrossRef]
175. Azmi, N.; Chee, S.H.; Mohd Fauzi, N.; Jasamai, M.; Kumolosasi, E. Viability and apoptotic effects of green tea (*Camellia sinensis*) methanol extract on human leukemic cell lines. *Acta Pol. Pharm. Drug Res.* **2018**, *75*, 51–58.
176. Yang, Y.; Xu, C.; Chen, Y.; Liang, J.J.; Xu, Y.; Chen, S.L.; Huang, S.; Yang, Q.; Cen, L.P.; Pang, C.P.; et al. Green tea extract ameliorates ischemia-induced retinal ganglion cell degeneration in rats. *Oxidative Med. Cell. Longev.* **2019**, *2019*, 8407206. [CrossRef]
177. Ren, J.L.; Yu, Q.X.; Liang, W.C.; Leung, P.Y.; Ng, T.K.; Chu, W.K.; Pang, C.P.; Chan, S.O. Green tea extract attenuates LPS-induced retinal inflammation in rats. *Sci. Rep.* **2018**, *8*, 429. [CrossRef]
178. Omar, M.S.; Adnan, N.N.; Kumolosasi, E.; Azmi, N.; Damanhuri, N.S.; Buang, F. Green tea (*Camellia sinensis*) extract reduces peptic ulcer induced by *Helicobacter pylori* in Sprague Dawley rats. *Sains Malays.* **2020**, *49*, 2793–2800. [CrossRef]
179. Zhang, W.; Chen, Y.; Gao, L.M.; Cao, Y.N. Neuroprotective role of epigallocatechin-3-gallate in acute glaucoma via the nuclear factor-κB signalling pathway. *Exp. Ther. Med.* **2021**, *22*, 1235. [CrossRef] [PubMed]
180. Shen, C.; Chen, L.; Jiang, L.; Lai, T.Y. Neuroprotective effect of epigallocatechin-3-gallate in a mouse model of chronic glaucoma. *Neurosci. Lett.* **2015**, *600*, 132–136. [CrossRef]
181. Xie, J.; Jiang, L.; Zhang, T.; Jin, Y.; Yang, D.; Chen, F. Neuroprotective effects of Epigallocatechin-3-gallate (EGCG) in optic nerve crush model in rats. *Neurosci. Lett.* **2010**, *479*, 26–30. [CrossRef]
182. Rivera-Perez, J.; Martinez-Rosas, M.; Conde-Castanon, C.A.; Toscano-Garibay, J.D.; Ruiz-Perez, N.J.; Flores, P.L.; Mera Jimenez, E.; Flores-Estrada, J. Epigallocatechin 3-Gallate has a neuroprotective effect in retinas of rabbits with ischemia/reperfusion through the activation of Nrf2/HO-1. *Int. J. Mol. Sci.* **2020**, *21*, 3716. [CrossRef]
183. Chen, F.; Jiang, L.; Shen, C.; Wan, H.; Xu, L.; Wang, N.; Jonas, J.B. Neuroprotective effect of epigallocatechin-3-gallate against N-methyl-D-aspartate-induced excitotoxicity in the adult rat retina. *Acta Ophthalmol.* **2012**, *90*, e609–e615. [CrossRef]

184. Patel, S.; Rauf, A. Adaptogenic herb ginseng (Panax) as medical food: Status quo and future prospects. *Biomed. Pharmacother.* **2017**, *85*, 120–127. [CrossRef]
185. Kang, J.Y.; Kim, D.Y.; Lee, J.S.; Hwang, S.J.; Kim, G.H.; Hyun, S.H.; Son, C.G. Korean red ginseng ameliorates fatigue via modulation of 5-HT and corticosterone in a sleep-deprived mouse model. *Nutrients* **2021**, *13*, 3121. [CrossRef] [PubMed]
186. Lee, K.; Yang, H.; Kim, J.Y.; Choi, W.; Seong, G.J.; Kim, C.Y.; Lee, J.M.; Bae, H.W. Effect of red ginseng on visual function and vision-related quality of life in patients with glaucoma. *J. Ginseng Res.* **2021**, *45*, 676–682. [CrossRef]
187. Bae, H.W.; Kim, J.H.; Kim, S.; Kim, M.; Lee, N.; Hong, S.; Seong, G.J.; Kim, C.Y. Effect of Korean red ginseng supplementation on dry eye syndrome in glaucoma patients—A randomized, double-blind, placebo-controlled study. *J. Ginseng Res.* **2015**, *39*, 7–13. [CrossRef]
188. Kim, N.R.; Kim, J.H.; Kim, C.Y. Effect of Korean red ginseng supplementation on ocular blood flow in patients with glaucoma. *J. Ginseng Res.* **2010**, *34*, 237–245. [CrossRef]
189. Mathiyalagan, R.; Yang, D.C. Ginseng nanoparticles: A budding tool for cancer treatment. *Nanomedicine* **2017**, *12*, 1091–1094. [CrossRef]
190. Zhong, H.; Yu, H.; Chen, B.; Guo, L.; Xu, X.; Jiang, M.; Zhong, Y.; Qi, J.; Huang, P. Protective effect of total Panax notoginseng saponins on retinal ganglion cells of an optic nerve crush injury rat model. *Biomed Res. Int.* **2021**, *2021*, 4356949. [CrossRef]
191. Wang, L.; Cao, T.; Chen, H. Treatment of glaucomatous optic nerve damage using ginsenoside Rg1 mediated by ultrasound targeted microbubble destruction. *Exp. Ther. Med.* **2018**, *15*, 300–304. [CrossRef] [PubMed]
192. Liu, Z.; Chen, J.; Huang, W.; Zeng, Z.; Yang, Y.; Zhu, B. Ginsenoside Rb1 protects rat retinal ganglion cells against hypoxia and oxidative stress. *Mol. Med. Rep.* **2013**, *8*, 1397–1403. [CrossRef] [PubMed]
193. O'Neill-Dee, C.; Spiller, H.A.; Casavant, M.J.; Kistamgari, S.; Chounthirath, T.; Smith, G.A. Natural psychoactive substance-related exposures reported to United States poison control centers, 2000–2017. *Clin. Toxicol.* **2019**, *58*, 813–820. [CrossRef]
194. Katz, J.; Costarides, A.P. Facts vs fiction: The role of cannabinoids in the treatment of glaucoma. *Curr. Ophthalmol. Rep.* **2019**, *7*, 177–181. [CrossRef]
195. Merritt, J.C.; Crawford, W.J.; Alexander, P.C.; Anduze, A.L.; Gelbart, S.S. Effect of marihuana on intraocular and blood pressure in glaucoma. *Ophthalmology* **1980**, *87*, 222–228. [CrossRef]
196. Mosaed, S.; Liu, J.H.K.; Minckler, D.S.; Fitzgerald, R.L.; Grelotti, D.; Sones, E.; Sheils, C.R.; Weinreb, R.N.; Marcotte, T.D. The effect of inhaled cannabis on intraocular pressure in healthy adult subjects. *Ophthalmology* **2021**, *15*, 33–37. [CrossRef]
197. Fischer, K.M.; Ward, D.A.; Hendrix, D.V. Effects of a topically applied 2% delta-9-tetrahydrocannabinol ophthalmic solution on intraocular pressure and aqueous humor flow rate in clinically normal dogs. *Am. J. Vet. Res.* **2013**, *74*, 275–280. [CrossRef] [PubMed]
198. Sweeney, C.; Dudhipala, N.; Thakkar, R.; Mehraj, T.; Marathe, S.; Gul, W.; ElSohly, M.A.; Murphy, B.; Majumdar, S. Effect of surfactant concentration and sterilization process on intraocular pressure-lowering activity of Delta(9)-tetrahydrocannabinol-valine-hemisuccinate (NB1111) nanoemulsions. *Drug Deliv. Transl. Res.* **2021**, *11*, 2096–2107. [CrossRef] [PubMed]
199. Muchtar, S.; Almog, S.; Torracca, M.T.; Saettone, M.F.; Benita, S. A submicron emulsion as ocular vehicle for delta-8-tetrahydrocannabinol: Effect on intraocular pressure in rabbits. *Ophthalmic Res.* **1992**, *24*, 142–149. [CrossRef]
200. Song, Z.H.; Slowey, C.A. Involvement of cannabinoid receptors in the intraocular pressure-lowering effects of WIN55212-2. *J. Pharmacol. Exp. Ther.* **2000**, *292*, 136–139.
201. Pinar-Sueiro, S.; Zorrilla Hurtado, J.A.; Veiga-Crespo, P.; Sharma, S.C.; Vecino, E. Neuroprotective effects of topical CB1 agonist WIN 55212-2 on retinal ganglion cells after acute rise in intraocular pressure induced ischemia in rat. *Exp. Eye Res.* **2013**, *110*, 55–58. [CrossRef]
202. Khoo, H.E.; Azlan, A.; Tang, S.T.; Lim, S.M. Anthocyanidins and anthocyanins: Colored pigments as food, pharmaceutical ingredients, and the potential health benefits. *Food Nutr. Res.* **2017**, *61*, 1361779. [CrossRef]
203. Eng Khoo, H.; Meng Lim, S.; Azlan, A. Evidence-Based Therapeutic Effects of Anthocyanins from Foods. *Pak. J. Nutr.* **2018**, *18*, 1–11. [CrossRef]
204. Ohguro, H.; Ohguro, I.; Katai, M.; Tanaka, S. Two-year randomized, placebo-controlled study of black currant anthocyanins on visual field in glaucoma. *Ophthalmologica* **2012**, *228*, 26–35. [CrossRef] [PubMed]
205. Ohguro, H.; Ohguro, I.; Yagi, S. Effects of black currant anthocyanins on intraocular pressure in healthy volunteers and patients with glaucoma. *J. Ocul. Pharmacol. Ther.* **2013**, *29*, 61–67. [CrossRef]
206. Yoshida, K.; Ohguro, I.; Ohguro, H. Black currant anthocyanins normalized abnormal levels of serum concentrations of endothelin-1 in patients with glaucoma. *J. Ocul. Pharmacol. Ther.* **2013**, *29*, 480–487. [CrossRef] [PubMed]
207. Chuang, L.H.; Wu, A.L.; Wang, N.K.; Chen, K.J.; Liu, L.; Hwang, Y.S.; Yeung, L.; Wu, W.C.; Lai, C.C. The intraocular staining potential of anthocyanins and their retinal biocompatibility: A preclinical study. *Cutan. Ocul. Toxicol.* **2018**, *37*, 359–366. [CrossRef] [PubMed]
208. Nakamura, O.; Moritoh, S.; Sato, K.; Maekawa, S.; Murayama, N.; Himori, N.; Omodaka, K.; Sogon, T.; Nakazawa, T. Bilberry extract administration prevents retinal ganglion cell death in mice via the regulation of chaperone molecules under conditions of endoplasmic reticulum stress. *Clin. Ophthalmol.* **2017**, *11*, 1825–1834. [CrossRef] [PubMed]
209. Wang, Y.; Zhao, L.; Lu, F.; Yang, X.; Deng, Q.; Ji, B.; Huang, F. Retinoprotective effects of bilberry anthocyanins via antioxidant, anti-inflammatory, and anti-apoptotic mechanisms in a visible light-induced retinal degeneration model in pigmented rabbits. *Molecules* **2015**, *20*, 22395–22410. [CrossRef] [PubMed]

210. Ramalingam, A.; Santhanathas, T.; Shaukat Ali, S.; Zainalabidin, S. Resveratrol supplementation protects against nicotine-induced kidney injury. *Int. J. Environ. Res Public Health* **2019**, *16*, 4445. [CrossRef]
211. Avotri, S.; Eatman, D.; Russell-Randall, K. Effects of Resveratrol on inflammatory biomarkers in glaucomatous human trabecular meshwork cells. *Nutrients* **2019**, *11*, 984. [CrossRef]
212. Pirhan, D.; Yuksel, N.; Emre, E.; Cengiz, A.; Kursat Yildiz, D. Riluzole- and resveratrol-induced delay of retinal ganglion cell death in an experimental model of glaucoma. *Curr. Eye Res.* **2016**, *41*, 59–69. [CrossRef]
213. Cao, K.; Ishida, T.; Fang, Y.; Shinohara, K.; Li, X.; Nagaoka, N.; Ohno-Matsui, K.; Yoshida, T. Protection of the retinal ganglion cells: Intravitreal injection of resveratrol in mouse model of ocular hypertension. *Investig. Ophthalmol. Vis. Sci.* **2020**, *61*, 13. [CrossRef]
214. Ye, M.J.; Meng, N. Resveratrol acts via the mitogen-activated protein kinase (MAPK) pathway to protect retinal ganglion cells from apoptosis induced by hydrogen peroxide. *Bioengineered* **2021**, *12*, 4878–4886. [CrossRef]
215. Ji, K.; Li, Z.; Lei, Y.; Xu, W.; Ouyang, L.; He, T.; Xing, Y. Resveratrol attenuates retinal ganglion cell loss in a mouse model of retinal ischemia reperfusion injury via multiple pathways. *Exp. Eye Res.* **2021**, *209*, 108683. [CrossRef]
216. Luo, H.; Zhuang, J.; Hu, P.; Ye, W.; Chen, S.; Pang, Y.; Li, N.; Deng, C.; Zhang, X. Resveratrol delays retinal ganglion cell loss and attenuates gliosis-related inflammation from ischemia-reperfusion injury. *Investig. Ophthalmol. Vis. Sci.* **2018**, *59*, 3879–3888. [CrossRef]
217. Xia, J.; Yang, X.; Chen, W. Resveratrol protects the retina from I/R injury by inhibiting RGCS apoptosis, glial activation and expression of inflammatory factors. *Trop. J. Pharm. Res.* **2020**, *19*, 1221–1226. [CrossRef]
218. Zhang, X.; Feng, Y.; Wang, Y.; Wang, J.; Xiang, D.; Niu, W.; Yuan, F. Resveratrol ameliorates disorders of mitochondrial biogenesis and dynamics in a rat chronic ocular hypertension model. *Life Sci.* **2018**, *207*, 234–245. [CrossRef] [PubMed]
219. Pang, Y.; Qin, M.; Hu, P.; Ji, K.; Xiao, R.; Sun, N.; Pan, X.; Zhang, X. Resveratrol protects retinal ganglion cells against ischemia induced damage by increasing Opa1 expression. *Int. J. Mol. Med.* **2020**, *46*, 1707–1720. [CrossRef] [PubMed]
220. Means, J.C.; Lopez, A.A.; Koulen, P. Resveratrol protects optic nerve head astrocytes from oxidative stress-induced cell death by preventing caspase-3 activation, tau dephosphorylation at Ser(422) and formation of misfolded protein aggregates. *Cell. Mol. Neurobiol.* **2020**, *40*, 911–926. [CrossRef]
221. Gandhi, G.R.; Vasconcelos, A.B.S.; Wu, D.T.; Li, H.B.; Antony, P.J.; Li, H.; Geng, F.; Gurgel, R.Q.; Narain, N.; Gan, R.Y. Citrus flavonoids as promising phytochemicals targeting diabetes and related complications: A systematic review of in vitro and in vivo studies. *Nutrients* **2020**, *12*, 2907. [CrossRef]
222. Himori, N.; Inoue Yanagimachi, M.; Omodaka, K.; Shiga, Y.; Tsuda, S.; Kunikata, H.; Nakazawa, T. The effect of dietary antioxidant supplementation in patients with glaucoma. *Clin. Ophthalmol.* **2021**, *15*, 2293–2300. [CrossRef] [PubMed]
223. Lu, B.; Wang, X.; Ren, Z.; Jiang, H.; Liu, B. Anti-glaucoma potential of hesperidin in experimental glaucoma induced rats. *AMB Express* **2020**, *10*, 94. [CrossRef]
224. Sato, K.; Sato, T.; Ohno-Oishi, M.; Ozawa, M.; Maekawa, S.; Shiga, Y.; Yabana, T.; Yasuda, M.; Himori, N.; Omodaka, K.; et al. CHOP deletion and anti-neuroinflammation treatment with hesperidin synergistically attenuate NMDA retinal injury in mice. *Exp. Eye Res.* **2021**, *213*, 108826. [CrossRef]
225. Maekawa, S.; Sato, K.; Fujita, K.; Daigaku, R.; Tawarayama, H.; Murayama, N.; Moritoh, S.; Yabana, T.; Shiga, Y.; Omodaka, K.; et al. The neuroprotective effect of hesperidin in NMDA-induced retinal injury acts by suppressing oxidative stress and excessive calpain activation. *Sci. Rep.* **2017**, *7*, 6885. [CrossRef]
226. Xin, X.; Li, Y.; Liu, H. Hesperidin ameliorates hypobaric hypoxia-induced retinal impairment through activation of Nrf2/HO-1 pathway and inhibition of apoptosis. *Sci. Rep.* **2020**, *10*, 19426. [CrossRef] [PubMed]
227. Md Isa, Z.; Anuar, A.A.; Danial Azmi, A.; Selvan, S.T.; Hisham, N.S.; Yong, Z.Q. Does caffeine intake influence mental health of medical students? *Malays. J. Public Health Med.* **2021**, *21*, 22–28. [CrossRef]
228. Tran, T.; Niyadurupola, N.; O'Connor, J.; Ang, G.S.; Crowston, J.; Nguyen, D. Rise of intraocular pressure in a caffeine test versus the water drinking test in patients with glaucoma. *Clin. Exp. Ophthalmol.* **2014**, *42*, 427–432. [CrossRef] [PubMed]
229. Chandra, P.; Gaur, A.; Varma, S. Effect of caffeine on the intraocular pressure in patients with primary open angle glaucoma. *Clin. Ophthalmol.* **2011**, *5*, 1623–1629. [CrossRef]
230. Vera, J.; Redondo, B.; Molina, R.; Bermudez, J.; Jimenez, R. Effects of caffeine on intraocular pressure are subject to tolerance: A comparative study between low and high caffeine consumers. *Psychopharmacology* **2019**, *236*, 811–819. [CrossRef] [PubMed]
231. Redondo, B.; Vera, J.; Molina, R.; Jimenez, R. Short-term effects of caffeine intake on anterior chamber angle and intraocular pressure in low caffeine consumers. *Graefes Arch. Clin. Exp. Ophthalmol.* **2020**, *258*, 613–619. [CrossRef] [PubMed]
232. Kim, J.; Aschard, H.; Kang, J.H.; Lentjes, M.A.H.; Do, R.; Wiggs, J.L.; Khawaja, A.P.; Pasquale, L.R.; Modifiable Risk Factors for Glaucoma Collaboration. Intraocular pressure, glaucoma, and dietary caffeine consumption: A gene-diet interaction study from the UK Biobank. *Ophthalmology* **2021**, *128*, 866–876. [CrossRef]
233. Nakano, E.; Miyake, M.; Hosoda, Y.; Mori, Y.; Suda, K.; Kameda, T.; Ikeda-Ohashi, H.; Tabara, Y.; Yamashiro, K.; Tamura, H.; et al. Relationship between intraocular pressure and coffee consumption in a Japanese population without glaucoma: The Nagahama study. *Ophthalmol. Glaucoma* **2021**, *4*, 268–276. [CrossRef]
234. Madeira, M.H.; Ortin-Martinez, A.; Nadal-Nicolas, F.; Ambrosio, A.F.; Vidal-Sanz, M.; Agudo-Barriuso, M.; Santiago, A.R. Caffeine administration prevents retinal neuroinflammation and loss of retinal ganglion cells in an animal model of glaucoma. *Sci. Rep.* **2016**, *6*, 27532. [CrossRef]

235. Boia, R.; Elvas, F.; Madeira, M.H.; Aires, I.D.; Rodrigues-Neves, A.C.; Tralhao, P.; Szabo, E.C.; Baqi, Y.; Muller, C.E.; Tome, A.R.; et al. Treatment with A_{2A} receptor antagonist KW6002 and caffeine intake regulate microglia reactivity and protect retina against transient ischemic damage. *Cell Death Dis.* 2017, 8, e3065. [CrossRef]
236. Conti, F.; Lazzara, F.; Romano, G.L.; Platania, C.B.M.; Drago, F.; Bucolo, C. Caffeine protects against retinal inflammation. *Front. Pharmacol.* 2022, 12, 824885. [CrossRef]
237. Zulfakar, M.H.; Chan, L.M.; Rehman, K.; Wai, L.K.; Heard, C.M. Coenzyme Q10-loaded fish oil-based bigel system: Probing the delivery across porcine skin and possible interaction with fish oil fatty acids. *AAPS PharmSciTech.* 2018, 19, 1116–1123. [CrossRef] [PubMed]
238. Ekeuku, S.O.; Ima-Nirwana, S.; Chin, K.Y. Skeletal protective effect of Coenzyme Q10: A review. *Int. J. Pharmacol.* 2020, 16, 181–190. [CrossRef]
239. Lee, D.; Kim, K.Y.; Shim, M.S.; Kim, S.Y.; Ellisman, M.H.; Weinreb, R.N.; Ju, W.K. Coenzyme Q10 ameliorates oxidative stress and prevents mitochondrial alteration in ischemic retinal injury. *Apoptosis* 2014, 19, 603–614. [CrossRef]
240. Lee, D.; Shim, M.S.; Kim, K.Y.; Noh, Y.H.; Kim, H.; Kim, S.Y.; Weinreb, R.N.; Ju, W.K. Coenzyme Q10 inhibits glutamate excitotoxicity and oxidative stress-mediated mitochondrial alteration in a mouse model of glaucoma. *Investig. Ophthalmol. Vis. Sci.* 2014, 55, 993–1005. [CrossRef] [PubMed]
241. Davis, B.M.; Tian, K.; Pahlitzsch, M.; Brenton, J.; Ravindran, N.; Butt, G.; Malaguarnera, G.; Normando, E.M.; Guo, L.; Cordeiro, M.F. Topical Coenzyme Q10 demonstrates mitochondrial-mediated neuroprotection in a rodent model of ocular hypertension. *Mitochondrion* 2017, 36, 114–123. [CrossRef]
242. Parisi, V.; Centofanti, M.; Gandolfi, S.; Marangoni, D.; Rossetti, L.; Tanga, L.; Tardini, M.; Traina, S.; Ungaro, N.; Vetrugno, M.; et al. Effects of coenzyme Q10 in conjunction with vitamin E on retinal-evoked and cortical-evoked responses in patients with open-angle glaucoma. *J. Glaucoma* 2014, 23, 391–404. [CrossRef] [PubMed]
243. Ekicier Acar, S.; Saricaoglu, M.S.; Colak, A.; Aktas, Z.; Sepici Dincel, A. Neuroprotective effects of topical coenzyme Q10 + vitamin E in mechanic optic nerve injury model. *Eur. J. Ophthalmol.* 2020, 30, 714–722. [CrossRef]
244. Wang, S.Y.; Singh, K.; Lin, S.C. Glaucoma and vitamins A, C, and E supplement intake and serum levels in a population-based sample of the United States. *Eye* 2013, 27, 487–494. [CrossRef]
245. Li, S.; Li, D.; Shao, M.; Cao, W.; Sun, X. Lack of association between serum vitamin B_6, vitamin B_{12}, and vitamin D levels with different types of glaucoma: A systematic review and meta-analysis. *Nutrients* 2017, 9, 636. [CrossRef]
246. Ramdas, W.D.; Schouten, J.; Webers, C.A.B. The effect of vitamins on glaucoma: A systematic review and meta-analysis. *Nutrients* 2018, 10, 359. [CrossRef] [PubMed]
247. Williams, P.A.; Harder, J.M.; Foxworth, N.E.; Cochran, K.E.; Philip, V.M.; Porciatti, V.; Smithies, O.; John, S.W. Vitamin B_3 modulates mitochondrial vulnerability and prevents glaucoma in aged mice. *Science* 2017, 355, 756–760. [CrossRef] [PubMed]
248. Chou, T.H.; Romano, G.L.; Amato, R.; Porciatti, V. Nicotinamide-rich diet in DBA/2J mice preserves retinal ganglion cell metabolic function as assessed by PERG adaptation to flicker. *Nutrients* 2020, 12, 1910. [CrossRef]
249. Hui, F.; Tang, J.; Williams, P.A.; McGuinness, M.B.; Hadoux, X.; Casson, R.J.; Coote, M.; Trounce, I.A.; Martin, K.R.; van Wijngaarden, P.; et al. Improvement in inner retinal function in glaucoma with nicotinamide (vitamin B_3) supplementation: A crossover randomized clinical trial. *Clin. Exp. Ophthalmol.* 2020, 48, 903–914. [CrossRef]
250. Vukovic Arar, Z.; Knezevic Pravecek, M.; Miskic, B.; Vatavuk, Z.; Vukovic Rodriguez, J.; Sekelj, S. Association between serum vitamin D level and glaucoma in women. *Acta Clin. Croat.* 2016, 55, 203–208. [CrossRef] [PubMed]
251. Lv, Y.; Yao, Q.; Ma, W.; Liu, H.; Ji, J.; Li, X. Associations of vitamin D deficiency and vitamin D receptor (Cdx-2, Fok I, Bsm I and Taq I) polymorphisms with the risk of primary open-angle glaucoma. *BMC Ophthalmol.* 2016, 16, 116. [CrossRef]
252. Kocaturk, T.; Bekmez, S.; Unubol, M. Effects of vitamin D deficiency on intraocular pressure values obtained by ocular response analyzer. *Int. Ophthalmol.* 2020, 40, 697–701. [CrossRef]
253. Kutuzova, G.D.; Gabelt, B.T.; Kiland, J.A.; Hennes-Beann, E.A.; Kaufman, P.L.; DeLuca, H.F. 1α,25-Dihydroxyvitamin D_3 and its analog, 2-methylene-19-nor-(20S)-1α,25-dihydroxyvitamin D_3 (2MD), suppress intraocular pressure in non-human primates. *Arch. Biochem. Biophys.* 2012, 518, 53–60. [CrossRef]
254. Lazzara, F.; Amato, R.; Platania, C.B.M.; Conti, F.; Chou, T.H.; Porciatti, V.; Drago, F.; Bucolo, C. 1α,25-dihydroxyvitamin D_3 protects retinal ganglion cells in glaucomatous mice. *J. Neuroinflamm.* 2021, 18, 206. [CrossRef]
255. Ko, M.L.; Peng, P.H.; Hsu, S.Y.; Chen, C.F. Dietary deficiency of vitamin E aggravates retinal ganglion cell death in experimental glaucoma of rats. *Curr. Eye Res.* 2010, 35, 842–849. [CrossRef]
256. Özmen, C.; Göçün, P.; Değim, Z.; Özkan, Y.; Onol, M.; Aktaş, Z. Retinal ganglion cell protection via topical and systemic alpha-tocopherol administration in optic nerve crush model of rat. *Turk. J. Ophthalmol.* 2013, 43, 161–166. [CrossRef]
257. Yellanki, S.K.; Anna, B.; Kishan, M.R. Preparation and in vivo evaluation of sodium alginate-poly (vinyl alcohol) electrospun nanofibers of forskolin for glaucoma treatment. *Pak. J. Pharm. Sci.* 2019, 32, 669–674. [PubMed]
258. Davis, B.M.; Pahlitzsch, M.; Guo, L.; Balendra, S.; Shah, P.; Ravindran, N.; Malaguarnera, G.; Sisa, C.; Shamsher, E.; Hamze, H.; et al. Topical curcumin nanocarriers are neuroprotective in eye disease. *Sci. Rep.* 2018, 8, 11066. [CrossRef] [PubMed]
259. Cheng, Y.H.; Ko, Y.C.; Chang, Y.F.; Huang, S.H.; Liu, C.J. Thermosensitive chitosan-gelatin-based hydrogel containing curcumin-loaded nanoparticles and latanoprost as a dual-drug delivery system for glaucoma treatment. *Exp. Eye Res.* 2019, 179, 179–187. [CrossRef] [PubMed]

260. Natesan, S.; Pandian, S.; Ponnusamy, C.; Palanichamy, R.; Muthusamy, S.; Kandasamy, R. Co-encapsulated resveratrol and quercetin in chitosan and peg modified chitosan nanoparticles: For efficient intra ocular pressure reduction. *Int. J. Biol. Macromol.* **2017**, *104*, 1837–1845. [CrossRef] [PubMed]
261. World Health Organization. *Research Guidelines for Evaluating the Safety and Efficacy of Herbal Medicines*; World Health Organization: Geneva, Switzerland, 1993; p. 89.
262. Suntar, I. Importance of ethnopharmacological studies in drug discovery: Role of medicinal plants. *Phytochem. Rev.* **2020**, *19*, 1199–1209. [CrossRef]
263. Vetrugno, M.; Uva, M.G.; Russo, V.; Iester, M.; Ciancaglini, M.; Brusini, P.; Centofanti, M.; Rossetti, L.M. Oral administration of forskolin and rutin contributes to intraocular pressure control in primary open angle glaucoma patients under maximum tolerated medical therapy. *J. Ocul. Pharmacol. Ther.* **2012**, *28*, 536–541. [CrossRef]
264. Nebbioso, M.; Rusciano, D.; Pucci, B.; Zicari, A.M.; Grenga, R.; Pescocolido, N. Treatment of glaucomatous patients by means of food supplement to reduce the ocular discomfort: A double blind randomized trial. *Eur. Rev. Med. Pharmacol. Sci.* **2013**, *17*, 1117–1122.
265. Nebbioso, M.; Belcaro, G.; Librando, A.; Rusciano, D.; Steigerwalt, R.D., Jr.; Pescosolido, N. Forskolin and rutin prevent intraocular pressure spikes after Nd:YAG laser iridotomy. *Panminerva Med.* **2012**, *54*, 77–82.
266. Mutolo, M.G.; Albanese, G.; Rusciano, D.; Pescosolido, N. Oral Administration of forskolin, homotaurine, carnosine, and folic acid in patients with primary open angle glaucoma: Changes in intraocular pressure, pattern electroretinogram amplitude, and foveal sensitivity. *J. Ocul. Pharmacol. Ther.* **2016**, *32*, 178–183. [CrossRef]
267. Rolle, T.; Dallorto, L.; Rossatto, S.; Curto, D.; Nuzzi, R. Assessing the Performance of daily intake of a homotaurine, carnosine, forskolin, vitamin B2, vitamin B6, and magnesium based food supplement for the maintenance of visual function in patients with primary open angle glaucoma. *J. Ophthalmol.* **2020**, *2020*, 7879436. [CrossRef] [PubMed]
268. Manabe, K.; Kaidzu, S.; Tsutsui, A.; Mochiji, M.; Matsuoka, Y.; Takagi, Y.; Miyamoto, E.; Tanito, M. Effects of French maritime pine bark/bilberry fruit extracts on intraocular pressure for primary open-angle glaucoma. *J. Clin. Biochem. Nutr.* **2021**, *68*, 67–72. [CrossRef]
269. Yadav, K.S.; Rajpurohit, R.; Sharma, S. Glaucoma: Current treatment and impact of advanced drug delivery systems. *Life Sci.* **2019**, *221*, 362–376. [CrossRef]
270. Gupta, R.; Patil, B.; Shah, B.M.; Bali, S.J.; Mishra, S.K.; Dada, T. Evaluating eye drop instillation technique in glaucoma patients. *J. Glaucoma* **2012**, *21*, 189–192. [CrossRef] [PubMed]
271. Rahic, O.; Tucak, A.; Omerovic, N.; Sirbubalo, M.; Hindija, L.; Hadziabdic, J.; Vranic, E. Novel drug delivery systems fighting glaucoma: Formulation obstacles and solutions. *Pharmaceutics* **2020**, *13*, 28. [CrossRef] [PubMed]
272. Li, J.; Jin, X.; Yang, Y.; Zhang, L.; Liu, R.; Li, Z. Trimethyl chitosan nanoparticles for ocular baicalein delivery: Preparation, optimization, in vitro evaluation, in vivo pharmacokinetic study and molecular dynamics simulation. *Int. J. Biol. Macromol.* **2020**, *156*, 749–761. [CrossRef] [PubMed]
273. Hsu, Y.T.; Youle, R.J. Nonionic detergents induce dimerization among members of the Bcl-2 family. *J. Biol. Chem.* **1997**, *272*, 13829–13834. [CrossRef]
274. Hsu, Y.T.; Youle, R.J. Bax in murine thymus is a soluble monomeric protein that displays differential detergent-induced conformations. *J. Biol. Chem.* **1998**, *273*, 10777–10783. [CrossRef]
275. Levin, L.A.; Schlamp, C.L.; Spieldoch, R.L.; Geszvain, K.M.; Nickells, R.W. Identification of the *bcl-2* family of genes in the rat retina. *Investig. Ophthalmol. Vis. Sci.* **1997**, *38*, 2545–2553.
276. Chen, S.T.; Garey, L.J.; Jen, L.S. Bcl-2 proto-oncogene protein immunoreactivity in normally developing and axotomised rat retinas. *Neurosci. Lett.* **1994**, *172*, 11–14. [CrossRef]

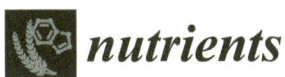

Article

Identification of Inhibitory Activities of Dietary Flavonoids against URAT1, a Renal Urate Re-Absorber: In Vitro Screening and Fractional Approach Focused on Rooibos Leaves

Yu Toyoda [1,†], Tappei Takada [1,*,†], Hiroki Saito [1,2,†], Hiroshi Hirata [2,†], Ami Ota-Kontani [2], Youichi Tsuchiya [2] and Hiroshi Suzuki [1]

[1] Department of Pharmacy, The University of Tokyo Hospital, 7-3-1 Hongo, Bunkyo-ku, Tokyo 113-8655, Japan; ytoyoda-tky@umin.ac.jp (Y.T.); hiroki.saito@sapporoholdings.co.jp (H.S.); suzukihi-tky@umin.ac.jp (H.S.)

[2] Frontier Laboratories for Value Creation, Sapporo Holdings Ltd., 10 Okatome, Yaizu, Shizuoka 425-0013, Japan; xjtpt341@gmail.com (H.H.); ami.ota@sapporoholdings.co.jp (A.O.-K.); yoichi.tsuchiya@sapporoholdings.co.jp (Y.T.)

* Correspondence: tappei-tky@umin.ac.jp; Tel.: +81-3-3815-5411 (ext. 37514)

† These authors contributed equally to this work.

Abstract: Hyperuricemia, a lifestyle-related disease characterized by elevated serum urate levels, is the main risk factor for gout; therefore, the serum urate-lowering effects of human diets or dietary ingredients have attracted widespread interest. As Urate transporter 1 (URAT1) governs most urate reabsorption from primary urine into blood, URAT1 inhibition helps decrease serum urate levels by increasing the net renal urate excretion. In this study, we used a cell-based urate transport assay to investigate the URAT1-inhibitory effects of 162 extracts of plant materials consumed by humans. Among these, we focused on *Aspalathus linearis*, the source of rooibos tea, to explore its active ingredients. Using liquid–liquid extraction with subsequent column chromatography, as well as spectrometric analyses for chemical characterization, we identified quercetin as a URAT1 inhibitor. We also investigated the URAT1-inhibitory activities of 23 dietary ingredients including nine flavanols, two flavanonols, two flavones, two isoflavonoids, eight chalcones, and a coumarin. Among the tested authentic chemicals, fisetin and quercetin showed the strongest and second-strongest URAT1-inhibitory activities, with IC_{50} values of 7.5 and 12.6 µM, respectively. Although these effects of phytochemicals should be investigated further in human studies, our findings may provide new clues for using nutraceuticals to promote health.

Keywords: SLC22A12; quercetin; fisetin; uricosuric activity; anti-hyperuricemia; functional food; transporter; uric acid; health promotion; rooibos tea

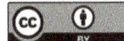

1. Introduction

Hyperuricemia is a lifestyle-related disease with an increasing global prevalence [1]. Sustained elevation of serum urate is a major risk factor for developing gout [2], the most common form of inflammatory arthritis. Therefore, serum urate management within appropriate ranges is important for health care. In the human body, uric acid is the end-product of purine metabolism because functional uricase (the urate-degrading enzyme) is genetically lost [3]. Consequently, serum urate levels are determined by the balance between the production and excretion of the urate—the predominant form of uric acid under physiological pH conditions. The kidney is responsible for the daily elimination of approximately two-thirds of urate [4]. However, the net proportion of urate secreted into the urine is only 3–10% of the urate filtered by the renal glomerulus [5]. This is because most of the filtered urate is re-absorbed from primary urine into the blood by renal proximal tubular cells through the urate transporter 1 (URAT1)-mediated pathway [6]. Therefore, inhibition of this route increases the net urinary excretion of urate, resulting in decreased serum urate.

URAT1, also known as SLC22A12, is a physiologically important renal urate reabsorber; its dysfunction causes renal hypouricemia type 1 [6,7], a genetic disorder characterized by impaired renal urate reabsorption, associated with extremely low serum urate levels (serum urate ≤ 2 mg/dL [8,9]; normal range: 3.0 to 7.0 mg/dL). Among the already identified urate reabsorption transporters that are expressed on the renal cell apical membrane, URAT1 has the highest influence on serum urate levels. Accordingly, in hyperuricemia, this urate transporter is considered a pharmacological target of some anti-hyperuricemic agents that promote renal urate excretion. The uricosuric effect based on URAT1 inhibition forms the mechanism of action for SUA-lowering drugs such as benzbromarone [6] and lesinurad [10]. Based on this information, daily consumption of food ingredients with URAT1-inhibitory activity may bring a beneficial effect on serum urate management in individuals with high serum urate levels. Hence, the exploration of URAT1-inhibitory ingredients in the human diet has received increasing attention. Previously, we and other groups have successfully identified food ingredients from *Citrus* flavonoids [11], coumarins [12], wood pigments [13], and fatty acids [14]. As just described, natural products are promising sources of URAT1-inhibitory compounds, encouraging us to explore such ingredients in various ordinary plants purchased in the market.

We herein investigated the URAT1-inhibitory activities of 162 dietary plant products employing a mammalian cell-based urate transport assay. Via screening plant extracts followed by liquid–liquid extraction and column chromatography, we successfully identified quercetin, a flavonol, as a novel URAT1 inhibitor with a half-maximal inhibitory concentration (IC$_{50}$) of 12.6 µM from rooibos (*Aspalathus linearis*) leaves. Focusing on other dietary flavonoids, we further investigated their effects on URAT1 function, and among the tested compounds in this study, we identified fisetin as the strongest URAT1 inhibitory ingredient with an IC$_{50}$ of 7.5 µM. The experimental procedures described below and the information obtained on URAT1-inhibitory activities in various plant extracts will be useful for further identification of natural product-derived URAT1 inhibitors.

2. Materials and Methods

2.1. Materials and Resources

The critical materials and resources are summarized in Table 1. All other chemicals were of analytical grade and were commercially available. All authentic chemicals were re-dissolved in dimethyl sulfoxide (DMSO) (Nacalai Tesque, Kyoto, Japan). Each inhibition assay was carried out with the same lot of the expression vector for URAT1 (URAT1 wild-type inserted in pEGFP-C1) or mock (empty vector, i.e., pEGFP-C1), derived from our previous study [14]. Urate transport assay (see below) using these vectors was used and validated in previous studies [11,14,15]. The plant materials (Table A1) were purchased, between July 2016 and July 2017, from local supermarkets in Shizuoka, Japan.

2.2. Preparation of Plant Ethanolic Extracts

Plant extracts were prepared as described in our previous studies [16,17], with some modifications. In brief, after fruits were cleaned, the peels and pulps were separated carefully. The fresh and dried materials (see Table A1) were chopped finely using a knife and ground using a mill (Crush Millser IFM-C20Gb) (Iwatani, Tokyo, Japan), respectively. In the next extraction step, the preprocessed plant material (approximately 50 g) was immersed in 100 mL of ethanol, sonicated for 5 min, and stirred for 30 min at room temperature, and the suspension was passed through a filter paper. Then, the filtrate was evaporated and dissolved in methanol. The extract was dried, weighed, dissolved in DMSO at 2 mg/mL (2000 ppm), and stored at $-20\,°C$ until use. Next, 5 µL of the resulting solution was mixed with 245 µL of Cl$^-$-free transport buffer (Buffer T2: 125 mM Na-gluconate, 25 mM HEPES, 5.6 mM D-glucose, 4.8 mM K-gluconate, 1.3 mM Ca-gluconate, 1.2 mM

MgSO$_4$, 1.2 mM KH$_2$PO$_4$, and pH 7.4), and this clear liquid (250 µL) was used for the urate transport assay (final concentration: 20 ppm with 1% DMSO) as described below.

Table 1. Key resources.

REAGENT or RESOURCE	SOURCE	IDENTIFIER
Chemicals		
Clear-sol II	Nacalai Tesque	Cat# 09136-83
[8-^{14}C]-Uric acid (53 mCi/mmol)	American Radiolabeled Chemicals	Cat# ARC0513
Dimethyl Sulfoxide	Nacalai Tesque	Cat# 13445-74; CAS: 67-68-5
Ethanol	FUJIFILM Wako Pure Chemical	057-00451; CAS: 64-17-5
Methanol	FUJIFILM Wako Pure Chemical	137-01823; CAS: 67-56-1
n-Hexane	FUJIFILM Wako Pure Chemical	085-00416; CAS: 110-54-3
Ethyl acetate	FUJIFILM Wako Pure Chemical	051-00356; CAS: 141-78-6
n-Butanol	FUJIFILM Wako Pure Chemical	026-03326; CAS: 71-36-3
Polyethelenimine "MAX"	Polysciences	Cat# 24765; CAS: 49553-93-7
2′-Hydroxychalcone	Tokyo Chemical Industry	Cat# H0385; CAS: 1214-47-7; Purity: >98%
3-Hydroxyflavone	Tokyo Chemical Industry	Cat# H0379; CAS: 577-85-5; Purity: ≥98%
4-Hydroxychalcone	Tokyo Chemical Industry	Cat# H0955; CAS: 20426-12-4; Purity: >96%
4′-Hydroxychalcone	Tokyo Chemical Industry	Cat# H0945; CAS: 2657-25-2; Purity: >95%
Aesculetin	FUJIFILM Wako Pure Chemical	Cat# A15393; CAS: 305-01-1; Purity: N/A
Apigenin	FUJIFILM Wako Pure Chemical	Cat# 016-18911; CAS: 520-36-5; Purity: ≥95%
Cardamonin	R&D systems	Cat# 2509/10; CAS: 19309-14-9; Purity: ≥98%
Daidzein	FUJIFILM Wako Pure Chemical	Cat# 043-28071; CAS: 486-66-8; Purity: ≥98%
Dihydromyricetin	EXTRASYNTHESE	Cat# 1351-10 mg; CAS: 27200-12-0; Purity: ≥95%
Fisetin	LKT Labs	Cat# F3473; CAS: 528-48-3; Purity: ≥97%
Galangin	ChromaDex	Cat# ASB-00007030-010; CAS: 548-83-4; Purity: N/A
Genistein	FUJIFILM Wako Pure Chemical	Cat# 073-05531; CAS: 446-72-0; Purity: ≥98%
Gossypetin	ChromaDex	Cat# ASB-00007390-010; CAS: 489-35-0; Purity: N/A
Isoliquiritigenin	Tokyo Chemical Industry	Cat# I0822; CAS: 961-29-5; Purity: ≥97%
Kaempferol	FUJIFILM Wako Pure Chemical	Cat# 110-00451; CAS: 520-18-3; Purity: ≥95%
Luteolin	Cayman Chemical	Cat# 10004161; CAS: 491-70-3; Purity: ≥98%
Morin	Combi-Blocks	Cat# QC-0527; CAS: 480-16-0; Purity: ≥98%
Myricetin	FUJIFILM Wako Pure Chemical	Cat# 137-16791; CAS: 529-44-2; Purity: ≥98%
Naringenin chalcone	ChromaDex	Cat# ASB-00014207-005; CAS: 73692-50-9; Purity: N/A
Phloretin	FUJIFILM Wako Pure Chemical	Cat# 160-17781; CAS: 60-82-2; Purity: ≥98%
Quercetagetin	ChromaDex	Cat# ASB-00017020-005; CAS: 90-18-6; Purity: N/A
Quercetin	ChromaDex	Cat# ASB-00017030-010; CAS: 117-39-5; Purity: ≥97%
Taxifolin	EXTRASYNTHESE	Cat# 1036; CAS: 17654-26-1; Purity: N/A
Xanthohumol	TOKIWA PHYTOCHEMICAL	Cat# P2217; CAS: 569-83-5; Purity: ≥98%
Critical Commercial Assays		
Pierce BCA Protein Assay Reagent A, B	Thermo Fisher Scientific	Cat# 23223, Cat# 23224
PureLink HiPure Plasmid Filter Midiprep Kit	Thermo Fisher Scientific	Cat# K210015
Recombinant DNA		
The complete human URAT1 cDNA in pEGFP-C1	Saito et al. 2020 [14]	NCBI Reference Sequence: NM_144585.3
Experimental Models: Cell Lines		
293A	Invitrogen	R70507

N/A, not available.

2.3. Cell Culture

Human embryonic kidney 293-derived 293A cells were maintained in DMEM—Dulbecco's Modified Eagle's Medium (Nacalai Tesque) supplemented with 10% fetal bovine serum (Biowest, Nuaillé, France), 2 mM L-Glutamine (Nacalai Tesque), 1 × Non-Essential Amino Acid (Life Technologies, Carlsbad, CA, USA), and 1% penicillin–streptomycin (Nacalai Tesque), at 37 °C in a humidified atmosphere of 5% (v/v) CO$_2$ in air.

As described previously [14], the plasmids for URAT1 expression or mock were transfected into 293A cells using polyethylenimine "MAX" (PEI-MAX) (Polysciences, Warrington, PA, USA). In brief, 293A cells were seeded onto twelve-well cell culture plates at a concentration of 0.92×10^5 cells/cm^2. After 24 h, each vector was transiently transfected into the cells (1 µg of plasmid/5 µL of PEI-MAX/well). At 24 h after transfection, the culture medium was replaced with fresh one.

2.4. Urate Transport Assay Using URAT1-Expressing 293A Cells

The urate transport assay using transiently URAT1-expressing 293A cells was conducted as described in our previous studies [11,14,18], with minor modifications. Briefly, 48 h after plasmid transfection, cells were washed twice with Buffer T2 and then pre-incubated in Buffer T2 for 15 min at 37 °C. Then, the buffer was exchanged with pre-warmed fresh Buffer T2 containing radiolabeled urate ([8-^{14}C]-uric acid; final concentration, 5 µM) with or without the test compound at the indicated concentrations (0, 0.3, 1, 3, 10, 30, 100, 300, or 500 µM); the cells were further incubated for 20 s at 37 °C; as vehicle control, 1% DMSO was used in this study. Subsequently, the cells were washed five times with ice-cold Buffer T2; then, the cells were lysed with 0.2 M NaOH solution (500 µL/well) on ice. The resulting lysates were neutralized with 1 M HCl solution (100 µL/well). The radioactivity in the lysate was then measured using a liquid scintillator (Tri-Carb 3110TR) (PerkinElmer, Waltham, MA, USA) for DPM (disintegrations per minute) counting. Using a Pierce BCA Protein Assay Kit (Thermo Fisher Scientific, Kanagawa, Japan), protein concentration was determined. Urate transport activity was calculated as the incorporated clearance (µL/mg protein/min): (incorporated level of urate [DPM/mg protein/min]/urate level in the incubation mixture [DPM/µL]). URAT1-dependent urate transport activity was calculated by subtracting the urate transport activity of mock (control) cells from that of URAT1-expressing cells.

Urate uptake was examined in the presence of several concentrations of each test compound to determine their IC$_{50}$ values. Then, URAT1-mediated transport activities were expressed as a percentage of the control (100%). Based on the calculated values, fitting curves were obtained according to the following formula using the least-squares method in Excel 2019 (Microsoft, Redmond, WA, USA):

$$\text{Predicted value } [\%] = 100 - \left(\frac{E_{max} \times C^n}{EC_{50}^n + C^n} \right) \tag{1}$$

where E_{max} is the maximum effect; EC_{50} is the half-maximal effective concentration; C is the concentration of the tested compound; n is the sigmoid-fit factor. Lastly, based on these results, the IC$_{50}$ value was calculated as previously described [11,14].

2.5. Fractionation of Rooibos Tea Leaves Extract

To purify the active ingredients for URAT1-inhibitory activity in the ethanolic extract of rooibos tea leaves, liquid–liquid extraction and column chromatography were conducted according to previous studies [16,17], with some modifications as described below.

First, the dried crude ethanolic extract of rooibos tea leaves was subjected to sequential liquid–liquid extraction using a solvent series with increasing polarity (*n*-hexane, ethyl acetate, and *n*-butanol). In brief, the ethanolic extract was mixed in approximately 500 mL of distilled water and added to a glass separatory funnel. Subsequently, an equal volume of *n*-hexane was added to the solution and mixed well for partitioning. After formation of the dual-phase, the *n*-hexane phase was collected; the remaining water phase was then shaken with the same volume of ethyl acetate. After the ethyl acetate phase was collected in a similar manner, the water phase was further partitioned with *n*-butanol. Finally, the *n*-butanol phase and bottom layer (aqueous phase residue) were collected separately. After evaporation process, the phases were reconstituted in an appropriate solvent prior to use in the urate transport assay for evaluation of URAT1-inhibitory activities and/or further separation by medium-pressure liquid chromatography (MPLC) as follows.

The ethyl acetate fraction, which was reconstituted in hexane and ethyl acetate for normal-phase chromatographic purification, was separated into 14 subfractions (Fr.#1–Fr.#14) by MPLC using a dual-channel automated flash chromatography system (EPCLC-W-Prep 2XY) (Yamazen, Osaka, Japan) on a disposable Silica-gel packed column with high throughput purification (Universal column premium Silicagel L, 40 g) (Yamazen, Osaka, Japan). Separation was conducted in the linear gradient elution mode with solvent A (hexane), solvent B (ethyl acetate), and solvent C (methanol) [solvent A:solvent B:solvent

C (v/v): 0–4 min 90:10:0, 4–8 min 90:10:0 to 60:40:0, 8–12 min 60:40:0, 12–32 min 60:40:0 to 0:100:0, 32–35.8 min 0:100:0, 35.8–36 min 0:0:100, 36–37 min 0:100:0, 37–53 min 0:100:0 to 0:50:50, 53–60 min 0:50:50] at a flow rate of 20 mL/min, with UV monitoring at 280 nm using an equipped UV detector. All subfractions obtained were evaporated to dryness and stored at −20 °C. Before use, they were reconstituted in DMSO (2 mg/mL).

2.6. Chemical Characterization

For qualitative determination of the isolated compounds, chromatographic separation and subsequent mass spectrometry (MS) (or MS/MS) analyses were performed using an LC-quadrupole time-of-flight (Q-TOF)-MS/MS system comprising an HPLC instrument [Agilent 1200 Series equipped with a diode array and multiple wavelength detector (DAD) (G1316A)] coupled with an Agilent 6510 Q-TOF (Agilent Technologies, Santa Clara, CA, USA) as described previously [16,17], with minor modifications. In brief, separation was performed on a Zorbax Eclipse Plus C18 column (1.8 μm, 2.1 mm × 100 mm; Agilent Technologies) maintained at 40 °C under gradient mobile conditions with a mixture of solvent C (0.1% formic acid in water) and solvent D (acetonitrile) (solvent C:solvent D (v/v): 0–8 min 95:5 to 5:95, 8–12 min 5:95) at a flow rate of 0.5 mL/min. The detection range of DAD was set from 190 to 400 nm; the MS detection system was operated in the positive ionization mode at an MS scan range of m/z 100–1100. Ionization was performed using a heated electrospray ionization probe with the following source parameters: gas temperature, 350 °C; drying gas, 12 L/min; nebulizer, 55 psi; Vcap, 3.5 kV. Peak analysis was conducted using the Agilent MassHunter Workstation software (version B.03.01; Agilent Technologies).

2.7. Statistical Analysis

We performed all statistical analyses using Excel 2019 with Statcel4 add-in software (OMS Publishing, Saitama, Japan). Different statistical tests were used for different experiments, as described in the figure legends, which include the number of biological replicates (n). In brief, when analyzing multiple groups, the similarity of variance between groups was compared using Bartlett's test. When passing the test for homogeneity of variance, a parametric Tukey–Kramer multiple-comparison test for all pairwise comparisons or a Dunnett's test for comparisons with a control group was used; otherwise, a non-parametric Steel test was used for comparisons with a control group. Likewise, to examine the concentration-dependent decrease in the URAT1 activity in the presence of extracts, a parametric Williams's multiple-comparison test or a non-parametric Shirley–Williams's multiple-comparison test was used. To investigate the inhibitory effect of each authentic chemical on URAT1 function (vs. the vehicle control indicated as 100%) in the screening stage, a one-sample t-test (two-sided) was employed. Statistical significance in this study was defined as $p < 0.05$ or 0.01.

Each experiment was designed to use the samples required to obtain informative results and sufficient material for subsequent procedures. All experiments were monitored in a non-blinded manner. No specific statistical test was employed to pre-determine the sample sizes which were empirically determined in the present study.

3. Results

3.1. Screening the URAT1-Inhibitory Activities of Plant Extracts

For the URAT1-inhibitory properties of natural products, we herein focused on various plants in the human diet including vegetables, fruits, and tea leaves. Each plant sample (Table A1) was extracted with ethanol, and a total of 162 ethanolic extracts were subjected to in vitro screening for URAT1-inhibitory activity at 20 ppm (Table A2). The top 40 samples (approximately 25%) of the tested extracts (Figure 1) included four kinds of herbal tea sources: rooibos tea (*Aspalathus linearis*), yacon tea (*Smallanthus sonchifolius*), Tartary buckwheat tea (*Fagopyrum tataricum*), and guava leaf tea (*Psidium guajava*). As the rooibos leaf extract was the most active among these, and because rooibos tea is globally consumed [19], we next explored the ingredients responsible for URAT1-inhibitory activity in rooibos tea leaves.

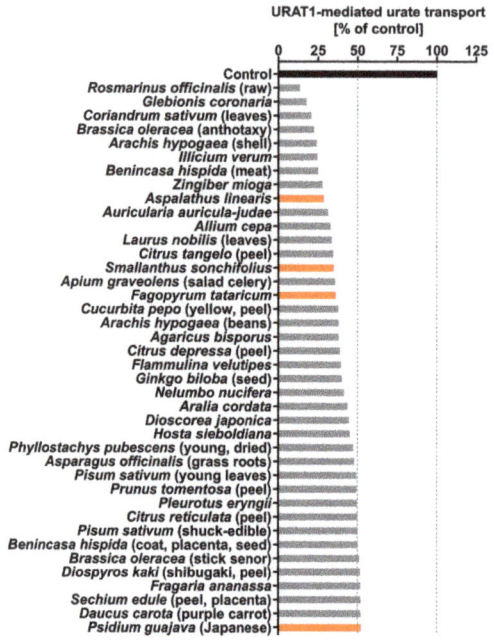

Figure 1. Screening of the inhibitory effects of various plant extracts on URAT1 function. The effects of each ethanolic extract (20 ppm), which was dried and finally dissolved in dimethyl sulfoxide (DMSO) at 2000 ppm (see Section 2.2.), on the URAT1-mediated [^{14}C]-urate transport was investigated using the cell-based urate transport assay; as the vehicle control, 1% DMSO was used. *Orange* indicates herbal tea sources. All data are expressed as % of the vehicle control (n = 1, each sample). This figure shows the results of the top 40 samples of the tested extracts (total 162); all data are listed in Table A2.

3.2. Fractionation and Isolation of the Aspalathus linearis (Rooibos Leaves) Extract

To determine the URAT1-inhibitory ingredients in the ethanolic extract of rooibos leaves, further fractionation was carried out using liquid–liquid extraction and subsequent column chromatography (Figure 2). For this purpose, 60 g of rooibos leaves were newly extracted using ethanol.

Prior to fractionation, we confirmed the concentration-dependent URAT1-inhibitory effect of the ethanolic extract (Figure 3a). The extract was then separated sequentially into *n*-hexane, ethyl acetate, *n*-butanol, and water-soluble fractions. Among the four fractions, the ethyl acetate fraction had the highest URAT1-inhibitory activity (Figure 3b). Both the *n*-hexane and water fractions showed little inhibitory activity, whereas the ethyl acetate fraction exhibited URAT1-inhibitory activity in a concentration-dependent manner. Additionally, the *n*-butanol fraction inhibited URAT1-mediated urate transport only at the maximum concentration employed in this study (40 ppm); however, its effect was weaker than that of the ethyl acetate fraction. Therefore, we further separated the ethyl acetate fraction by column chromatography to obtain a total of 14 subfractions (Fr.#1–#14) based on the monitored absorbance chromatogram (Figure 4a), as described in the *Materials and Methods* section (Section 2.5). The URAT1-inhibitory activity of each subfraction was then analyzed; among the 14 subfractions, Fr.#11 showed the highest URAT1-inhibitory activity (Figure 4b). Therefore, we focused on this subfraction for further analyses.

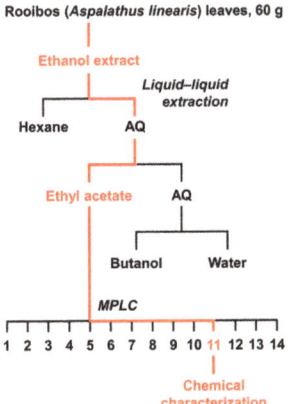

Figure 2. A flow chart of extraction and isolation for rooibos (*Aspalathus linearis*) leaves. In each separation procedure, the fraction with the highest URAT1-inhibitory activity is colored in red. AQ, aqueous layer; MPLC, medium pressure liquid chromatography.

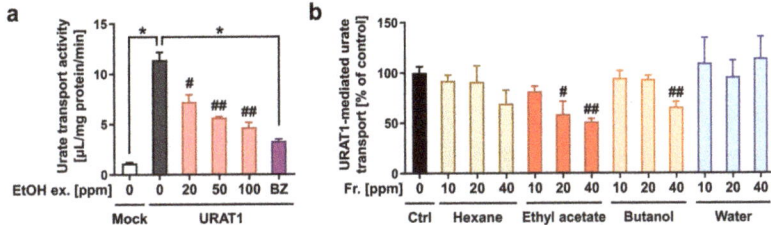

Figure 3. URAT1-inhibitory activity of the ethanolic extraction of rooibos leaves and each fraction obtained by liquid–liquid extraction; 1% dimethyl sulfoxide was used as the vehicle control. (**a**) Concentration-dependent URAT1 inhibitory activity of the ethanolic extraction (EtOH ex.); 0 ppm means only vehicle treatment. Mock, empty vector-transfected cells for the detection of background activity for urate transport; BZ, benzbromarone (final concentration 2.5 µM), a well-known URAT1 inhibitor, was used as the positive control. All data are expressed as the mean ± S.E.M., $n = 4$. #, $p < 0.05$; ##, $p < 0.01$ with concentration-dependent decreasing tendency vs. the control (Shirley–Williams's multiple-comparison test); *, $p < 0.05$ between the indicated groups (Steel test) (**b**) URAT1 inhibitory activity of each fraction (Fr.). All data are expressed as % of the vehicle control (Ctrl) and the mean ± S.E.M., $n = 3$–4. #, $p < 0.05$; ##, $p < 0.01$ with a concentration-dependent decreasing tendency vs. the control (Williams' test in each fraction category).

3.3. Structural Characterization of the Putative URAT1 Inhibitor Derived from Rooibos Leaves

We used spectrometric analyses to determine the purity of the target subfraction (Fr.#11) and to obtain structural information about the candidate active ingredients (Figure 5). The results of LC-DAD analyses supported that the ingredient yielding the main peak in the chromatogram of Fr.#11 was almost completely isolated from the other subfractions (Figure 5a, left); subsequent LC-Q-TOF-MS analyses revealed that based on the obtained accurate mass information (m/z 303.0506 in the positive ion mode with a retention time of 5.298 min), the elemental composition of the target analyte was determined as $C_{15}H_{10}O_7$ ($\Delta -2.14$ ppm from $[M+H]^+$) (Figure 5a, right). Based on the polarity of ethyl acetate, the sub-fractionation source (ethyl acetate fraction) was considered to contain flavonoids characterized by a 15-carbon skeleton (C_6-C_3-C_6). Moreover, the compositional formula ($C_{15}H_{10}O_7$) was consistent with that of quercetin, and a previous study has identified quercetin in rooibos leaves [20]. Based on this information, we hypothesized that the main component of Fr.#11 could be quercetin (Figure 5b). To test this hypothesis, we conducted spectroscopic analyses and found that Fr.#11 and authentic quercetin were identical in their photoabsorption spectrum (Figure 5c), retention time, the accurate mass of the parent ion (Figure 5d), and MS/MS spectrum (Figure 5e). Thus, the isolated substance should be quercetin.

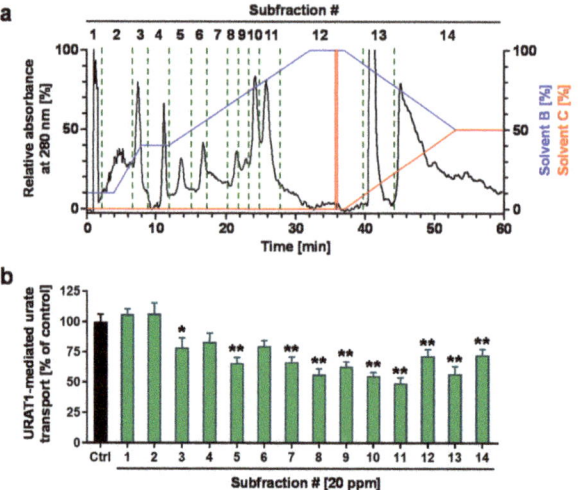

Figure 4. URAT1-inhibitory activity of each subfraction from the ethyl acetate fraction of the ethanolic extract of rooibos leaves. (**a**) A preparative MPLC chromatogram for separating the ethyl acetate fraction. The chromatogram was recorded at 280 nm. Blue and red lines indicate the linear gradients of solvent B (ethyl acetate) and solvent C (methanol), respectively. (**b**) URAT1-inhibitory activity profile of each subfraction (20 ppm) obtained from the column chromatography; 1% dimethyl sulfoxide was used for the vehicle control. All data are expressed as % of the vehicle control and the mean ± S.E.M.; n = 9 (Ctrl, control), 5 (the others). #, fraction number; *, $p < 0.05$; **, $p < 0.01$ vs. control (Dunnett's test).

3.4. Identification of Quercetin as an Active Ingredient with URAT1-Inhibitory Activity

To determine whether quercetin could be responsible for inhibiting URAT1 function, we investigated the effect of quercetin on the urate transport activity of URAT1 (Figure 6). As expected, at the experimentally maximum concentration (300 μM), quercetin inhibited URAT1 (Figure 6a). Further investigation of its concentration-dependent inhibitory effects revealed an IC_{50} of 12.6 μM (Figure 6b). Based on these results and the determined structural characteristics (Figure 5), we concluded that quercetin was an active ingredient in Fr.#11.

3.5. URAT1-Inhibitory Activities of Various Dietary Flavonoids

Finally, we investigated whether other dietary flavonoids of interest, including nine flavanols, two flavanonols, two flavones, two isoflavonoids, and eight chalcones, have URAT1-inhibitory activities (Figure 7). Additionally, we also tested aesculetin, a coumarin identified in rooibos leaves [20]. The chemical structures of the selected natural compounds are summarized in Figure A1. At 100 μM, eight of the tested authentic chemicals (fisetin, gossypetin, morin, myricetin, quercetagetin, luteolin, genistein, and naringenin chalcone) lowered the URAT1-mediated urate transport to less than 50% of that in the control group. Our results were qualitatively consistent with a previous report showing that morin is a URAT1 inhibitor [13]. Moreover, based on our previous study, the URAT1-mediated urate transport activity in the presence of 100 μM naringenin chalcone (44.0 ± 7.1% of that of the control) (Figure 7) was higher than that in the presence of 100 μM naringenin (17.9 ± 7.7%) [11], suggesting that naringenin chalcone has a weaker URAT1-inhibitory activity than naringenin, a metabolite of naringenin chalcone. Thus, we focused on the other six flavonoids in our subsequent analyses.

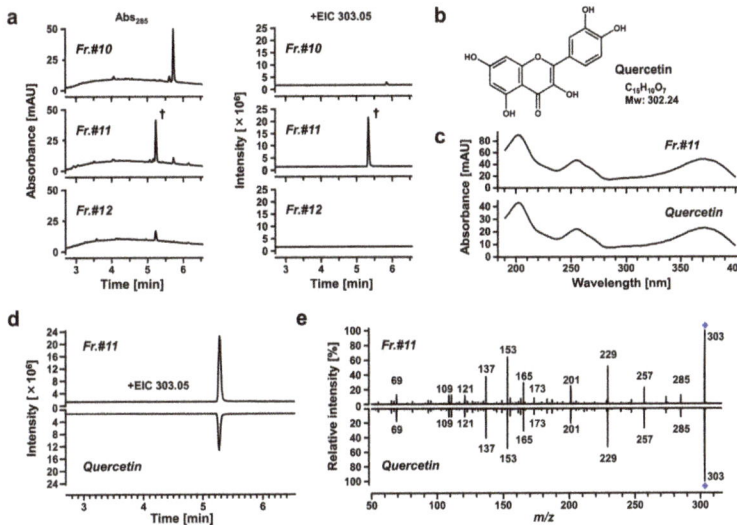

Figure 5. Chemical characterization of a URAT1-inhibitory activity-guided fraction from the ethanolic extract of rooibos leaves. Each subfraction and authentic quercetin (lower panels in (c–e)) were analyzed using a high-performance liquid chromatography instrument coupled with a diode array and multiple wavelength detector (LC-DAD), and a quadrupole time-of-flight-mass spectrometry system (LC-Q-TOF-MS). (a) Purity verification of the isolated ingredient in Subfraction #11 (Fr.#11) by spectrometric analyses. *Left panels*, UV chromatograms recorded at 285 nm. *Right panels*, LC-Q-TOF-MS extracted ion chromatograms (EICs; at *m/z* 303.0506 in the positive ESI spectrum). †, a specific peak in Fr.#11 with a retention time of 5.298 min. (b) Chemical structure of quercetin. (c–e) Comparison of obtained data between Fr.#11 and quercetin; (c) DAD spectrum; (d) EIC; (e) information regarding the fragment ions derived from MS/MS analyses.

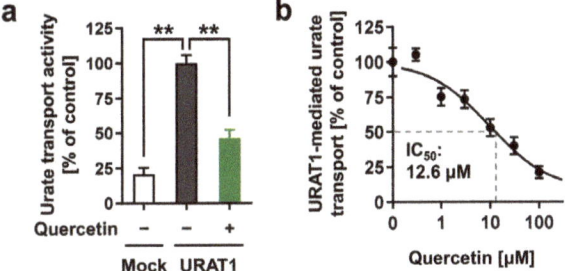

Figure 6. Effects of quercetin on the URAT1 function. (a) Inhibitory effects of quercetin (300 μM) on URAT1-mediated urate transport. (b) Concentration-dependent inhibition. All data are expressed as % of the vehicle control (1% dimethyl sulfoxide) and the mean ± S.E.M.; $n = 4$. **, $p < 0.05$ (Tukey–Kramer multiple-comparison test).

Further investigation of the concentration-dependent inhibitory effects of the six flavonoids on URAT1 determined their IC_{50} values (Figure 8). Genistein exhibited the highest IC_{50} value among the tested samples, and its value was consistent with the results of flavonoid screening (Figure 7). Based on these IC_{50} values and that of quercetin, fisetin was the strongest URAT1 inhibitor among the seven dietary flavonoids examined (Figure 8a), whereas quercetin was second to fisetin (Figure 6b). Based on the structural difference between fisetin and quercetin (Figure A1), the presence of a hydroxyl group at the 5-position of the flavanol skeleton could somewhat negatively affect the URAT1-inhibitory effect. Interestingly, a contrasting effect was observed in the case of the isoflavone skeleton, as shown for daidzein and genistein (Figure 7). Although further studies are needed to clarify the quantitative structure–activity relationship, our findings provide a better understanding of small molecule-dependent URAT1 inhibition.

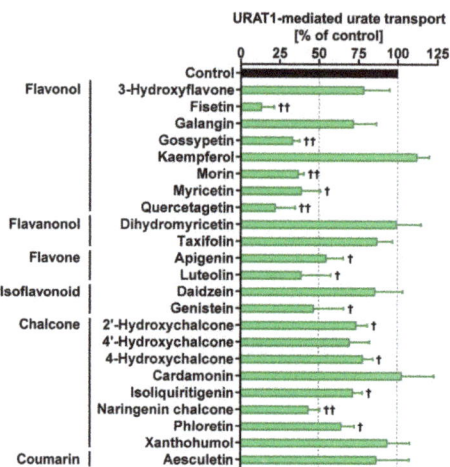

Figure 7. URAT1-inhibitory activities of each food ingredient at 100 µM; 1% dimethyl sulfoxide was used as the vehicle control. All data are expressed as % of the vehicle control and the mean ± S.D.; $n = 3$. †, $p < 0.05$; ††, $p < 0.01$ vs. vehicle control (two-sided one-sample t-test).

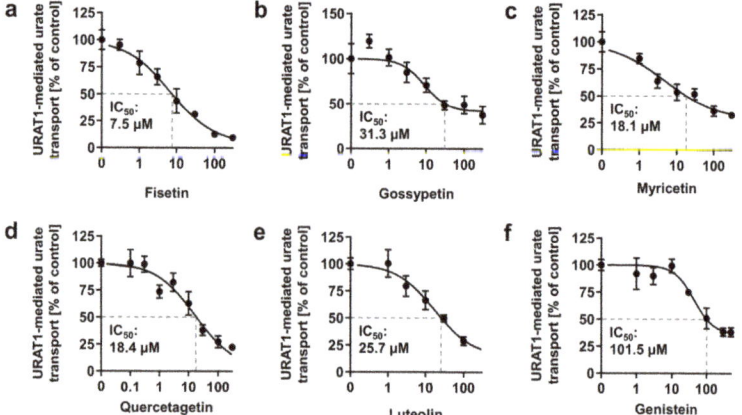

Figure 8. Concentration-dependent inhibition of URAT1-mediated urate transport by (**a**) fisetin; (**b**) gossypetin; (**c**) myricetin; (**d**) quercetagetin; (**e**) luteolin; (**f**) genistein. The x-axis indicates drug concentrations (µM). All data are expressed as % of the vehicle control and the mean ± S.E.M.; $n = 4$ (**a**–**e**), 3 (**f**).

4. Discussion

In this study, we screened the inhibitory effects of the ethanolic extracts of various dietary plant materials on the function of URAT1 as a urate transporter (Figure 1). Among the plants, we focused on rooibos leaves and identified quercetin as an active ingredient responsible for the URAT1-inhibitory activity in the extract (Figures 2–6). Moreover, to extend our understanding of the interaction between URAT1 and flavonoids, 24 dietary flavonoids were further investigated (Figures 7 and 8). Although some previous studies have examined the effect of certain flavonoids with respect to their effect on URAT1-mediated urate transport [11,13], to the best of our knowledge, this is the first study to comprehensively address the inhibitory effect of dietary flavonoids on URAT1 function.

Flavonoids are well-known ingredients of natural products and have received considerable attention for their health-promoting and/or potential therapeutic properties in many diseases based on a broad spectrum of biological functions including anti-oxidative, anti-inflammatory, neuroprotective, and anti-cancer activities [21,22]. Although the present study was limited to in vitro evaluations, our findings regarding the potential uricosuric activities of flavonoids may extend the possibilities of their nutraceutical application. In particular, fisetin and quercetin, which exhibited the smallest and second-smallest IC_{50} values against urate transport by URAT1, respectively, are relatively well studied and are some of the most prevalent plant flavonoids [23–25]. However, to our knowledge, few studies have investigated their effects on the renal handling of endogenous substances such as urate. Further studies are thus required to deepen our understanding of this issue. Further, fisetin and quercetin are abundantly found in fruits and vegetables such as apples and onions [23]; fisetin is also abundant in strawberries and teas [24]. Hence, the effects of dietary habits including such plant-based foods on serum urate levels and renal urate handling are of significant interest.

Although little information is available on the effects of quercetin on urate handling in humans, a human study (randomized, double-blinded, placebo-controlled, crossover four-week intervention trial) demonstrated that daily supplementation with 500 mg quercetin as a single tablet, which contained the bioavailable amount of quercetin as present in approximately 100 g of red onions, significantly reduced (mean difference, -0.45 mg/dL) the plasma uric acid concentrations (mean, 5.5 mg/dL) in healthy males [26]. In contrast, the previous study confirmed the urinary excretion of quercetin, but did not sufficiently investigate the effect of quercetin on renal urate handling—no parameters on renal urate clearance or fractional excretion of uric acid were reported; only the urinary uric acid output over a 24-h period (24 h-UUA) was documented. Given that no significant difference in the amount of 24 h-UUA was found between before and after the quercetin treatment, despite the serum urate-lowering effect, renal urate clearance might have been influenced by quercetin. Based on the inhibitory activity of quercetin against xanthine oxidoreductase (XOD, an essential enzyme of uric acid formation) [27], the serum urate-lowering effect was considered to have been mainly associated with suppressed uric acid production; however, quercetin might also have enhanced renal urate excretion. Although such a dual inhibitory activity will be welcome, it is necessary to understand the activity that majorly contributes to the serum urate-lowering effect in the context of combination with serum urate-lowering drugs (urate synthesis inhibitors or uricosuric agents), for a more effective application.

Our findings also highlight the potential health benefits of rooibos-based food products. Today, especially for health-conscious people, the global popularity of rooibos tea seems to depend on its caffeine-free status, comparatively low tannin content, and anti-oxidative activity as potential health-promoting properties [28]. The influence of continuous consumption of rooibos tea on the serum urate levels and the risk of urate-related diseases remains to be elucidated; however, in addition to our findings demonstrating URAT1-inhibitory activity in rooibos extract (Figure 1) and rooibos flavonoids (Figures 6 and 7), a previous study reported that aspalathin, a C-glycosyl dihydrochalcone contained in rooibos, inhibits XOD [29]. Given this information, additional human studies and/or epidemiological studies will be helpful to address the serum urate-lowering potential of rooibos extracts.

Some limitations of this study and possible future directions are described below. First, although we successfully identified quercetin as an active compound for URAT1-inhibitory activity in rooibos extract, other ingredients may have contributed to the activity based on the results of the bioactivity-guided fractionation approach (Figures 3 and 4). Some of these might overlap with the dietary flavonoids tested in this study. Second, the other plant extracts that we could not handle further in this study may be good sources for exploring additional compounds for URAT1-inhibition. Third, to extrapolate our findings to humans, bioavailability and in vivo levels in nutraceutical-achievable situations as well as the effects of metabolic conversion on the URAT1-inhibitory activities of dietary flavonoids should be examined. Despite the need for further studies, as most previous studies were conducted to find plant-derived bioactive compounds with potential anti-hyperuricemia activity in the context of XOD inhibition [30], our study focusing on their potential uricosuric activity will facilitate progress in nutrition research, contributing to the treatment and prevention of hyperuricemia.

5. Conclusions

We found that the ethanolic extract of rooibos leaves inhibited the urate transport activity of URAT1. From this plant extract, we successfully identified quercetin, a natural compound considered safe for humans, as an active ingredient. Moreover, we expanded our understanding of the inhibitory effects of dietary flavonoids and chalcones on URAT1 function in a comprehensive manner. These effects of phytochemicals need further investigation in human studies; however, our findings may provide new clues for promoting health through appropriate serum urate maintenance.

6. Patents

Yu Toyoda, Tappei Takada, Hiroki Saito, Hiroshi Hirata, Ami Ota-Kontani, and Hiroshi Suzuki have a patent pending related to the work reported in this article.

Author Contributions: Conceptualization, Y.T. (Yu Toyoda), T.T., H.S. (Hiroki Saito) and H.H.; Data curation, H.S. (Hiroki Saito); Formal analysis, Y.T. (Yu Toyoda) and H.S. (Hiroki Saito); Funding acquisition, Y.T. (Yu Toyoda) and T.T.; Investigation, Y.T. (Yu Toyoda), H.S. (Hiroki Saito), H.H. and A.O.-K.; Methodology, Y.T. (Yu Toyoda) and H.H.; Project administration, Y.T. (Yu Toyoda), T.T. and H.H.; Resources, H.H.; Supervision, Y.T. (Youichi Tsuchiya) and H.S. (Hiroshi Suzuki); Validation, Y.T. (Yu Toyoda) and H.S. (Hiroki Saito); Visualization, Y.T. (Yu Toyoda) and H.S. (Hiroki Saito); Writing—original draft, Y.T. (Yu Toyoda); Writing—review and editing, Y.T. (Yu Toyoda), T.T., H.S. (Hiroki Saito) and H.H. All authors have read and agreed to the published version of the manuscript.

Funding: This study was supported by JSPS KAKENHI Grant Numbers 21H03350 [to Y.T. (Yu Toyoda)] and 20H00568; 16H01808 (to T.T.). T.T. received research grants from "Gout and uric acid foundation of Japan"; "Mochida Memorial Foundation for Medical and Pharmaceutical Research"; "Suzuken Memorial Foundation"; "Takeda Science Foundation"; "The Pharmacological Research Foundation, Tokyo".

Institutional Review Board Statement: Not applicable because this study did not involve humans or animals.

Informed Consent Statement: Not applicable because this study did not involve humans.

Data Availability Statement: Data supporting the findings of this study are included in this published article or are available from the corresponding author on reasonable request.

Acknowledgments: The authors sincerely appreciate Naoyuki Kobayashi for his support for this study, as well as his continuous encouragement, Takeshi Amiya for providing help in checking the data of plant materials, and Chie Umatani for her technical support in visualization.

Conflicts of Interest: H.S. (Hiroki Saito), H.H., A.O.-K. (Ami Ota-Kontani), and Y.T. (Youichi Tsuchiya) were the employees of Sapporo Holdings Ltd.; Y.T. (Yu Toyoda), T.T., H.S. (Hiroki Saito), H.H., Ami Ota-Kontani, and Hiroshi Suzuki have a patent-pending related to the work reported in this article. The funders had no role in the design of the study; in the collection, analyses, or interpretation of data; in the writing of the manuscript; or in the decision to publish the results.

Appendix A

Table A1. Tested plant materials.

Descriptions in This Study	Common Names	Academic Names	Details of Material *
Abelmoschus esculentus (beniokura)	Beniokura	*Abelmoschus esculentus*	Fresh
Agaricus bisporus	Common mushroom	*Agaricus bisporus*	Fresh
Allium cepa	Onion	*Allium cepa*	Fresh
Allium oschaninii	Shallot	*Allium oschaninii*	Fresh
Allium sativum	Garlic	*Allium sativum*	Fresh
Allium sativum (sprout)	Garlic shoots	*Allium sativum*	Fresh sprout
Allium tuberosum	Chinese chive	*Allium tuberosum*	Fresh
Ananas comosus (coat)	Pineapple	*Ananas comosus*	Fresh coat
Apium graveolens	Celery	*Apium graveolens*	Fresh
Apium graveolens (salad celery)	Salad celery	*Apium graveolens*	Fresh
Arachis hypogaea (beans)	Peanut	*Arachis hypogaea*	Fresh beans
Arachis hypogaea (shell)	Peanut	*Arachis hypogaea*	Fresh shell
Aralia cordata	Udo	*Aralia cordata*	Fresh
Aralia elata (sprout)	Fatsia sprouts	*Aralia elata*	Fresh sprout
Arctium lappa	Edible burdock	*Arctium lappa*	Fresh root
Arctium lappa (burdock tea)	Burdock root tea	*Arctium lappa*	Dried root for tea
Aspalathus linearis	Rooibos tea leaves	*Aspalathus linearis*	Dried leaves for tea
Asparagus officinalis (grass roots)	Asparagus	*Asparagus officinalis*	Fresh grass roots
Asparagus spp.	Asparagus	*Asparagus* spp.	Fresh stalk
Auricularia auricula-judae	Jew's ear fungus	*Auricularia auricula-judae*	Fresh
Barley (*Hordeum vulgare*) Miso	Barley Miso	*Hordeum vulgare* [#]	Japanese traditional fermented product
Basella alba	Indian spinach	*Basella alba*	Fresh
Benincasa hispida (coat, placenta, seed)	Winter melon	*Benincasa hispida*	Fresh coat, placenta and seeds
Benincasa hispida (meat)	Winter melon	*Benincasa hispida*	Fresh meat
Brassica chinensis	Green pak choi	*Brassica rapa var. chinensis*	Fresh
Brassica oleracea (broccoli, anthotaxy)	Broccoli	*Brassica oleracea var. italica*	Fresh anthotaxy
Brassica oleracea (broccoli, sprout)	Broccoli	*Brassica oleracea var. italica*	Fresh sprout
Brassica oleracea (broccoli, stem)	Broccoli	*Brassica oleracea var. italica*	Fresh stem
Brassica oleracea (kohlrabi, peel)	German turnip or turnip cabbage	*Brassica oleracea var. gongylodes*	Fresh peel
Brassica oleracea (red cabbage, sprout)	Red cabbage	*Brassica oleracea var. capitata F. rubra*	Fresh sprout
Brassica oleracea (romanesco broccoli, stem)	Romanesco broccoli	*Brassica oleracea var. botrytis*	Fresh stem
Brassica oleracea (soft kale)	Soft kale	*Brassica oleracea var. acephala*	Fresh stems and leaves
Brassica oleracea (stick senor)	Stick senor	*Brassica oleracea var. italica*	Fresh
Brassica oleracea (wild cabbage, flower)	Romanesco broccoli	*Brassica oleracea var. botrytis*	Fresh flower
Brassica rapa (ayameyuki-kabu)	Ayameyuki-kabu	*Brassica rapa*	Fresh leaves
Brassica rapa (ayameyuki-kabu, meat)	Ayameyuki-kabu	*Brassica rapa*	Fresh meat
Brassica rapa (nabana)	Chinese colza	*Brassica rapa L. var. nippo-oleifera*	Fresh leaves
Brassica rapa (nabana, flower)	Chinese colza	*Brassica rapa L. var. nippo-oleifera*	Fresh flower
Brassica rapa (red)	Red potherb mustard	*Brassica rapa var. laciniifolia*	Fresh
Brassica rapa (santo-sai)	Santo-sai	*Brassica rapa L. var. pekinensis*	Fresh
Capsicum annuum (redpepper)	Chili pepper	*Capsicum annuum L.*	Fresh
Capsicum annuum (sweet pepper)	Sweet pepper	*Capsicum annuum L. 'grossum'*	Fresh
Capsicum annuum (red)	Red bell pepper	*Capsicum annuum L. 'grossum'*	Fresh
Capsicum annuum (shishitou)	Shishitou	*Capsicum annuum L.*	Fresh
Capsicum annuum (yellow)	Yellow bell pepper	*Capsicum annuum L. 'grossum'*	Fresh
Capsicum frutescens	Shima pepper	*Capsicum frutescens L.*	Fresh
Carica papaya (immature, meat)	Green papaya	*Carica papaya L.*	Fresh meat
Carica papaya (immature, peel, placenta, seed)	Green papaya	*Carica papaya L.*	Fresh peel, placenta and seed

Table A1. *Cont.*

Descriptions in This Study	Common Names	Academic Names	Details of Material *
Caulerpa lentillifera	Sea grape	*Caulerpa lentillifera*	Fresh
Citrus aurantiifolia (peel)	Lime	*Citrus aurantiifolia*	Peel
Citrus depressa (peel)	Shikuwasa	*Citrus depressa*	Peel
Citrus junos (peel)	Yuzu	*Citrus junos*	Peel
Citrus maxima (peel)	Pomelo	*Citrus maxima*	Peel
Citrus maxima (placenta)	Pomelo	*Citrus maxima*	Inner white and soft tissue layer
Citrus natsudaidai (peel)	Suruga elegant	*Citrus natsudaidai*	Peel
Citrus paradisi (peel)	Grapefruit	*Citrus paradisi*	Peel
Citrus reticulata (peel)	Ponkan	*Citrus reticulata*	Peel
Citrus sinensis (blood orange, peel)	Blood orange	*Citrus sinensis*	Peel
Citrus sinensis (navel)	Navel	*Citrus sinensis*	Peel
Citrus sphaerocarpa (peel)	Kabosu	*Citrus sphaerocarpa*	Peel
Citrus sudachi (peel)	Sudachi	*Citrus sudachi*	Peel
Citrus tangelo (peel)	Mineola orange (tangelo)	*Citrus tangelo*	Peel
Cocos nucifera (young)	Young coconut	*Cocos nucifera*	Fresh
Colocasia esculenta	Eddoe	*Colocasia esculenta* L. schott	Fresh
Coriandrum sativum	Coriander	*Coriandrum sativum*	Fresh leaves
Coriandrum sativum (leaves)	Coriander	*Coriandrum sativum*	Fresh leaves
Cucumis melo (coat)	Melon	*Cucumis melo*	Fresh coat
Cucurbita (meat)	Squash	*Cucurbita*	Fresh meat, without seeds
Cucurbita (peel)	Squash	*Cucurbita*	Fresh peel
Cucurbita pepo (yellow, peel)	Zucchini	*Cucurbita pepo*	Fresh peel
Curcuma longa	Turmeric	*Curcuma longa* L.	Dried powder
Cyperus esculentus (powder)	Yellow nutsedge	*Cyperus esculentus*	Milled powder of stem
Daucus carota	Carrot	*Daucus carota* subsp. *sativus*	Fresh
Daucus carota (purple carrot)	Purple carrot	*Daucus carota* subsp. *sativus*	Fresh
Dioscorea japonica	Japanese yam	*Dioscorea japonica*	Fresh
Diospyros kaki (shibugaki, meat)	Kaki persimmon	*Diospyros kaki*	Fresh
Diospyros kaki (shibugaki, peel)	Kaki persimmon	*Diospyros kaki*	Fresh
Eriobotrya japonica (peel)	Loquat	*Eriobotrya japonica*	Fresh
Eutrema japonicum	Japanese horseradish	*Eutrema japonicum*	Fresh root
Eutrema japonicum (stem)	Japanese horseradish	*Eutrema japonicum*	Fresh stem
Fagopyrum tataricum	Tartary buckwheat	*Fagopyrum tataricum*	Dried seed
Ficus carica	Fig tree	*Ficus carica*	Fresh fruit
Flammulina velutipes	Enoki mushroom	*Flammulina velutipes*	Fresh
Fortunella (peel)	Kumquat	*Fortunella*	Peel
Fragaria ananassa	Strawberry	*Fragaria ananassa*	Fresh
Ginkgo biloba (seed)	Ginkgo	*Ginkgo biloba*	Fresh
Glebionis coronaria	Crown daisy	*Glebionis coronaria*	Fresh
Glycine max	Soybeans (yellow soybean)	*Glycine max*	Dried product
Glycine max (hidenmame)	Soybeans (green soybean)	*Glycine max*	Dried product
Glycine max (immature)	Immature soybeans	*Glycine max*	Fresh
Glycine max (immature, shuck)	Immature soybeans	*Glycine max*	Fresh shuck
Glycine max × *Bacillus subtilis*	Natto	*Glycine max*	Commercially available Japanese traditional fermented product
Grifola frondosa	Hen-of-the-woods	*Grifola frondosa*	Fresh
Hibiscus rosa-sinensis	Chinese hibiscus	*Hibiscus rosa-sinensis*	Fresh
Hosta sieboldiana	Hosta	*Hosta sieboldiana*	Fresh young leaves
Houttuynia cordata	Fish mint	*Houttuynia cordata*	Dried leaves and stem
Humulus lupulus (cone)	Hop	*Humulus lupulus*	Frozen hop cone
Hylocereus undatus (peel)	Dragon fruit	*Hylocereus undatus*	Fresh peel
Hypsizygus marmoreus	Shimeji mushroom	*Hypsizygus marmoreus*	Fresh
Ilex paraguariensis (roasted)	Yerba mate tea leaves	*Ilex paraguariensis*	Dried and roasted leaves for tea
Illicium verum	Star anise	*Illicium verum*	Dried fruit
Ipomoea aquatica	Water morning glory	*Ipomoea aquatica*	Fresh
Jasminum sambac	Jasmine tea leaves	*Jasminum sambac*	Dried leaves for tea
Lactuca sativa	Stem lettuce	*Lactuca sativa* L. var. *crispa*	Fresh
Laminaria longissima (tororomekonbu)	Tororomekonbu	*Laminaria longissima*	Dried product
Laurus nobilis (leaves)	Laurel	*Laurus nobilis*	Fresh leaves
Lentinula edodes	Shiitake mushroom	*Lentinula edodes*	Fresh
Lycopersicum esculentum (yellow)	Cherry tomato	*Solanum lycopersicum* L.	Fresh
Matricaria recutita	Chamomile	*Matricaria recutita*	Dried herb product

Table A1. *Cont.*

Descriptions in This Study	Common Names	Academic Names	Details of Material *
Matteuccia struthiopteris (young)	Ostrich fern	*Matteuccia struthiopteris*	Fresh young leaves
Mesembryanthemum crystallinum	Common ice plant	*Mesembryanthemum crystallinum*	Fresh
Momordica charantia (coat)	Bitter melon	*Momordica charantia*	Fresh coat
Musa spp. (peel)	Banana	*Musa* spp.	Fresh peel
Musa spp. (peel, Ecuador)	Banana	*Musa* spp.	Fresh peel
Nasturtium officinale	Watercress	*Nasturtium officinale*	Fresh
Nelumbo nucifera	Lotus root	*Nelumbo nucifera*	Fresh root
Ocimum basilicum	Basil	*Ocimum basilicum*	Fresh
Ocimum basilicum (purple)	Purple basil	*Ocimum basilicum*	Fresh
Oryza sativa (black)	Brack rice	*Oryza sativa*	Fresh
Perilla frutescens	Perilla	*Perilla frutescens*	Fresh
Persea americana (coat)	Avocado	*Persea americana*	Fresh coat
Persea americana (seed)	Avocado	*Persea americana*	Fresh seed
Petasites japonicus	Giant butterbur	*Petasites japonicus*	Fresh
Petroselinum crispum (leaves)	Parsley	*Petroselinum crispum*	Fresh leaves
Phaseolus vulgaris	Common bean	*Phaseolus vulgaris*	Fresh
Phaseolus vulgaris (Moroccan kidney beans)	Moroccan kidney beans	*Phaseolus vulgaris*	Fresh
Pholiota microspora	Butterscotch mushroom	*Pholiota microspora*	Fresh
Phyllostachys pubescens (young, dried)	Bamboo shoot	*Phyllostachys pubescens*	Dried young stem
Pisum sativum	Pea	*Pisum sativum*	Fresh
Pisum sativum (shelled)	Shelled pea	*Pisum sativum*	Fresh
Pisum sativum (shuck-edible)	Shuck-edible pea	*Pisum sativum*	Fresh
Pisum sativum (young leaves)	Pea young leaves	*Pisum sativum*	Fresh
Pleurotus cornucopiae	Golden oyster mushroom	*Pleurotus cornucopiae var. citrinopileatus*	Fresh
Pleurotus eryngii	King trumpet mushroom	*Pleurotus eryngii*	Fresh
Pleurotus ostreatus	Oyster mushroom	*Pleurotus ostreatus*	Fresh
Prunus domestica (extract)	Prune extract	*Prunus domestica*	Product of prune pulp extract ‡
Prunus domestica (meat)	Prune	*Prunus domestica*	Product of prune pulp without seed
Prunus tomentosa (peel)	Cherry	*Prunus tomentosa*	Fresh peel
Psidium guajava (Chinese)	Guava tea leaves	*Psidium guajava*	Dried leaves for tea cultivated in China
Psidium guajava (Japanese)	Guava tea leaves	*Psidium guajava*	Dried leaves for tea cultivated in Japan
Psophocarpus tetragonolobus	Winged bean	*Psophocarpus tetragonolobus*	Fresh
Pteridium aquilinum	Western bracken fern	*Pteridium aquilinum*	Fresh
Pyrus communis (peel)	Pear	*Pyrus communis*	Fresh peel
Raphanus sativus (leaves)	Radish	*Raphanus sativus* L. var. *sativus*	Fresh leaves
Raphanus sativus (meat)	Radish	*Raphanus sativus* L. var. *sativus*	Fresh meat
Raphanus sativus (radish sprout)	Radish sprout	*Raphanus sativus*	Fresh
Rice (*Oryza sativa*) Miso	Rice Miso	*Oryza sativa* #	Japanese traditional fermented product
Rosmarinus officinalis (raw)	Rosemary	*Rosmarinus officinalis*	Fresh
Sechium edule (meat)	Chayote	*Sechium edule*	Fresh meat
Sechium edule (peel, placenta)	Chayote	*Sechium edule*	Fresh peel and placenta
Sesamum indicum	Sesame	*Sesamum indicum*	Dried seeds
Siranuhi, (*Citrus unshiu* × *C. sinensis*) × *C. reticulata* (peel)	Siranuhi	(*Citrus unshiu* × *C. sinensis*) × *C. reticulata*	Fresh peel
Smallanthus sonchifolius	Yacón tea	*Smallanthus sonchifolius*	Dried tea powder
Smallanthus sonchifolius (meat)	Yacón	*Smallanthus sonchifolius*	Fresh meat
Smallanthus sonchifolius (peel)	Yacón	*Smallanthus sonchifolius*	Fresh peel
Solanum melongena (peel)	Aubergine	*Solanum melongena*	Fresh peel
Vitis labruscana (peel)	Delaware grapes	*Vitis labruscana*	Fresh peel
Zanthoxylum bungeanum	Sichuan pepper	*Zanthoxylum bungeanum*	Dried powder
Zea mays (baby corn)	Baby corn	*Zea mays*	Fresh
Zea mays (kiritani)	Kiritani	*Zea mays*	Fresh
Zingiber mioga	Myoga	*Zingiber mioga*	Fresh
Zingiber officinale	Ginger	*Zingiber officinale*	Fresh

*, Unless otherwise indicated, fresh material was used. #, Academic name of main material of Miso product. ‡, After defatting via liquid–liquid partition with an equal volume of ethyl acetate, the obtained water phase of extract was subjected to lyophilization.

Table A2. Screening of the inhibitory effects of tested plant extracts (20 ppm) on URAT1 function.

Descriptions in This Study	% *	Descriptions in This Study	% *	Descriptions in This Study	% *
Abelmoschus esculentus (beniokura)	57.3	*Citrus natsudaidai* (peel)	74.5	*Matricaria recutita*	126.1
Agaricus bisporus	38.1	*Citrus paradisi* (peel)	92.4	*Matteuccia struthiopteris* (young)	116.6
Allium cepa	32.9	*Citrus reticulata* (peel)	50.2	*Mesembryanthemum crystallinum*	97.4
Allium oschaninii	59.5	*Citrus sinensis* (blood orange, peel)	65.2	*Momordica charantia* (coat)	97.8
Allium sativum	92.1	*Citrus sinensis* (navel)	81.4	*Musa* spp. (peel)	62.2
Allium sativum (sprout)	117.9	*Citrus sphaerocarpa* (peel)	119.1	*Musa* spp. (peel, Ecuador)	94.8
Allium tuberosum	77.7	*Citrus sudachi* (peel)	59.3	*Nasturtium officinale*	107.7
Ananas comosus (coat)	108.1	*Citrus tangelo* (peel)	34.7	*Nelumbo nucifera*	41.4
Apium graveolens	68.7	*Cocos nucifera* (young)	100.2	*Ocimum basilicum*	100.0
Apium graveolens (salad celery)	35.8	*Colocasia esculenta*	58.5	*Ocimum basilicum* (purple)	79.4
Arachis hypogaea (beans)	38.0	*Coriandrum sativum*	130.2	*Oryza sativa* (black)	67.8
Arachis hypogaea (shell)	24.3	*Coriandrum sativum* (leaves)	20.8	*Perilla frutescens*	81.6
Aralia cordata	43.9	*Cucumis melo* (coat)	67.3	*Persea americana* (coat)	106.7
Aralia elata (sprout)	86.4	*Cucurbita* (meat)	91.5	*Persea americana* (seed)	63.8
Arctium lappa	59.9	*Cucurbita* (peel)	66.5	*Petasites japonicus*	64.3
Arctium lappa (burdock tea)	97.4	*Cucurbita pepo* (yellow, peel)	37.8	*Petroselinum crispum* (leaves)	75.7
Aspalathus linearis	29.0	*Curcuma longa*	83.7	*Phaseolus vulgaris*	132.6
Asparagus officinalis (grass roots)	48.1	*Cyperus esculentus* (powder)	99.2	*Phaseolus vulgaris* (Moroccan kidney beans)	140.3
Asparagus spp.	77.0	*Daucus carota*	55.1	*Pholiota microspora*	55.4
Auricularia auricula-judae	31.4	*Daucus carota* (purple carrot)	52.0	*Phyllostachys pubescens* (young, dried)	47.4
Barley (*Hordeum vulgare*) Miso	105.5	*Dioscorea japonica*	44.8	*Pisum sativum*	62.2
Basella alba	63.5	*Diospyros kaki* (shibugaki, meat)	112.0	*Pisum sativum* (shelled)	107.8
Benincasa hispida (coat, placenta, seed)	50.3	*Diospyros kaki* (shibugaki, peel)	51.7	*Pisum sativum* (shuck-edible)	50.2
Benincasa hispida (meat)	25.2	*Eriobotrya japonica* (peel)	109.7	*Pisum sativum* (young leaves)	49.3
Brassica chinensis	93.8	*Eutrema japonicum*	73.7	*Pleurotus cornucopiae*	90.7
Brassica oleracea (broccoli, anthotaxy)	22.7	*Eutrema japonicum* (stem)	102.2	*Pleurotus eryngii*	49.9
Brassica oleracea (broccoli, sprout)	61.4	*Fagopyrum tataricum*	36.5	*Pleurotus ostreatus*	73.1
Brassica oleracea (broccoli, stem)	68.5	*Ficus carica*	79.1	*Prunus domestica* (extract)	84.4
Brassica oleracea (kohlrabi, peel)	73.4	*Flammulina velutipes*	39.7	*Prunus domestica* (meat)	96.3
Brassica oleracea (red cabbage, sprout)	106.2	*Fortunella* (peel)	62.5	*Prunus tomentosa* (peel)	49.5
Brassica oleracea (romanesco broccoli, stem)	109.8	*Fragaria ananassa*	52.0	*Psidium guajava* (Chinese)	73.4
Brassica oleracea (soft kale)	94.4	*Ginkgo biloba* (seed)	40.2	*Psidium guajava* (Japanese)	52.5
Brassica oleracea (stick senor)	51.2	*Glebionis coronaria*	17.9	*Psophocarpus tetragonolobus*	90.7
Brassica oleracea (wild cabbage, flower)	60.0	*Glycine max*	66.4	*Pteridium aquilinum*	192.2
Brassica rapa (ayameyuki-kabu)	108.2	*Glycine max* (hidenmame)	104.0	*Pyrus communis* (peel)	58.8
Brassica rapa (ayameyuki-kabu, meat)	85.2	*Glycine max* (immature)	64.6	*Raphanus sativus* (leaves)	70.8
Brassica rapa (nabana)	86.1	*Glycine max* (immature, shuck)	96.1	*Raphanus sativus* (meat)	64.7
Brassica rapa (nabana, flower)	64.2	*Glycine max* × *Bacillus subtilis*	60.6	*Raphanus sativus* (radish sprout)	79.6
Brassica rapa (red)	52.6	*Grifola frondosa*	69.5	Rice (*Oryza sativa*) Miso	58.6
Brassica rapa (santo-sai)	72.2	*Hibiscus rosa-sinensis*	97.5	*Rosmarinus officinalis* (raw)	13.6
Capsicum annuum (redpepper)	83.0	*Hosta sieboldiana*	45.2	*Sechium edule* (meat)	130.0
Capsicum annuum (sweet pepper)	107.8	*Houttuynia cordata*	84.0	*Sechium edule* (peel, placenta)	52.0
Capsicum annuum (red)	80.3	*Humulus lupulus* (cone)	78.9	*Sesamum indicum*	158.6
Capsicum annuum (shishitou)	73.0	*Hylocereus undatus* (peel)	120.0	Siranuhi, (*Citrus unshiu* × *C. sinensis*) × *C. reticulata* (peel)	52.7
Capsicum annuum (yellow)	81.4	*Hypsizygus marmoreus*	58.1	*Smallanthus sonchifolius*	35.4
Capsicum frutescens	58.8	*Ilex paraguariensis* (roasted)	69.1	*Smallanthus sonchifolius* (meat)	74.3
Carica papaya (immature, meat)	78.5	*Illicium verum*	24.6	*Smallanthus sonchifolius* (peel)	110.5
Carica papaya (immature, peel, placenta, seed)	94.3	*Ipomoea aquatica*	75.5	*Solanum melongena* (peel)	133.8
Caulerpa lentillifera	65.5	*Jasminum sambac*	66.5	*Vitis labruscana* (peel)	150.9
Citrus aurantiifolia (peel)	185.5	*Lactuca sativa*	91.6	*Zanthoxylum bungeanum*	57.2
Citrus depressa (peel)	38.9	*Laminaria longissima* (tororomekonbu)	112.2	*Zea mays* (baby corn)	65.3
Citrus junos (peel)	61.6	*Laurus nobilis* (leaves)	33.6	*Zea mays* (kiritani)	78.1
Citrus maxima (peel)	64.7	*Lentinula edodes*	62.8	*Zingiber mioga*	28.0
Citrus maxima (placenta)	68.9	*Lycopersicum esculentum* (yellow)	60.6	*Zingiber officinale*	57.3

*, Data for URAT1-mediated urate transport are expressed as % of the vehicle control (1% dimethyl sulfoxide) (*n* = 1, each sample). Results for the top 40 samples are shown in Figure 1.

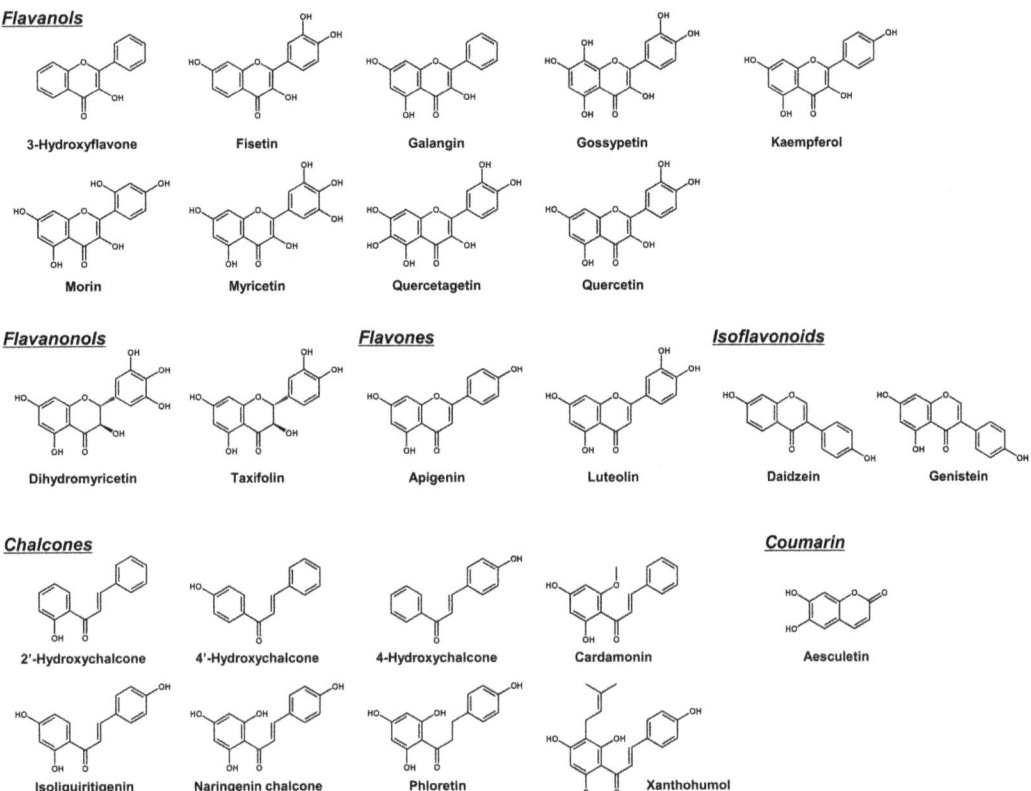

Figure A1. Chemical structures of authentic chemicals tested in this study.

References

1. Dalbeth, N.; Merriman, T.R.; Stamp, L.K. Gout. *Lancet* **2016**, *388*, 2039–2052. [CrossRef]
2. Dalbeth, N.; Choi, H.K.; Joosten, L.A.B.; Khanna, P.P.; Matsuo, H.; Perez-Ruiz, F.; Stamp, L.K. Gout. *Nat. Rev. Dis. Primers* **2019**, *5*, 69. [CrossRef] [PubMed]
3. Wu, X.W.; Muzny, D.M.; Lee, C.C.; Caskey, C.T. Two independent mutational events in the loss of urate oxidase during hominoid evolution. *J. Mol. Evol.* **1992**, *34*, 78–84. [CrossRef] [PubMed]
4. Bobulescu, I.A.; Moe, O.W. Renal transport of uric acid: Evolving concepts and uncertainties. *Adv. Chronic Kidney Dis.* **2012**, *19*, 358–371. [CrossRef]
5. Hyndman, D.; Liu, S.; Miner, J.N. Urate Handling in the Human Body. *Curr. Rheumatol. Rep.* **2016**, *18*, 34. [CrossRef]
6. Enomoto, A.; Kimura, H.; Chairoungdua, A.; Shigeta, Y.; Jutabha, P.; Cha, S.H.; Hosoyamada, M.; Takeda, M.; Sekine, T.; Igarashi, T.; et al. Molecular identification of a renal urate anion exchanger that regulates blood urate levels. *Nature* **2002**, *417*, 447–452. [CrossRef]
7. Kawamura, Y.; Toyoda, Y.; Ohnishi, T.; Hisatomi, R.; Higashino, T.; Nakayama, A.; Shimizu, S.; Yanagi, M.; Kamimaki, I.; Fujimaru, R.; et al. Identification of a dysfunctional splicing mutation in the SLC22A12/URAT1 gene causing renal hypouricaemia type 1: A report on two families. *Rheumatology* **2020**, *59*, 3988–3990. [CrossRef]
8. Nakayama, A.; Matsuo, H.; Ohtahara, A.; Ogino, K.; Hakoda, M.; Hamada, T.; Hosoyamada, M.; Yamaguchi, S.; Hisatome, I.; Ichida, K.; et al. Clinical practice guideline for renal hypouricemia (1st edition). *Hum. Cell* **2019**, *32*, 83–87. [CrossRef]
9. Nakayama, A.; Kawamura, Y.; Toyoda, Y.; Shimizu, S.; Kawaguchi, M.; Aoki, Y.; Takeuchi, K.; Okada, R.; Kubo, Y.; Imakiire, T.; et al. Genetic-epidemiological analysis of hypouricemia from 4,993 Japanese on nonfunctional variants of URAT1/SLC22A12 gene. *Rheumatology* **2021**. [CrossRef]
10. Miner, J.N.; Tan, P.K.; Hyndman, D.; Liu, S.; Iverson, C.; Nanavati, P.; Hagerty, D.T.; Manhard, K.; Shen, Z.; Girardet, J.L.; et al. Lesinurad, a novel, oral compound for gout, acts to decrease serum uric acid through inhibition of urate transporters in the kidney. *Arthritis Res. Ther.* **2016**, *18*, 214. [CrossRef]
11. Toyoda, Y.; Takada, T.; Saito, H.; Hirata, H.; Ota-Kontani, A.; Kobayashi, N.; Tsuchiya, Y.; Suzuki, H. Inhibitory effect of Citrus flavonoids on the in vitro transport activity of human urate transporter 1 (URAT1/SLC22A12), a renal re-absorber of urate. *NPJ Sci. Food* **2020**, *4*, 3. [CrossRef] [PubMed]
12. Tashiro, Y.; Sakai, R.; Hirose-Sugiura, T.; Kato, Y.; Matsuo, H.; Takada, T.; Suzuki, H.; Makino, T. Effects of Osthol Isolated from Cnidium monnieri Fruit on Urate Transporter 1. *Molecules* **2018**, *23*, 2837. [CrossRef] [PubMed]
13. Yu, Z.; Fong, W.P.; Cheng, C.H. Morin (3,5,7,2′,4′-pentahydroxyflavone) exhibits potent inhibitory actions on urate transport by the human urate anion transporter (hURAT1) expressed in human embryonic kidney cells. *Drug Metab. Dispos. Biol. Fate Chem.* **2007**, *35*, 981–986. [CrossRef] [PubMed]
14. Saito, H.; Toyoda, Y.; Takada, T.; Hirata, H.; Ota-Kontani, A.; Miyata, H.; Kobayashi, N.; Tsuchiya, Y.; Suzuki, H. Omega-3 Polyunsaturated Fatty Acids Inhibit the Function of Human URAT1, a Renal Urate Re-Absorber. *Nutrients* **2020**, *12*, 1601. [CrossRef]
15. Toyoda, Y.; Kawamura, Y.; Nakayama, A.; Nakaoka, H.; Higashino, T.; Shimizu, S.; Ooyama, H.; Morimoto, K.; Uchida, N.; Shigesawa, R.; et al. Substantial anti-gout effect conferred by common and rare dysfunctional variants of URAT1/SLC22A12. *Rheumatology* **2021**, *60*, 5224–5232. [CrossRef]
16. Saito, H.; Toyoda, Y.; Hirata, H.; Ota-Kontani, A.; Tsuchiya, Y.; Takada, T.; Suzuki, H. Soy Isoflavone Genistein Inhibits an Axillary Osmidrosis Risk Factor ABCC11: In Vitro Screening and Fractional Approach for ABCC11-Inhibitory Activities in Plant Extracts and Dietary Flavonoids. *Nutrients* **2020**, *12*, 2452. [CrossRef]
17. Hirata, H.; Takazumi, K.; Segawa, S.; Okada, Y.; Kobayashi, N.; Shigyo, T.; Chiba, H. Xanthohumol, a prenylated chalcone from Humulus lupulus L., inhibits cholesteryl ester transfer protein. *Food Chem.* **2012**, *134*, 1432–1437. [CrossRef]
18. Miyata, H.; Takada, T.; Toyoda, Y.; Matsuo, H.; Ichida, K.; Suzuki, H. Identification of Febuxostat as a New Strong ABCG2 Inhibitor: Potential Applications and Risks in Clinical Situations. *Front Pharmacol.* **2016**, *7*, 518. [CrossRef]
19. McKay, D.L.; Blumberg, J.B. A review of the bioactivity of South African herbal teas: Rooibos (*Aspalathus linearis*) and honeybush (*Cyclopia intermedia*). *Phytother Res.* **2007**, *21*, 1–16. [CrossRef]
20. Shimamura, N.; Miyase, T.; Umehara, K.; Warashina, T.; Fujii, S. Phytoestrogens from Aspalathus linearis. *Biol. Pharm. Bull.* **2006**, *29*, 1271–1274. [CrossRef]
21. Panche, A.N.; Diwan, A.D.; Chandra, S.R. Flavonoids: An overview. *J. Nutr. Sci.* **2016**, *5*, e47. [CrossRef] [PubMed]
22. Vauzour, D.; Vafeiadou, K.; Rodriguez-Mateos, A.; Rendeiro, C.; Spencer, J.P. The neuroprotective potential of flavonoids: A multiplicity of effects. *Genes Nutr.* **2008**, *3*, 115–126. [CrossRef] [PubMed]
23. Kashyap, D.; Garg, V.K.; Tuli, H.S.; Yerer, M.B.; Sak, K.; Sharma, A.K.; Kumar, M.; Aggarwal, V.; Sandhu, S.S. Fisetin and Quercetin: Promising Flavonoids with Chemopreventive Potential. *Biomolecules* **2019**, *9*, 174. [CrossRef] [PubMed]
24. Sundarraj, K.; Raghunath, A.; Perumal, E. A review on the chemotherapeutic potential of fisetin: In vitro evidences. *Biomed. Pharmacother.* **2018**, *97*, 928–940. [CrossRef]
25. Boots, A.W.; Haenen, G.R.; Bast, A. Health effects of quercetin: From antioxidant to nutraceutical. *Eur. J. Pharmacol.* **2008**, *585*, 325–337. [CrossRef]
26. Shi, Y.; Williamson, G. Quercetin lowers plasma uric acid in pre-hyperuricaemic males: A randomised, double-blinded, placebo-controlled, cross-over trial. *Br. J. Nutr.* **2016**, *115*, 800–806. [CrossRef]
27. Day, A.J.; Bao, Y.; Morgan, M.R.A.; Williamson, G. Conjugation position of quercetin glucuronides and effect on biological activity. *Free Radic. Biol. Med.* **2000**, *29*, 1234–1243. [CrossRef]

28. Joubert, E.; de Beer, D. Rooibos (*Aspalathus linearis*) beyond the farm gate: From herbal tea to potential phytopharmaceutical. *S. Afr. J. Bot.* **2011**, *77*, 869–886. [CrossRef]
29. Kondo, M.; Hirano, Y.; Nishio, M.; Furuya, Y.; Nakamura, H.; Watanabe, T. Xanthine oxidase inhibitory activity and hypouricemic effect of aspalathin from unfermented rooibos. *J. Food Sci.* **2013**, *78*, H1935–H1939. [CrossRef]
30. Jiang, L.L.; Gong, X.; Ji, M.Y.; Wang, C.C.; Wang, J.H.; Li, M.H. Bioactive Compounds from Plant-Based Functional Foods: A Promising Choice for the Prevention and Management of Hyperuricemia. *Foods* **2020**, *9*, 973. [CrossRef]

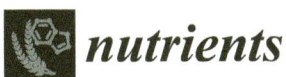

Article

Mokko Lactone Alleviates Doxorubicin-Induced Cardiotoxicity in Rats via Antioxidant, Anti-Inflammatory, and Antiapoptotic Activities

Alaa Sirwi [1], Rasheed A. Shaik [2], Abdulmohsin J. Alamoudi [2], Basma G. Eid [2], Mahmoud A. Elfaky [1,3], Sabrin R. M. Ibrahim [4,5], Gamal A. Mohamed [1], Hossam M. Abdallah [1,6] and Ashraf B. Abdel-Naim [2,*]

[1] Department of Natural Products, Faculty of Pharmacy, King Abdulaziz University, Jeddah 21589, Saudi Arabia; asirwi@kau.edu.sa (A.S.); melfaky@kau.edu.sa (M.A.E.); gahussein@kau.edu.sa (G.A.M.); hmafifi@kau.edu.sa (H.M.A.)
[2] Department of Pharmacology and Toxicology, Faculty of Pharmacy, King Abdulaziz University, Jeddah 21589, Saudi Arabia; rashaikh1@kau.edu.sa (R.A.S.); ajmalamoudi@kau.edu.sa (A.J.A.); beid@kau.edu.sa (B.G.E.)
[3] Centre for Artificial Intelligence in Precision Medicines, King Abdulaziz University, Jeddah 21589, Saudi Arabia
[4] Department of Chemistry, Preparatory Year Program, Batterjee Medical College, Jeddah 21442, Saudi Arabia; sabrin.ibrahim@bmc.edu.sa
[5] Department of Pharmacognosy, Faculty of Pharmacy, Assiut University, Assiut 71526, Egypt
[6] Department of Pharmacognosy, Faculty of Pharmacy, Cairo University, Cairo 11562, Egypt
* Correspondence: aaabdulalrahman1@kau.edu.sa; Tel.: +966-55-6814781

Abstract: Doxorubicin (DOX), a commonly utilized anthracycline antibiotic, suffers deleterious side effects such as cardiotoxicity. Mokko lactone (ML) is a naturally occurring guainolide sesquiterpene with established antioxidant and anti-inflammatory actions. This study aimed at investigating the protective effects of ML in a DOX-induced cardiotoxicity model in rats. Our results indicated that ML exerted protection against cardiotoxicity induced by DOX as indicated by ameliorating the rise in serum troponin and creatine kinase-MB levels and lactate dehydrogenase activity. Histological assessment showed that ML provided protection against pathological alterations in heart architecture. Furthermore, treatment with ML significantly ameliorated DOX-induced accumulation of malondialdehyde and protein carbonyl, depletion of glutathione, and exhaustion of superoxide dismutase and catalase. ML's antioxidant effects were accompanied by increased nuclear translocation of NF-E2-related factor 2 (Nrf2) and heme oxygenase-1 (HO-1) expression. Moreover, ML exhibited significant anti-inflammatory activities as evidenced by lowered nuclear factor κB, interleukin-6, and tumor necrosis factor-α expression. ML also caused significant antiapoptotic actions manifested by modulation in mRNA expression of Bax, Bcl-2, and caspase-3. This suggests that ML prevents heart injury induced by DOX via its antioxidant, anti-inflammatory, and antiapoptotic activities.

Keywords: doxorubicin; mokko lactone; heart

Citation: Sirwi, A.; Shaik, R.A.; Alamoudi, A.J.; Eid, B.G.; Elfaky, M.A.; Ibrahim, S.R.M.; Mohamed, G.A.; Abdallah, H.M.; Abdel-Naim, A.B. Mokko Lactone Alleviates Doxorubicin-Induced Cardiotoxicity in Rats via Antioxidant, Anti-Inflammatory, and Antiapoptotic Activities. *Nutrients* **2022**, *14*, 733. https://doi.org/10.3390/nu14040733

Academic Editor: Md Soriful Islam

Received: 28 December 2021
Accepted: 7 February 2022
Published: 9 February 2022

Publisher's Note: MDPI stays neutral with regard to jurisdictional claims in published maps and institutional affiliations.

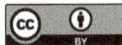

Copyright: © 2022 by the authors. Licensee MDPI, Basel, Switzerland. This article is an open access article distributed under the terms and conditions of the Creative Commons Attribution (CC BY) license (https:// creativecommons.org/licenses/by/ 4.0/).

1. Introduction

Doxorubicin (DOX) is a commonly utilized anthracycline antibiotic for treating several types of cancer, including breast cancer and lymphomas [1]. However, its clinical applications are relatively restricted due to its detrimental side effects that include cardiotoxicity [2]. It was reported that the incidence of acute DOX cardiotoxicity is around 11%, which can be characterized on the electrocardiogram by decreased amplitude of QRS complexes and nonspecific ST changes [3,4]. This toxic damage to the cardiomyocytes induced by DOX can lead to the development of tachycardia, arrhythmia, pericarditis, myocarditis, left ventricular function transient depression, late-onset refractory cardiomyopathy, and, eventually, congestive heart failure [5,6]. Unfortunately, the development of congestive heart failure with DOX therapy indicates a poor prognosis of cancer patients, as it is associated with nearly 50% mortality in 1 year [7]. DOX cardiomyopathy is characterized histopathologically by patchy interstitial fibrosis and myocyte vacuolar degeneration [8,9]. DOX cardiotoxicity is usually accompanied by raised troponin, creatine kinase isoenzyme MB (CK-MB), and lactate dehydrogenase (LDH) levels in the serum [10]. DOX can induce dose-related cardiomyopathy through multiple mechanisms that involve increased oxidative stress, as shown by the increased cardiac generation of oxygen free radicals and lipid peroxidation products [11–13].

Since DOX is a useful chemotherapy drug in cancer, different approaches have been adopted to alleviate its toxic side effects that include dosage optimization, combination therapy, and the development of analogs. However, no satisfactory results have been achieved out of these ongoing efforts [14]. Therefore, cardioprotection during DOX treatment is required to reduce the incidence of DOX-induced heart damage; hence, it is necessary to discover new drugs that can be utilized as cardioprotective agents with DOX therapy. In this regard, natural products remain an attractive source of bioactive lead compounds that can tackle this problem [15]. With regards to disease treatment and prevention, natural products are still considered one of the best sources of novel bioactive molecules. The potential of research efforts in this field is highlighted by the fact that 16% of the US-FDA drug approvals in 2018 were for new drugs classified as natural products [16]. Phytoconstituents are considered a source of bioactive compounds that could lead to new drugs. In this regard, rhizomes of *Costus speciosus* (*Zingiberaceae*) are traditionally utilized in Indian folk medicine for their anti-inflammatory, antispasmodic, hepatoprotective, antidiabetic, antihyperlipidemic, antimicrobial, and anthelmintic activities. Moreover, it was shown that the rhizomes of this plant exert cardioprotective effects against oxidative stress in atherosclerotic [17]. The rhizomes are rich in different phytoconstituents, mainly guaianolides sesquiterpene lactones [18,19]. Guaianolides have several reported pharmacological effects that include antioxidant, anti-inflammatory, and antimicrobial activities [20]. Mokko lactone (ML, dihydrodehydrocostus lactone) is a major guaianolide in *C. speciosus* that possesses notable anti-inflammatory action, as it has been shown to significantly reduce the release of TNF-α and IL-6 from stimulated human peripheral blood mononuclear cells [21]. ML has also demonstrated significant antioxidant and hepatoprotective effects in rats challenged with DOX [22]. Thus, this work aimed at examining the possible protection offered by ML, extracted from the rhizomes of *C. speciosus*, against acute cardiotoxicity induced by DOX in rats.

2. Materials and Methods

2.1. Chemicals

ML (purity > 98%) was isolated from *Costus speciosus* rhizomes extract (Supplementary Materials). DOX HCl was obtained from Sigma-Aldrich (St. Louis, MO, USA). Remaining chemicals conformed with the highest available commercial purity.

2.2. Animals

Twenty-four Wistar rats (males, 200–230 g) were purchased from the animal facility, Faculty of Pharmacy, King Abdulaziz University. Animals were kept on a 12-h light/dark cycle at ambient temperature (22 $\pm$ 3 °C) with humidity (60–70%), with access to food and water. Research Ethics Committee, Faculty of Pharmacy, King Abdulaziz University approved the experimental protocol (Reference # PH-1443-13).

2.3. Toxicity Study

Acute oral toxicity of ML was assessed according to OECD guideline number 423. Briefly, rats were given a single oral dose of 2000 mg/kg. After treatment, animals were individually observed at least one time during the first hour and regularly for the upcoming 24 h, with particular attention during the first 4 h. Since all rats survived, the experiment was repeated using three additional male rats.

2.4. Experimental Protocol

Animals were placed in groups of four in a random fashion (n = 6): controls, the DOX group, the first treatment group was given 15 mg/kg ML and DOX while the second treatment group was given 30 mg/kg ML and DOX. The doses of ML were chosen after carrying out a pilot study and were consistent with those in the literature [22]. Control and DOX groups were given 0.5% carboxymethyl cellulose (CMC) orally one time daily for 10 days consecutively. ML was suspended in CMC and was administered to both treatment groups orally for 10 days at the mentioned doses. On the tenth day, controls were given an intraperitoneal (IP) injection of 0.9% saline, 60 min after ML administration. Similarly, on the tenth day and 60 min after ML the remaining groups were administered an IP dose of 15 mg/kg DOX dissolved in 0.9% saline. Volume used for dosing all animals was 10 mL/kg. Twenty-four hours post last injection, animals were given 50 mg/kg ketamine and 5 mg/kg xylazine IP for anesthesia. Electrocardiogram (ECG) measurements were then performed on the animals. The retroorbital plexus was used for collecting blood samples. Blood was kept for 15 min and then centrifuged for 10 min at 3000 RPM and 4 °C to obtain serum. Decapitation was performed, and hearts were dissected out, gently rinsed with saline (ice-cooled), and blotted between filter paper. Part of the heart was placed in 10% formalin for histopathological and immunohistochemical studies. Remaining sections of the hearts were placed in RNAProtect Tissue Reagent (Cat. No. 76106, Qiagen, MD, USA). The remaining parts were flash-frozen with liquid nitrogen and held together with serum at −80 °C for analysis.

2.5. Electrocardiography

At the end of the treatment protocol, animals were given a combination of ketamine (100 mg/kg; i.p.) + xylazine (10 mg/kg; i.p.) for anesthesia. During electrocardiography, rectal temperatures were kept at 37.5 °C by a thermostatically controlled heating blanket. In all animals, 10 min after anesthesia, three needle electrodes were placed below the skin of the animals. Electrodes were placed in the right hind and front limbs and the left hind limb. A PowerLab, model 8/35 (ADInstruments, Sydney, Australia), was used to record the ECG. ECG parameters were recorded. The changes in duration of P wave (ms), QRS complex (ms), QRS amplitude (µV), QT interval (ms), PR interval (ms), RR interval (ms), and amplitude of ST segment (µV) were determined.

2.6. Biochemical Assays and Measurements of Cardiac Enzymes

Serum was collected from blood samples by centrifugation for 10 min at 3000 rpm and placed in Eppendorf tubes for biochemical analysis of creatine kinase myocardial band (CK-MB), cardiac troponin levels, and lactate dehydrogenase (LDH), and were assessed using colorimetric kits (SEA479Ra, SEA478Ra, and SEB370Ra, Cloud-Clone, Houston, TX, USA, respectively).

2.7. Histopathological Study

Heart tissues were fixed in 10% neutral formalin, and then paraffinization was performed. Tissues were cut into slices (5 µm). Hematoxylin and eosin (H&E) was used to stain the sections, which were then photographed using light microscopy (Nikon Eclipse TE2000-U, Nikon, Tokyo, Japan). This examination was carried out by a pathologist in a blind manner.

2.8. Assessment of Oxidative and Inflammatory Markers

Homogenization of heart tissues was carried out in a 10-fold volume of ice-cooled phosphate-buffered saline (PBS) (ice-cooled, pH 7.4). Following centrifugation at $10,000 \times g$ for 20 min and 4 °C, the supernatant was then collected for analysis of oxidative and inflammatory markers. ELISA kits were used in the assessment of the hearts' content of malondialdehyde (MDA), reduced glutathione (GSH), enzymatic activities of superoxide dismutase (SOD), catalase (CAT) (Cat. No. MD 2529, GR 2511, SD 2521, and CA 2517,

Biodiagnostic, Giza, Egypt, respectively), and protein carbonyl, interlukin-6 (IL-6), and tumor necrosis factor α (TNF-α) (Cat. No. ab238536, ab234570, and ab100785, Abcam, Cambridge, UK, respectively).

Nuclear fractions of tissue homogenates were obtained using NE-PER nuclear and cytoplasmic extraction kit (Cat. No. 78833, Thermo Fisher Scientific, Waltham, MA, USA). Protein content of the nuclear extracts was determined, and a volume equivalent to 80 µg was employed in the assessment of the DNA-binding activity of NF-kB p65 using NF-κB p65 ELISA Kit (Cat. No. ab133112, Abcam, Cambridge, UK). Results are expressed as fold change of control.

2.9. Tissue Staining for Immunohistochemistry

Tissue sections were deparaffinized, and then ethanol serial dilutions were employed for tissue rehydration before boiling in 0.1 M citrate buffer (pH 6.0) for 10 min. A 2-hour incubation period in 5% bovine serum albumin (BSA) in tris buffered saline (TBS) was subsequently followed. Primary antibodies were then used in the tissue incubation for 12 h at 4 °C, namely: TNFα (Cat. No. ab220210, Abcam®, Cambridge, UK), IL-6, (Cat. No. ab9324, Abcam®, Cambridge, UK), NFκB (Cat. No. sc-8414, Santa Cruz, TX, USA), and Nrf2 (Cat. No. MBS9608128, MyBioSource, San Diego, CA, USA). After tissue flushing using TBS, another incubation was carried out in either antimouse or antirabbit biotinylated secondary antibody based on the primary antibody reactivity (Cell & Tissue Staining Kit, Cat. No. CTS002, CTS006, R&D systems, Minneapolis, MN, USA). Quantification was performed with an image analysis software (Image J, 1.8.0, NIH, Bethesda, MD, USA).

2.10. Quantitative Real-Time Polymerase Chain Reaction (PCR)

TRIzol was used for isolation of total RNA from the tissues of the heart. A260/A280 ratio was employed in assessing RNA purity. Samples with a ratio greater than 1.7 were included in the synthesis of cDNA. Omniscript RT kit (Cat. No. 205113, Qiagen, MD, USA) was used for first-strand cDNA synthesis. A SYBR Green Master Mix (Cat. No. 180830, Qiagen, MD, USA) with forward and reverse primers was used for quantification of mRNA using qPCR. The following sequences represented the forward primers for Nrf2, HO-1, Bax, Bcl-2, caspase-3, and β-actin: 5′TTTGTAGATGACCATGAGTCGC,5′TCTGCAGGGGAGA ATCTTGC, 5′CCTGAGCTGACCTTGGAGCA, 5′TGATAACCGGGAGATCGTGA, 5′CTCG GTCTGGTACAGATGTCGATG, and 5′TCCGTCGCCGGTCCACACCC, respectively. The following sequences represented the reverse primers for Nrf2, HO-1, Bax, Bcl-2, caspase-3 and β-actin: 5′TGTCCTGCTGTATGCTGCTT, 5′TTGGTGACGGAAATGTGCCA, 5′GGTG GTTGCCCTTTTCTACT, 5′AAAGCACATCCAATAAAAAGC, 5′GGTTAACCCGGGTAAG AATGTGCA, and 5′TCACCAACTGGGACGATATG, respectively. The primers sequences were taken from references that have been already validated in our laboratory [22]. Data were analyzed by the ΔΔCT method, and β-actin was used for normalization [23].

2.11. Statistics

Data are represented as means ± SD. One-way ANOVA followed by Tukey's multiple comparison test was used for assessing results. GraphPad Prism (Prism 8.1, GraphPad Software, Inc., La Jolla, CA, USA) was used for all analyses. $p < 0.05$ was considered significant.

3. Results

3.1. Assessment of Acute Toxicity of ML

At 24 h of oral ML dose of 2000 mg/kg to rats, no deaths were observed in three tested male animals. A further study was carried out in three male animals utilizing the same dose, which, similarly, resulted in no deaths after 24 h.

3.2. Assessment of Heart Electrical Activities

Electrocardiographic patterns (P wave duration, QRS complex duration, QRS amplitude, QT interval, PR interval duration, RR interval duration, ST segment amplitude) of the control and experimental groups are displayed in Table 1 and Figure 1. The values of ECG indices are given in Table 1. Control rats had normal ECG findings, while the DOX-challenged rats demonstrated a markedly lowered P wave and QRS complex. Furthermore, DOX injection induced a significant increase in the QT, PR, and RR intervals and ST segment relative to controls. However, these pathological changes in P wave magnitude and QRS amplitude and complexes were prevented by ML in a dose-related manner. ML also resulted in a significant restoration of the QT, PR, and RR intervals and ST segment.

Table 1. Effect of ML on DOX-induced alterations in electrocardiographic (ECG) indices.

	Control	DOX	DOX + ML (15 mg/kg)	DOX + ML (30 mg/kg)
P wave (duration, ms)	30 ± 1 (29–30)	22 ± 5 [a] (17–27)	26 ± 1 (25–27)	34 ± 1 [b] (33–35)
QRS complex (duration, ms)	63 ± 2 (61–65)	30 ± 1 [a] (29–31)	40 ± 2 (38–42)	65 ± 1 [b] (64–66)
QRS amplitude (µV)	82 ± 2 (80–84)	140 ± 10 [a] (130–150)	60 ± 2 [b] (58–62)	80 ± 1 [b] (79–81)
QT interval (duration, ms)	50 ± 1 (49–51)	72 ± 3 [a] (69–75)	60 ± 1 (59–61)	54 ± 1 [b] (53–55)
PR interval (duration, ms)	20 ± 1 (19–21)	25 ± 1 [a] (24–26)	22 ± 1 (21–23)	19 ± 1 [b] (18–20)
RR interval (duration, ms)	150 ± 1 (149–151)	260 ± 1 [a] (259–261)	220 ± 3 (217–223)	130 ± 3 [b] (127–133)
ST segment amplitude (µV)	51 ± 3 (48–54)	180 ± 3 [a] (177–183)	100 ± 3 (97–103)	55 ± 1 [b] (54–56)

Results are displayed as mean ± SD ($n = 6$) and range of values in each group is shown between brackets; DOX = Doxorubicin, ML = Mokko Lactone, [a] significantly different from control ($p < 0.05$); [b] significantly different from DOX ($p < 0.05$).

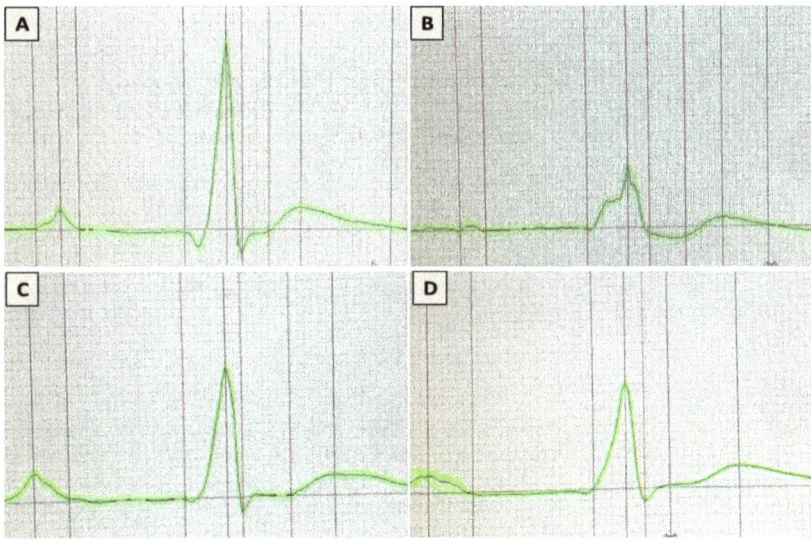

Figure 1. Effect of ML on DOX-induced on ECG patterns: (**A**) control group; (**B**) DOX group; (**C**) DOX + ML (15 mg/kg); and (**D**) DOX + ML (30 mg/kg), DOX = Doxorubicin, ML = Mokko Lactone.

3.3. Histopathological Assessment

Microscopic examination of heart sections from the control group revealed a normal histological structure of cardiac architecture (Figure 2A). However, the DOX group revealed marked cardiotoxicity that was characterized by scattered degeneration of cardiac myofibers, mononuclear inflammatory cells infiltration, myocarditis, and extensive cytoplasmic vacuolization (Figure 2B). Sections from DOX + ML (15 mg/kg) showed moderate enhancement of the cardiac histology with fewer inflammatory areas and degenerated cardiomyocytes (Figure 2C). Rats given DOX + ML (30 mg/kg) showed the highest protection that revealed an apparently normal structure in most examined sections (Figure 2D).

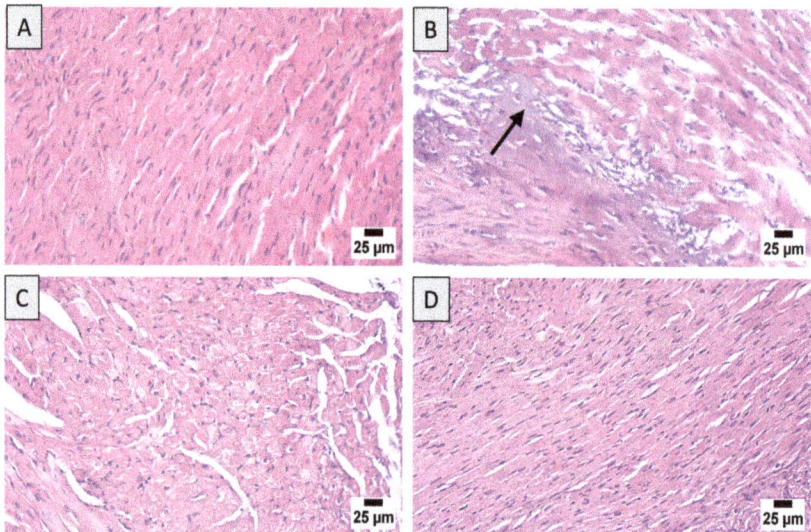

Figure 2. Effect of ML on DOX-induced histopathological changes on cardiac tissues: (**A**) control group demonstrating normal architecture of the heart tissues; (**B**) DOX group exhibiting mononuclear inflammatory cells infiltration and widespread necrosis of cardiac tissues (black arrow); (**C**) DOX + ML (15 mg/kg) treated group showing limited inflammatory areas and degenerated cardiomyocytes; (**D**) DOX + ML (30 mg/kg) treated group with restoration of a nearly normal cardiac histology. DOX = Doxorubicin, ML = Mokko Lactone.

Data in Table 2 show semi-quantitatively the cardiac injury induced by DOX. The pathological alterations included severe disruption of cardiac muscles architecture, interstitial edema, inflammatory cellular infiltrate, apoptosis, and necrosis, as evidenced by nuclear pyknosis, karyorrhexis, and/or karyolysis. Both doses of ML obviously ameliorated such deleterious effects to the borderline score in cardiac myocyte death in animals treated with the 30 mg/kg ML.

3.4. Effect of ML on Serum Cardiac Markers

The protective activity of ML against DOX-induced heart injury was confirmed based on the levels of serum markers of cardiotoxicity, namely, troponin, CK-MB, and LDH. As can be observed in Figure 3A,B, rats challenged with DOX showed raised troponin and CK-MB levels in the serum compared with control rats. However, treatment with ML significantly ameliorated and prevented this DOX-induced increase in both markers at 15 mg/kg and 30 mg/kg, respectively. The data in Figure 3C reveal that prior treatment with ML at 15 mg/kg to DOX-challenged rats significantly ameliorated the increase in serum LDH activity by approximately 32%; this increase was significantly inhibited at an ML dose level of 30 mg/kg.

Table 2. Histopathological semi-quantitative scoring showing the effects of ML on DOX-induced severity of histopathologic lesions in DOX-treated rats.

	Control	DOX	DOX + ML (15 mg/kg)	DOX + ML (30 mg/kg)
Disruption of cardiac muscles	-	+++	++	+
Interstitial edema	-	+++	++	+
Inflammatory cellular infiltrate	-	+++	++	+
Apoptosis	-	++	+	±
Necrosis (nuclear pyknosis, karyolysis, karyorrhexis)	-	++	+	±

Score values are obtained from tissue sections of six animals of each group, five fields/section (X 100): scores of -, normal; ±, borderline; +, mild; ++, moderate; +++, severe. DOX = Doxorubicin, ML = Mokko Lactone.

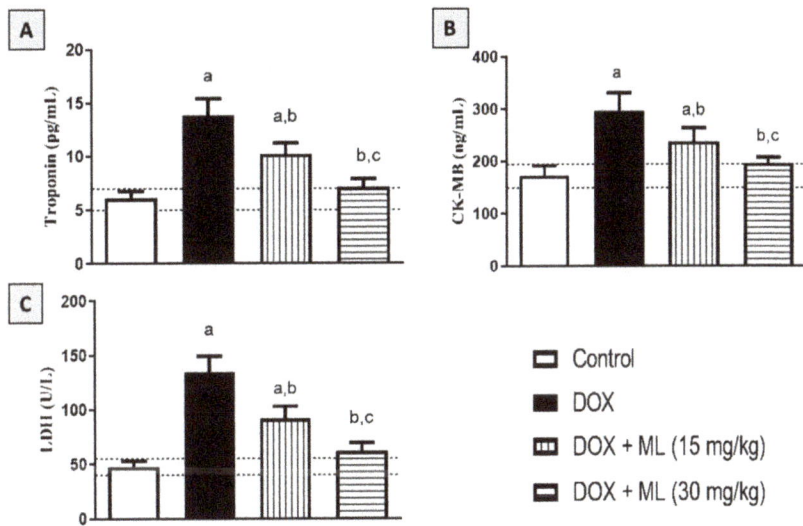

Figure 3. Effect of ML on serum cardiac markers in DOX-treated rats: (A) serum troponin level; (B) serum CK-MB level; (C) serum LDH activity. Background dotted lines represent range of corresponding control values. Data are displayed as mean ± SD ($n = 6$). DOX = Doxorubicin, ML = Mokko Lactone. a, significantly different than control ($p < 0.05$); b, significantly different than DOX ($p < 0.05$); c, significantly different than DOX + ML (15 mg/kg) ($p < 0.05$).

3.5. Effect of ML on Cardiac Oxidative Stress

The antioxidant activity of ML was also examined in rats following acute DOX exposure. Figure 4A shows that DOX resulted in increased oxidative stress, as shown by the increased contents of MDA. Nonetheless, treatment with ML significantly ameliorated the increase in MDA by around 20% and 33% at 15 mg/kg and 30 mg/kg, respectively. It can also be observed in Figure 4B–D that the DOX challenge led to significant GSH depletion and CAT and SOD exhaustion. However, treatment with ML at both doses tested significantly attenuated the depletion of GSH, increasing the values by 92.3% and 151.9% relative to the DOX group, respectively. ML also significantly ameliorated the exhaustion of CAT and SOD associated with DOX-induced oxidative stress at both doses tested in a concentration-related manner. In addition, ML significantly ameliorated the increase in protein carbonyl associated with DOX-induced oxidative stress at both doses tested in a dose-related manner (Figure 4E).

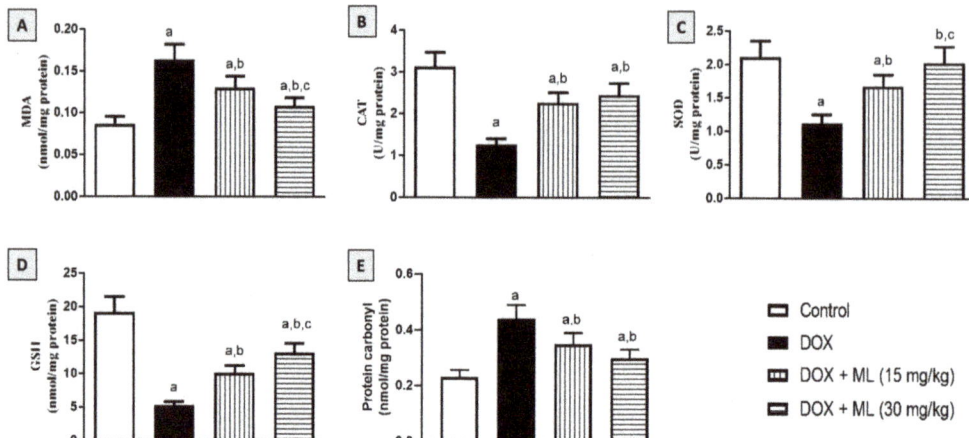

Figure 4. Effect of ML on oxidative status of on DOX-induced cardiotoxicity in rats: (**A**) cardiac MDA content; (**B**) cardiac CAT activity; (**C**) cardiac SOD activity; (**D**) cardiac GSH; and (**E**) cardiac protein carbonyl content. Data are displayed as mean ± SD (n = 6). DOX = Doxorubicin, ML = Mokko Lactone. a, significantly different compared with control ($p < 0.05$); b, significantly different compared with DOX ($p < 0.05$); c, significantly different compared with DOX + ML (15 mg/kg) ($p < 0.05$).

3.6. Effect of ML on Nrf2 and HO-1 Expression

To confirm the antioxidant activity and to assess the anti-inflammatory potential of ML, the cardiac expression of Nrf2 was examined following ML and DOX treatments. As it can be observed in Figure 5A–E, DOX caused a marked lowering of Nrf2 expression in comparison to the control value. Interestingly, treatment with ML not only ameliorated this decrease in Nrf2 at 15 mg/kg by approximately 50% but also significantly prevented it at 30 mg/kg. In addition, these data were confirmed by assessing Nrf2 and HO-1 mRNA expression, which were significantly downregulated by DOX challenge. However, both doses of ML ameliorated such effects and significantly inhibited the decrease in mRNA expression of Nrf2 and HO-1 (Figure 5F,G).

3.7. Effect of ML on Expression of Heart Inflammatory Markers

The inflammatory status of cardiac tissues was examined immunohistochemically in DOX-challenged rats following ML treatment. DOX challenge significantly induced the expression of NF-κb, while ML treatment significantly attenuated the increased expression of NF-κb at 15 mg/kg and 30 mg/kg by 33.8% and 44.7%, respectively. Moreover, the expression of IL-6 and TNF-α was also increased with DOX and this was significantly ameliorated by ML at 15 mg/kg by 28.9% and 26.7%, respectively. ML at 30 mg/kg resulted in an even further decrease in the expression of IL-6 by 36.3% and TNF-α by 38.0% compared with DOX alone (Figure 6A). These data were confirmed using the ELISA technique that indicated the ability of DOX to activate NF-κb and the cardiac content of IL-6 and TNF-α. The same protective actions of both doses of ML were observed. ML treatment was associated with the significant amelioration of NF-κb DNA-binding activity and prevented the rise in IL-6 and TNF-α content (Figure 6B).

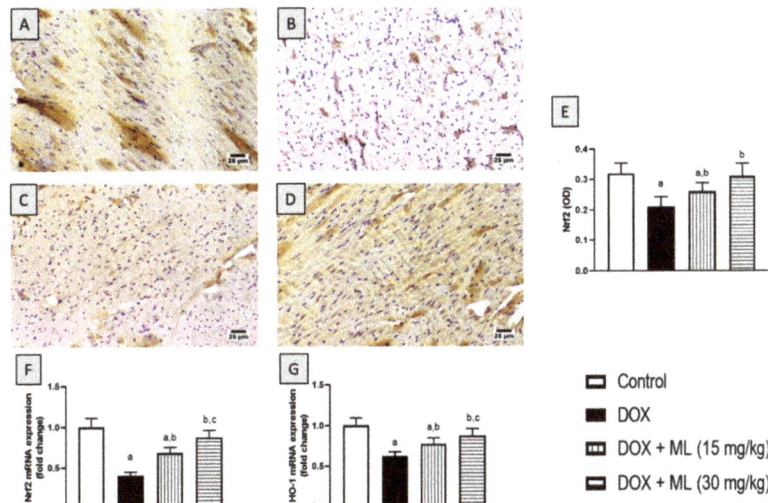

Figure 5. Effect of ML on Nrf2 expression as determined immunohistochemically (**A–E**) and mRNA expression of Nrf2 (**F**) and HO-1 (**G**) in cardiac tissues of DOX-treated rats. Data shown as bar charts are mean ± SD ($n = 6$). DOX = Doxorubicin, ML = Mokko Lactone. a, b, or c: statistically different from control, DOX, or DOX + ML (15 mg/kg), respectively ($p < 0.05$).

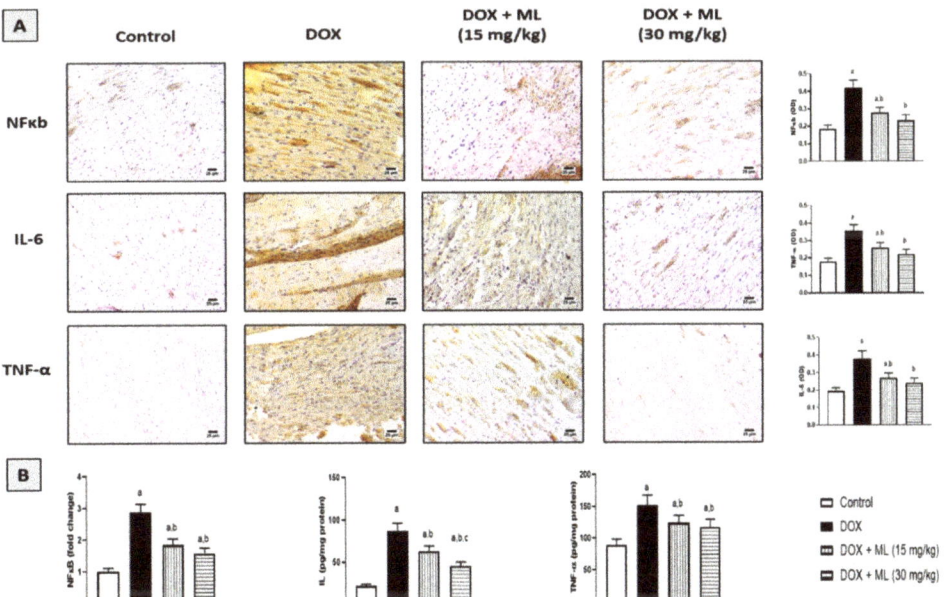

Figure 6. Effect of ML on NFκB, IL-6, and TNF-α, as determined by immunohistochemistry (**A**) or ELISA (**B**) in cardiac tissues of DOX-treated rats. Data in bar charts are mean ± SD ($n = 6$). DOX = Doxorubicin, ML = Mokko Lactone. a, b or c: statistically significant compared with control, DOX, or DOX + ML (15 mg/kg), respectively ($p < 0.05$).

3.8. Effect of ML on Bax, Bcl-2, and Caspase-3 mRNA Expression

ML's antiapoptotic effects were examined based on the Bax, Bcl2, and caspase-3 mRNA expression in cardiac tissues of rats who received a single DOX injection. As demonstrated in Figure 7A, DOX resulted in a significant increase in the mRNA expression of the proapoptotic regulator Bax. However, ML markedly ameliorated this rise by 21.2% and 33.3% at 15 mg/kg and 30 mg/kg, respectively. Regarding the antiapoptotic Bcl-2, DOX significantly decreased Bcl-2 mRNA expression while ML significantly ameliorated this change, as it enhanced its values by more than one- and two-fold at 15 mg/kg and 30 mg/kg, respectively (Figure 7B). In addition, DOX showed significant apoptotic activities, as evidenced by enhanced mRNA expression of caspase-3. ML markedly ameliorated this rise by approximately 18% and 25% at 15 mg/kg and 30 mg/kg, respectively (Figure 7C).

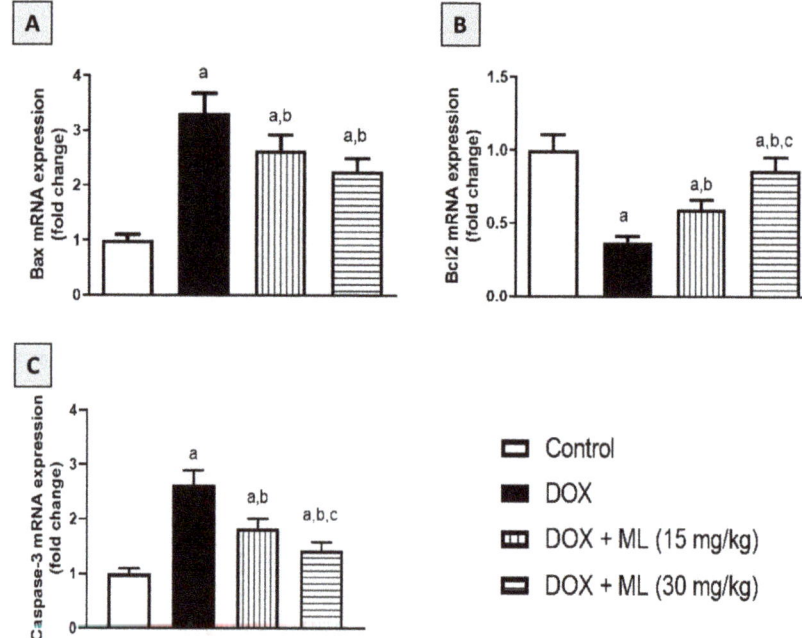

Figure 7. Effect of ML on cardiac mRNA expression of Bax (**A**), Bcl-2 (**B**), and caspase-3 (**C**) in DOX-treated rats. Data shown in bar charts are mean ± SD (n = 6). DOX = Doxorubicin, ML = Mokko Lactone. a, b or c: statistically significant compared with control, DOX, or DOX + ML (15 mg/kg), respectively ($p < 0.05$).

4. Discussion

Cardiotoxicity associated with doxorubicin is acute, occurring within 2 days of its administration, and acute cardiotoxicity occurs in approximately 11% of cases [24]. However, DOX is frequently utilized in anticancer treatment protocols because of the high rates of complete remission associated with this agent compared with many other drugs [25]. DOX-induced cardiotoxicity mechanism is complex and multifaceted and involves the induction of oxidative stress [26]. ML is a sesquiterpene lactone obtained from the rhizomes of *Costus speciosus*, which has been shown to have significant antioxidant and anti-inflammatory properties [20,27]. Hence, we aimed at investigating the possible protective actions of ML due to DOX-induced cardiotoxicity in rats.

Oral LD50 examination of ML in rats indicated almost no toxicity of the compound. On the experiments of electrical potential generated by the heart, our data demonstrated that DOX challenge in rats induced acute cardiotoxicity, as indicated by the alterations in

ECG indices [28]. The administration of ML significantly ameliorated these changes in P wave, QRS complex, QT/RR intervals, and ST segments at 15 mg/kg and prevented them at 30 mg/kg. Moreover, ML inhibited cardiac myopathy, as indicated by the histopathological examination of heart tissues, as ML treatment was associated with relatively preserved cardiomyocytes and almost normal cardiac architecture, indicating a protective activity of ML. According to these functional and histological parameters, it appears that ML can prevent DOX-induced cardiac toxicity in a dose-related manner. Cardiac dysfunction associated with DOX occurs via varied mechanisms that primarily include the induction of oxidative stress leading to severe cellular injury [29]. The results obtained in the current work indicate significant antioxidant activity of ML, as evidenced by the amelioration of pathological changes induced by DOX to the oxidative stress markers MDA, CAT, SOD, GSH, and carbonyl in cardiac tissues. These antioxidant effects could be attributed to the α-methylene-γ-lactone moiety in the chemical structure of ML that confers the ability to interact with the cysteine sulfhydryl groups of many cellular peptides and proteins [30]. These results are consistent with the reported antioxidant activity of ML in DOX-induced hepatotoxicity [22]. Hence, these results indicate that ML decreases oxidative stress and cellular injury in cardiac tissues.

Nrf2 expression analysis further confirmed the antioxidant activity of ML against DOX-induced oxidative stress in cardiac tissues. DOX challenge significantly reduced the cardiac expression of Nrf2. However, treatment with ML significantly prevented this decrease in Nrf2 induced by the DOX challenge. Nrf2 is known to be heavily involved in mediating cellular resistance to oxidative stress in DOX-induced cardiotoxicity [31–33]. Hence, the antioxidant action associated with ML administration be positively regulated by Nrf2 expressed in cardiomyocytes. Furthermore, Nrf2 is also known to reduce inflammatory injury via the regulation of inflammatory cytokines and antioxidant enzymes [34].

The finding of the current study showed increased expression of proinflammatory mediators and cytokines with DOX challenge, while this increase was prevented with ML treatment in a dose-related manner. It has been suggested that cardiac inflammation plays a significant role in DOX-related cardiotoxicity. Inhibiting inflammation has even been shown to facilitate recovering heart dysfunction following DOX administration [35]. These findings are in harmony with other findings in the literature demonstrating the significant anti-inflammatory activity of ML, as evidenced by the reduced release of proinflammatory cytokines, including IL-6 and TNF-α, from activated human peripheral blood mononuclear cells [21]. Thus, this observed anti-inflammatory activity could contribute to the protective effects of ML against cardiotoxicity induced by DOX.

It is documented that DOX cardiotoxicity was likened to the increased apoptotic potential of cardiomyocytes [36]. In this regard, ML was found in the current study to protect against the apoptosis of cardiac tissues in rats who received DOX. Interestingly, the observed antiapoptotic changes in expression of Bax, Bcl2, and caspase-3 caused by ML may be due to Nrf2 dependent mechanisms. It is known that Nrf2 enhances resistance to apoptotic stimuli by upregulating the antiapoptotic protein Bcl2 [37]. It has also been shown that a structurally related compound, costunolide, protects against apoptosis mediated by oxidative stress in a defense mechanism that is dependent on Nrf2 expression and involves antiapoptotic changes in the expression of Bax and Bcl2 [38–40]. Taken together, the generated findings in the current study highlight the importance of the antioxidant, anti-inflammatory, and antiapoptotic activities of ML in mediating resistance to the acute cardiotoxic effects of DOX in rats.

Supplementary Materials: The following supporting information can be downloaded at: https://www.mdpi.com/article/10.3390/nu14040733/s1, Figure S1: Chemical structure of mokko lactone, Figure S2: ESIMS of mokko lactone, Figure S3: 1H NMR spectrum of mokko lactone in CDCl3 (600 MHz), Figure S4: 13C NMR spectrum of mokko lactone in CDCl3 (150 MHz).

Author Contributions: Conceptualization, A.S., A.J.A., and A.B.A.-N.; methodology, A.S., R.A.S., M.A.E., G.A.M., S.R.M.I., and H.M.A.; software, A.J.A., G.A.M., S.R.M.I., and B.G.E.; validation, A.S.,

A.J.A., M.A.E., and R.A.S.; formal analysis, A.S., R.A.S., B.G.E., and A.J.A.; investigation, A.S., R.A.S., B.G.E., A.B.A.-N., and H.M.A.; resources, A.S. and B.G.E.; data curation, R.A.S., M.A.E., G.A.M., S.R.M.I., and B.G.E.; writing—original draft preparation, A.S., A.J.A., G.A.M., and S.R.M.I.; writing—review and editing, A.B.A.-N., B.G.E., A.J.A., and H.M.A.; visualization, A.S., B.G.E., A.J.A., and H.M.A.; supervision, A.S., A.B.A.-N., and H.M.A.; project administration, A.S. and M.A.E.; funding acquisition, A.S. All authors have read and agreed to the published version of the manuscript.

Funding: This project was funded by the Deanship of Scientific Research (DSR) at King Abdulaziz University, Jeddah, under grant no. (G: 234-249-1440). The authors, therefore, acknowledge and give thanks to DSR for technical and financial support.

Institutional Review Board Statement: The study was conducted according to the guidelines of the Declaration of Helsinki and approved by the Research Ethics Committee, Faculty of Pharmacy, King Abdulaziz University (Approval Reference # PH-1443-13).

Informed Consent Statement: Not applicable.

Data Availability Statement: Data are contained within the article and the Supplementary Materials.

Acknowledgments: This project was funded by the Deanship of Scientific Research (DSR) at King Abdulaziz University, Jeddah, under grant no. (G: 234-249-1440). The authors, therefore, acknowledge and give thanks to DSR for technical and financial support. In addition, the authors are grateful to Gamal S. Abd El-Aziz, Department of Anatomy, Faculty of Medicine, King Abdulaziz University, for his help in the histopathological examinations.

Conflicts of Interest: The authors declare no conflict of interest.

References

1. Jain, D.; Aronow, W. Cardiotoxicity of cancer chemotherapy in clinical practice. *Hosp. Pract.* **2019**, *47*, 6–15. [CrossRef] [PubMed]
2. Cai, F.; Luis, M.A.F.; Lin, X.; Wang, M.; Cai, L.; Cen, C.; Biskup, E. Anthracycline-induced cardiotoxicity in the chemotherapy treatment of breast cancer: Preventive strategies and treatment (Review). *Mol. Clin. Oncol.* **2019**, *11*, 15–23. [CrossRef] [PubMed]
3. Syahputra, R.A.; Harahap, U.; Dalimunthe, A.; Pandapotan, M.; Satria, D. Protective effect of Vernonia amygdalina Delile against doxorubicin-induced cardiotoxicity. *Heliyon* **2021**, *7*, e07434. [CrossRef] [PubMed]
4. Bennink, R.J.; van der Hoff, M.J.; Van Hemert, F.J.; De Bruin, K.M.; Spijkerboer, A.L.; Vanderheyden, J.-L.; Steinmetz, N.; Van Eck-Smit, B.L. Annexin V imaging of acute doxorubicin cardiotoxicity (apoptosis) in rats. *J. Nucl. Med.* **2004**, *45*, 842–848.
5. Zhao, L.; Tao, X.; Qi, Y.; Xu, L.; Yin, L.; Peng, J. Protective effect of dioscin against doxorubicin-induced cardiotoxicity via adjusting microRNA-140-5p-mediated myocardial oxidative stress. *Redox Biol.* **2018**, *16*, 189–198. [CrossRef] [PubMed]
6. Christiansen, S.; Autschbach, R. Doxorubicin in experimental and clinical heart failure. *Eur. J. Cardio-Thoracic Surg.* **2006**, *30*, 611–616. [CrossRef] [PubMed]
7. Von Hoff, D.D.; Layard, M.W.; Basa, P.; Davis, H.L., Jr.; Von Hoff, A.L.; Rozencweig, M.; Muggia, F.M. Risk Factors for Doxorubicin-Induced Congestive Heart Failure. *Ann. Intern. Med.* **1979**, *91*, 710–717. [CrossRef] [PubMed]
8. Billingham, M.E.; Mason, J.W.; Bristow, M.R.; Daniels, J.R. Anthracycline cardiomyopathy monitored by morphologic changes. *Cancer Treat. Rep.* **1978**, *62*, 865–872. [PubMed]
9. Buja, L.M.; Ferrans, V.J.; Mayer, R.J.; Roberts, W.C.; Henderson, E.S. Cardiac ultrastructural changes induced by daunorubicin therapy. *Cancer* **1973**, *32*, 771–788. [CrossRef]
10. Zilinyi, R.; Czompa, A.; Czegledi, A.; Gajtko, A.; Pituk, D.; Lekli, I.; Tosaki, A. The Cardioprotective Effect of Metformin in Doxorubicin-Induced Cardiotoxicity: The Role of Autophagy. *Molecules* **2018**, *23*, 1184. [CrossRef] [PubMed]
11. El-Agamy, D.S.; Ibrahim, S.R.M.; Ahmed, N.; Khoshhal, S.; Abo-Haded, H.M.; Elkablawy, M.A.; Aljuhani, N.; Mohamed, G.A. Aspernolide F, as a new cardioprotective butyrolactone against doxorubicin-induced cardiotoxicity. *Int. Immunopharmacol.* **2019**, *72*, 429–436. [CrossRef] [PubMed]
12. McGowan, J.V.; Chung, R.; Maulik, A.; Piotrowska, I.; Walker, J.M.; Yellon, D.M. Anthracycline Chemotherapy and Cardiotoxicity. *Cardiovasc. Drugs Ther.* **2017**, *31*, 63–75. [CrossRef]
13. Lipshultz, S.E.; Alvarez, J.A.; Scully, R. Anthracycline associated cardiotoxicity in survivors of childhood cancer. *Heart* **2007**, *94*, 525–533. [CrossRef] [PubMed]
14. Injac, R.; Strukelj, B. Recent Advances in Protection against Doxorubicin-induced Toxicity. *Technol. Cancer Res. Treat.* **2008**, *7*, 497–516. [CrossRef] [PubMed]
15. Quiles, J.L.; Huertas, J.R.; Battino, M.; Mataix, J.; Ramirez-Tortosa, M.C. Antioxidant nutrients and adriamycin toxicity. *Toxicology* **2002**, *180*, 79–95. [CrossRef]
16. De La Torre, B.G.; Albericio, F. The Pharmaceutical Industry in 2018. An Analysis of FDA Drug Approvals from the Perspective of Molecules. *Molecules* **2019**, *24*, 809. [CrossRef] [PubMed]

17. El-Far, A.; Shaheen, H.M.; Alsenosy, A.E.-W.; El-Sayed, Y.; Al Jaouni, S.K.; Mousa, S. Costus speciosus: Traditional uses, phytochemistry, and therapeutic potentials. *Pharmacogn. Rev.* **2018**, *12*, 120. [CrossRef]
18. Ivanescu, B.; Miron, A.; Corciova, A. Sesquiterpene Lactones fromArtemisiaGenus: Biological Activities and Methods of Analysis. *J. Anal. Methods Chem.* **2015**, *2015*, 247685. [CrossRef]
19. Morgan, E.D.; Wilson, I.D. ChemInform Abstract: Insect Hormones and Insect Chemical Ecology. *ChemInform* **2001**, *32*, 263–375. [CrossRef]
20. Ramawat, K.G.; Mérillon, J.-M. *Natural Products: Phytochemistry, Botany and Metabolism of Alkaloids, Phenolics and Terpenes*; Springer: Berlin/Heidelberg, Germany, 2013.
21. Al-Attas, A.A.; El-Shaer, N.S.; Mohamed, G.A.; Ibrahim, S.R.; Esmat, A. Anti-inflammatory sesquiterpenes from Costus speciosus rhizomes. *J. Ethnopharmacol.* **2015**, *176*, 365–374. [CrossRef]
22. Sirwi, A.; Shaik, R.A.; Alamoudi, A.J.; Eid, B.G.; Kammoun, A.K.; Ibrahim, S.R.M.; Mohamed, G.A.; Abdallah, H.M.; Abdel-Naim, A.B. Mokko Lactone Attenuates Doxorubicin-Induced Hepatotoxicity in Rats: Emphasis on Sirt-1/FOXO1/NF-κB Axis. *Nutrients* **2021**, *13*, 4142. [CrossRef]
23. Livak, K.J.; Schmittgen, T.D. Analysis of Relative Gene Expression Data Using Real-Time Quantitative PCR and the $2^{-\Delta\Delta CT}$ Method. *Methods* **2001**, *25*, 402–408. [CrossRef] [PubMed]
24. Chatterjee, K.; Zhang, J.; Honbo, N.; Karliner, J.S. Doxorubicin Cardiomyopathy. *Cardiology* **2010**, *115*, 155–162. [CrossRef] [PubMed]
25. Singal, P.K.; Iliskovic, N. Doxorubicin-Induced Cardiomyopathy. *N. Engl. J. Med.* **1998**, *339*, 900–905. [CrossRef]
26. Kalivendi, S.V.; Konorev, E.A.; Cunningham, S.; Vanamala, S.K.; Kaji, E.H.; Joseph, J.; Kalyanaraman, B. Doxorubicin activates nuclear factor of activated T-lymphocytes and Fas ligand transcription: Role of mitochondrial reactive oxygen species and calcium. *Biochem. J.* **2005**, *389*, 527–539. [CrossRef] [PubMed]
27. Ibrahim, S.R.M.; Ahmed El-Shaer, N.S.A.; Asfour, H.Z.; Elshali, K.Z.; Awad Shaaban, M.I.; Al-Attas, A.A.M.; Allah Mo-hamed, G.A. Antimicrobial, antiquorum sensing, and antiproliferative activities of sesquiterpenes from Costus speciosus rhizomes. *Pak. J. Pharm. Sci.* **2019**, *32*, 109–115. [PubMed]
28. Lim, K.H.; Ko, D.; Kim, J.-H. Cardioprotective potential of Korean Red Ginseng extract on isoproterenol-induced cardiac injury in rats. *J. Ginseng Res.* **2013**, *37*, 273–282. [CrossRef] [PubMed]
29. Kaul, N.; Siveski-Iliskovic, N.; Hill, M.; Slezak, J.; Singal, P.K. Free radicals and the heart. *J. Pharmacol. Toxicol. Methods* **1993**, *30*, 55–67. [CrossRef]
30. Kim, D.Y.; Choi, B.Y. Costunolide—A Bioactive Sesquiterpene Lactone with Diverse Therapeutic Potential. *Int. J. Mol. Sci.* **2019**, *20*, 2926. [CrossRef]
31. Ma, Q. Role of Nrf2 in Oxidative Stress and Toxicity. *Annu. Rev. Pharmacol. Toxicol.* **2013**, *53*, 401–426. [CrossRef]
32. Guo, Z.; Yan, M.; Chen, L.; Fang, P.; Li, Z.; Wan, Z.; Cao, S.; Hou, Z.; Wei, S.; Li, W.; et al. Nrf2-dependent antioxidant response mediated the protective effect of tanshinone IIA on doxorubicin-induced cardiotoxicity. *Exp. Ther. Med.* **2018**, *16*, 3333–3344. [CrossRef] [PubMed]
33. Li, S.; Wang, W.; Niu, T.; Wang, H.; Li, B.; Shao, L.; Lai, Y.; Li, H.; Janicki, J.S.; Wang, X.L.; et al. Nrf2 Deficiency Exaggerates Doxorubicin-Induced Cardiotoxicity and Cardiac Dysfunction. *Oxidative Med. Cell. Longev.* **2014**, *2014*, 748524. [CrossRef]
34. Xue, W.-L.; Bai, X.; Zhang, L. rhTNFR:Fc increases Nrf2 expression via miR-27a mediation to protect myocardium against sepsis injury. *Biochem. Biophys. Res. Commun.* **2015**, *464*, 855–861. [CrossRef]
35. Zhang, S.; You, Z.-Q.; Yang, L.; Li, L.-L.; Wu, Y.-P.; Gu, L.-Q.; Xin, Y.-F. Protective effect of Shenmai injection on doxorubicin-induced cardiotoxicity via regulation of inflammatory mediators. *BMC Complement. Altern. Med.* **2019**, *19*, 317. [CrossRef]
36. Zhang, Y.-W.; Shi, J.; Li, Y.-J.; Wei, L. Cardiomyocyte death in doxorubicin-induced cardiotoxicity. *Arch. Immunol. Ther. Exp.* **2009**, *57*, 435–445. [CrossRef] [PubMed]
37. Niture, S.K.; Jaiswal, A.K. Nrf2 Protein Up-regulates Antiapoptotic Protein Bcl-2 and Prevents Cellular Apoptosis. *J. Biol. Chem.* **2012**, *287*, 9873–9886. [CrossRef]
38. Peng, S.; Hou, Y.; Yao, J.; Fang, J. Activation of Nrf2 by costunolide provides neuroprotective effect in PC12 cells. *Food Funct.* **2019**, *10*, 4143–4152. [CrossRef]
39. Cheong, C.-U.; Yeh, C.-S.; Hsieh, Y.-W.; Lee, Y.-R.; Lin, M.-Y.; Chen, C.-Y.; Lee, C.-H. Protective Effects of Costunolide against Hydrogen Peroxide-Induced Injury in PC12 Cells. *Molecules* **2016**, *21*, 898. [CrossRef]
40. Mao, J.; Yi, M.; Wang, R.; Huang, Y.; Chen, M. Protective Effects of Costunolide Against D-Galactosamine and Lipopolysaccharide-Induced Acute Liver Injury in Mice. *Front. Pharmacol.* **2018**, *9*, 1469. [CrossRef] [PubMed]

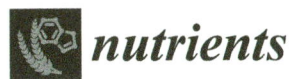

Article

Rubi Fructus Water Extract Alleviates LPS-Stimulated Macrophage Activation via an ER Stress-Induced Calcium/CHOP Signaling Pathway

Do-Hoon Kim [1,†], Ji-Young Lee [2,†], Young-Jin Kim [2], Hyun-Ju Kim [2] and Wansu Park [2,*]

- [1] Department of Medical Classics and History, College of Korean Medicine, Gachon University, Seongnam 13120, Korea; chulian@gachon.ac.kr
- [2] Department of Pathology, College of Korean Medicine, Gachon University, Seongnam 13120, Korea; oxygen1119@naver.com (J.-Y.L.); godsentry@naver.com (Y.-J.K.); eternity0304@daum.net (H.-J.K.)
- * Correspondence: pws98@gachon.ac.kr; Tel.: +82-31-750-8821
- † These authors contributed equally to this work.

Received: 16 October 2020; Accepted: 20 November 2020; Published: 22 November 2020

Abstract: Despite the availability of antibiotics and vaccines, many intractable infectious diseases still threaten human health across the globe. Uncontrolled infections can lead to systemic inflammatory response syndrome and the excessive production of inflammatory cytokines, known as a cytokine storm. As cytokines also play necessary and positive roles in fighting infections, it is important to identify nontoxic and anti-inflammatory natural products that can modulate cytokine production caused by infections. Rubi Fructus, the unripe fruits of *Rubus coreanus* Miquel, are known to possess antioxidative properties. In this study, the effect of the water extract of Rubi Fructus (RF) on the lipopolysaccharide (LPS)-induced inflammatory response in RAW 264.7 macrophages was investigated using biochemical and cell biology techniques. Our data indicated that RF inhibits p38 phosphorylation, intracellular calcium release, and the production of nitric oxide (NO), interleukin (IL)-6, monocyte chemotactic activating factor (MCP)-1, tumor necrosis factor (TNF)-α, leukemia inhibitory factor (LIF), lipopolysaccharide-induced CXC chemokine (LIX), granulocyte-colony stimulating factor (G-CSF), granulocyte macrophage colony-stimulating factor (GM-CSF), vascular endothelial growth factor (VEGF), macrophage colony-stimulating factor (M-CSF), macrophage inflammatory protein (MIP)-1α, MIP-1β, MIP-2, and regulated on activation, normal T cell expressed and secreted (RANTES) in LPS-treated macrophages. In addition, we observed decreasing mRNA expression of *Chop*, *Camk2a*, *Stat1*, *Stat3*, *Jak2*, *Fas*, *c-Jun*, *c-Fos*, *Nos2*, and *Ptgs2* without cytotoxic effects. We concluded that RF demonstrated immunoregulatory activity on LPS-stimulated macrophages via an endoplasmic reticulum (ER) stress-induced calcium/CCAAT-enhancer-binding protein homologous protein (CHOP) pathway and the Janus kinase (JAK)/signal transducers and activators of transcription (STAT) pathway.

Keywords: Rubi Fructus; Rubus coreanus; lipopolysaccharide; macrophage; ER stress; calcium; chop; STAT; cytokine; nitric oxide

1. Introduction

Inflammatory reactions in response to pathogenic infections are essential for human survival [1]. These inflammatory cascades are regulated by immune cells, such as neutrophils, monocytes, macrophages, dendritic cells, eosinophils, basophils, T-lymphocytes, and B-lymphocytes [2]. Among these cell types, macrophages are one of the major regulators of the innate immune system response to infectious pathogens [3]. Macrophages are well known to identify and destroy intrusive microorganisms (i.e., gram-negative bacteria) via the upregulation of inflammatory mediators, such as nitric oxide

(NO), cytokines, chemokines, growth factors, prostaglandins, leukotrienes, and blood coagulation factors [4]. One of major pathways induced by endotoxins, such as lipopolysaccharide (LPS), is the endoplasmic reticulum (ER) stress-induced calcium/CCAAT-enhancer-binding protein homologous protein (CHOP) pathway, which consists of calcium release from the NO-stressed ER and activation of CHOP, calcium/calmodulin dependent protein kinase II alpha (CAMK2a), signal transducers and activators of transcription (STAT), and Fas proteins [5]. However, although necessary for the removal of invasive pathogens, macrophage activation can lead to a cytokine storm (hypercytokinemia), or the excessive production of cytokines, commonly observed in systemic inflammatory response syndrome (SIRS), resulting in multiple organ dysfunction [6]. As there are no effective therapies for cytokine storm, it is important to search for nontoxic and anti-inflammatory natural products that can modulate cytokine production caused by infections.

Traditional medicines can be beneficial for human health, as reported by Tu Youyou, who was awarded the 2015 Nobel Prize for Physiology or Medicine for the discovery of artemisinin from *Artemisia apiacea* [7]. Rubi Fructus (Black Raspberry), the unripe fruits of *Rubus coreanus* Miquel, has traditionally been used as a medical drug in East Asia, including Korea and China [8,9]. Rubi Fructus is also well known to have antioxidative properties [10] and contain large quantities of polyphenolic compounds [11]. Concretely, Seo et al. reported in 2019 that the ethanol extract of Rubi Fructus (ERF) demonstrated that high radical scavenging activity and inhibited the production of inflammatory mediators via the nuclear factor (NF)-κB signaling pathway in RAW 264.7 macrophages stimulated by lipopolysaccharide (LPS) [12]. In 2014, Lee et al. reported that ERF reduced the production of inflammatory mediators, such as NO, prostaglandin E2 (PGE2), tumor necrosis factor (TNF)-α, interleukin (IL)-1β, and IL-6 via suppression of NF-κB and mitogen-activated protein kinase (MAPK) activation in LPS-stimulated RAW 264.7 cells [13]. In 2013, Kim et al. reported that the water extract of Rubi Fructus (WRF) also suppressed NF-κB activation, reactive oxygen species (ROS) production, and inflammatory and phase II gene expression in LPS-stimulated RAW 264.7 macrophages [14].

In the previous study, we reported that *Angelica sinensis* root water extract has an anti-inflammatory effect on LPS-stimulated RAW 264.7 via calcium-mediated Janus kinase (JAK)-STAT pathway [15]. Since Rubi Fructus has antioxidative properties, such as *Angelica sinensis* root, we set the hypothesis that Rubi Fructus modulates inflammatory reactions in LPS-stimulated macrophages via calcium-STAT signaling pathway and conducted related experiments to evaluate effects of the WRF (RF) on the inflammatory cascade in LPS-stimulated RAW 264.7. Experimental data showed that RF inhibited p38 MAPK phosphorylation, intracellular calcium release, and production of NO and various cytokines, chemokines, and growth factors in LPS-stimulated RAW 264.7 cells. We also detected decreased mRNA expressions of *Chop, Camk2a, Stat1, Stat3, Jak2, Fas, c-Jun, c-Fos, Nos2,* and *Ptgs2* without cytotoxic effect. These results indicate that RF possesses immunoregulatory activity in LPS-stimulated macrophages via ER stress-induced calcium/CHOP pathway and the JAK/STAT pathway.

2. Materials and Methods

2.1. Materials

Dulbecco's modified Eagle medium (DMEM), LPS (0.1~1 µg/mL), baicalein (25 µM), and other cell culture reagents were obtained from Millipore (Billerica, MA, USA). Phospho-p38 MAPK Antibody (T180/Y182) (eBioscience 17-9078-42) and Mouse immunoglobulin G2b (IgG2b) kappa Isotype Control (eBioscience 12-4732-81) were obtained from Life Technologies Corporation (Carlsbad, CA, USA).

2.2. Preparation of RF

Commercial Rubi Fructus were obtained from Omniherb (Daegu, Korea) and authenticated by Professor W. Park of Gachon University in July 2016. A voucher specimen (no. 2016-0012) was deposited at the Department of Pathology in Gachon University's College of Korean Medicine. As herbal drugs have been traditionally extracted using water, in the present study, Rubi Fructus were extracted with boiling water for 2 h, filtered, and then lyophilized (yield: 17.42%). The powdered extract (25~200 mg/mL) was dissolved in saline and then filtered through a 0.22 μm syringe filter [15].

2.3. Total Flavonoid Content of RF

The total flavonoid content of RF was determined using the diethylene glycol colorimetric method. Briefly, the sample solution (20 μL of 2 mg/mL RF) was mixed with 200 μL of diethylene glycol and 20 μL of 1 N NaOH. The sample absorbance was read at 405 nm after 1 h incubation at 37 °C. Rutin was used as a reference standard, and total flavonoid content was expressed as milligrams of rutin equivalents (mg RE/g extract) [16].

2.4. Effects of RF on Cell Viability of RAW 264.7

RAW 264.7 mouse macrophages were purchased from the Korea Cell Line Bank (Seoul, Korea). RAW 264.7 cells were cultured in DMEM supplemented with 10% fetal bovine serum containing 100 U/mL of penicillin and 100 μg/mL of streptomycin at 37 °C in a 5% CO_2 humidified incubator. Cell viability was evaluated using a modified MTT assay in 96-well plates (1×10^4 cells/well). Optical density (OD) was determined at 540 nm with a microplate reader (Bio-Rad, Hercules, CA, USA) [15]. In order to determine the toxicity of RF, RF at concentrations of 25, 50, 100, or 200 μg/mL were used for the dose response experiments.

2.5. Effects of RF on NO Production in RAW 264.7 Macrophages Stimulated with LPS

The concentration of NO in culture medium was determined using a Griess reaction assay. Specifically, after incubation of cells in 96-well plates (1×10^4 cells/well) for 24 h with LPS (1 μg/mL) and RF, 100 μL of supernatant from each well was collected and mixed with 100 μL of Griess reagent in a new 96-well plate. After an incubation of 15 min at room temperature, OD was determined at 540 nm with a microplate reader (Bio-Rad) [15].

2.6. Effects of RF on Intracellular Calcium Release in RAW 264.7 Stimulated by LPS

After RAW 264.7 cells were seeded in 96-well plates (1×10^5 cells/well), LPS (1 μg/mL) and RF were added to the culture medium and incubated for 18 h at 37 °C. Thereafter, the medium was removed and cells were incubated with 100 μL of the Fluo-4 dye loading solution (Molecular Probes, Eugene, OR, USA) for 30 min at 37 °C. After 30 min incubation, cells were incubated for a further 30 min at room temperature. Then, the fluorescence intensity of each well was determined using a spectrofluorometer (Dynex, West Sussex, UK) at excitation and emission wavelengths of 485 nm and 535 nm, respectively [15].

2.7. Effects of RF on Cytokine Production in RAW 264.7 Cells Stimulated by LPS

RAW 264.7 cells were seeded in 96-well plates (1×10^4 cells/well) and treated with LPS (1 μg/mL) and RF [15]. After 24 h treatment, levels of the following cytokines in each well were analyzed: interleukin (IL)-6; monocyte chemoattractant protein (MCP)-1; tumor necrosis factor (TNF)-α; leukemia inhibitory factor (LIF); lipopolysaccharide-induced CXC chemokine (LIX; CXCL5); granulocyte colony-stimulating factor (G-CSF); granulocyte macrophage colony-stimulating factor (GM-CSF); macrophage colony-stimulating factor (M-CSF); vascular endothelial growth factor (VEGF); macrophage inflammatory proteins (MIP)-1α, MIP-1β, MIP-2; RANTES (CCL5; regulated on activation, normal T cell expressed and secreted); and interferon gamma-induced protein 10 (IP-10; CXCL10). Cytokines were measured using a Luminex assay based on xMAP technology with MILLIPLEX MAP Mouse Cytokine/Chemokine Magnetic Bead Panel kits (Millipore) and a Bio-Plex 200 suspension array system (Bio-Rad), as described previously [15]. The assay used in this experiment was designed for the multiplexed quantitative measurement of multiple cytokines in a single well, using as little as 25 μL of cell culture supernatant. Standard curves for each cytokine were generated using the kit-supplied reference cytokine samples. Briefly, the following procedure was performed: after pre-wetting the 96-well plate with Wash Buffer, Wash Buffer in each well was removed using a Handheld Magnetic Separation Block (HMSB). Next, cell culture supernatants from each well were incubated with antibody-conjugated beads on a plate shaker for 2 h at room temperature. After incubation, well contents were gently removed with a HMSB, and the 96-well plate was washed 2 times. Then, 25 µL of detection antibodies were added to each well and incubated with agitation on a plate shaker for 1 h at room temperature. Subsequently, 25 µL Streptavidin–Phycoerythrin was added to each well containing the detection antibodies and incubated for 30 min with agitation on a plate shaker at room temperature. After incubation, the well contents were gently removed and washed 2 times using a HMSB. Then, 150 µL of Sheath Fluid was added to all wells, and the beads bound to each cytokine were analyzed with a Bio-Plex 200 instrument (Bio-Rad). Raw data (fluorescence intensity) were analyzed using Bio-Plex Manager software (Bio-Rad). Baicalein (25 µM), a well-known anti-inflammatory flavonoid, was used as a positive control.

2.8. Effects of RF on mRNA Expression in RAW 264.7 Cells Stimulated by LPS

2.8.1. Isolation of RNA

RAW 264.7 cells were incubated with LPS (1 µg/mL) and RF for 18 h in 6-well plates (1×10^6 cells/well). After 18 h incubation, total RNA of each well was isolated using NucleoSpin RNA kit (Macherey-Nagel, Duren, Germany). Briefly, 350 µL Lysis Buffer RA1 and 3.5 µL β-mercaptoethanol was added to the cell pellet and vortexed vigorously to lyse cells. Lysate was cleared by filtration using a NucleoSpin® Filter, and then 350 µL ethanol (70%) was added, and mixed by vortexing. The lysate was loaded into the NucleoSpin® RNA Column, and 350 µL Membrane Desalting Buffer was added and centrifuged. A total of 95 µL DNase reaction mixture was applied directly to the center of the silica membrane of the column, followed by incubation at room temperature for 15 min. Samples were washed with Wash Buffer RA2 and Wash Buffer RA3, and silica membrane was dried. RNA was eluted in 60 µL RNase-free water and centrifuged [15].

2.8.2. Determination of RNA Concentration

RNA concentration was measured using Experion RNA StdSens Analysis kit (Bio-Rad) with the Experion Automatic Electrophoresis System (Bio-Rad). First, the electrodes were cleaned using a cleaning chip filled with 900 µL DEPC-treated water. Then, the Gel-Stain solution was prepared, 9 µL was added into labeled wells, and the chip was primed. Samples and RNA ladder were loaded into the chip, which was vortexed using the Experion vortex station for 1 min. Then the chip was loaded into the electrophoresis platform and the RNA StdSens Analysis program was run [15].

2.8.3. cDNA Synthesis

cDNA of the RNA samples was produced using iScript cDNA Synthesis kit (Bio-Rad) [15]. Briefly, 20 µL complete reaction mixes were prepared with 5× iScript Reaction Mix (4 µL), iScript Reverse Transcriptase (1 µL), Nuclease-free water (variable), and RNA template (variable, 1 µg total RNA). The reaction mix (20 µL) was incubated in a thermal cycler (C1000 Thermal Cycler, Bio-Rad) according to the manufacturer's protocol (priming at 25 °C for 5 min, reverse transcription at 46 °C for 20 min, and RT inactivation at 95 °C for 1 min).

2.8.4. RT-qPCR Analysis

Gene expression was measured using quantitative polymerase chain reaction with iQ SYBR Green Supermix (Bio-Rad) using the CFX96 Real-Time PCR Detection System (Bio-Rad) [15]. Briefly, a master mix was prepared for all reactions by adding iQ SYBR Green Supermix and Forward/Reverse primers for each target gene. This master mix was thoroughly mixed to ensure homogeneity, and 7 µL was dispensed into the wells of a qPCR plate. A total of 3 µL of cDNA was added to each well; any air bubbles in the vessel bottom were removed, and the PCR plate was loaded into the real-time PCR instrument. PCR was performed using the following protocol: denaturation of DNA at 95 °C for 3 min, followed by 40 cycles of 95 °C for 10 sec and 55 °C for 30 sec. The $2^{-\Delta\Delta Ct}$ cycle threshold method was used to normalize the relative mRNA expression levels to the internal control, β-actin. The primers used in this assay are listed in Table 1.

Table 1. Primers used for quantitative PCR.

Name [1]	Forward Primer (5′–3′)	Reverse Primer (5′–3′)
Chop	CCACCACACCTGAAAGCAG	TCCTCATACCAGGCTTCCA
Camk2a	AGCCATCCTCACCACTAT	ATTCCTTCACGCCATCATT
Stat1	TGAGATGTCCCGGATAGTGG	CGCCAGAGAGAAATTCGTGT
Stat3	GTCTGCAGAGT TCAAGCACCT	TCCTCAGTCACGATCAAGGAG
Jak2	TTGGTTTTGAATTATGGTGTCTGT	TCCAAATTTTACAAATTCTTGAACC
Fas	CGCTGTTTTCCCTTGCTG	CCTTGAGTATGAACTCTTAACTGTGAG
c-Jun	ACTGGGTTGCGACCTGAC	CAATAGGCCGCTGCTCTC
c-Fos	AGAGCGGGAATGGTGAAGA	TCTTCCTCTTCAGGAGATAGCTG
Nos2	TGGAGGTTCTGGATGAGAGC	AATGTCCAGGAAGTAGGTGAGG
Ptgs2	TCAAACAGTTTCTCTACAACAACTCC	ACATTTCTTCCCCCAGCAA
β-actin	CTAAGGCCAACCGTGAAAAG	ACCAGAGGCATACAGGGACA

[1] Primer's names; C/EBP homologous protein (Chop), calcium/calmodulin dependent protein kinase II alpha (Camk2a), signal transducers and activators of transcription 1 (Stat1), Stat3, Janus kinase 2 (Jak2), first apoptosis signal receptor (Fas), c-Jun, c-Fos, nitric oxide synthase 2 (Nos2), prostaglandin-endoperoxide synthase 2 (Ptgs2), and β-actin.

2.9. Effects of RF on Phosphorylation of p38 MAPK in RAW 264.7 Cells Stimulated by LPS

Flow cytometry was performed to detect phosphorylated p38 MAPK in RAW 264.7 cells using an Attune NxT flow cytometer (Thermo Fisher Scientific) [17]. Briefly, RAW 264.7 macrophages were seeded in 6-well plates (1×10^6 cells/well) and incubated with LPS (0.1 µg/mL) and RF for 30 min. After incubation, cells were harvested and washed with Flow Cytometry Staining Buffer (SB). Prior to antibody staining, cells were fixed with the pre-warmed Fix Buffer I for 10 min. Then, cells were washed with SB and permeabilized with Perm Buffer III on the ice for 30 min. Then, cells were stained with 5 µg/mL of phospho-p38 MAPK Antibody (T180/Y182) (eBioscience 17-9078-42), or 1.2 µg/mL of Mouse IgG2b kappa Isotype Control (eBioscience 12-4732-81), and analyzed on the Attune NxT flow cytometer (Thermo Fisher Scientific) using Attune NxT software (Thermo Fisher Scientific).

2.10. Statistics

Data are presented as means ± SD. All data were analyzed by one-way analysis of variance (ANOVA) test followed by Tukey's multiple comparison test using GraphPad Prism (version 4; GraphPad Software, San Diego, CA, USA).

3. Results

3.1. Determination of the Total Flavonoid Content of RF

We found that the total flavonoid content of RF was 9.15 mg RE/g extract.

3.2. Effects of RF on Cell Viability

In this study, RF at concentrations of 25, 50, 100, or 200 µg/mL did not decrease cell viability of RAW 264.7 cells after 24 h (108.00 ± 7.84%, 103.84 ± 3.71%, 104.47 ± 4.77%, and 103.19 ± 0.83% of the normal group (Nor) treated with media only, respectively). These results indicated that RF does not exert any cytotoxic effect on macrophages at concentrations of up to 200 µg/mL, which were used in all subsequent experiments (Figure 1A).

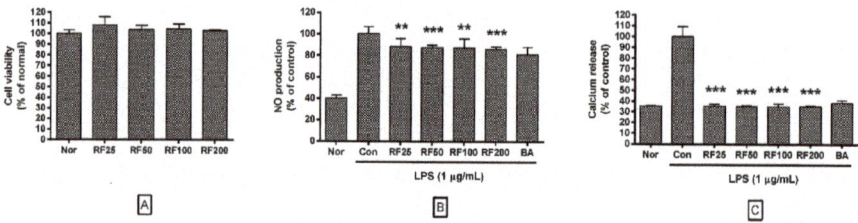

Figure 1. Effects of Rubi Fructus water extract (RF) on (**A**) cell viability, (**B**) nitric oxide (NO) production, and (**C**) intracellular calcium release. Cells were treated with RF and LPS for 24 h (**A,B**) or 18 h (**C**). "Nor" indicates the group treated with media only. "Con" indicates the group treated with 1 μg/mL of lipopolysaccharide (LPS) alone. RF25, RF50, RF100, and RF200 indicate 25, 50, 100, and 200 μg/mL of RF, respectively. "BA" indicates treatment with baicalein (25 μM). Values represent means ± SD of three independent experiments ($n = 3$). Statistical significance was calculated by one-way ANOVA and a Tukey multiple comparison test. ** $p < 0.01$ vs. Con; *** $p < 0.001$ vs. Con.

3.3. NO Production in RAW 264.7 Cells

Data showed that RF significantly inhibited NO production from RAW 264.7 cells stimulated by 24 h treatment with LPS. NO production in RAW 264.7 cells incubated with RF at concentrations of 25, 50, 100, and 200 μg/mL were 88.29 ± 7.33%, 87.6 ± 2.22%, 87.22 ± 8.5%, and 86.26 ± 1.98% of that treated with LPS alone (Figure 1B). These data indicated that RF might modulate excessive NO-induced inflammatory signaling.

3.4. Calcium Release in RAW 264.7 Cells

Data showed that RF significantly inhibited calcium release in RAW 264.7 cells stimulated by 18 h LPS treatment. Calcium release in RAW 264.7 cells incubated with RF at concentrations of 25, 50, 100, and 200 μg/mL were 35.25 ± 1.86%, 34.91 ± 1.12%, 34.72 ± 2.6%, and 34.94 ± 1.08% of that induced by LPS treatment alone (Figure 1C). Our results indicated that RF might exert a regulatory effect over the calcium-related ER stress response pathway.

3.5. Cytokine Production in RAW 264.7 Cells

RF significantly reduced the production of cytokines in RAW 264.7 cells stimulated by LPS for 24 h. In particular, RF reduced productions of IL-6, MCP-1, G-CSF, LIF, LIX, MIP-1α, MIP-1β, MIP-2, VEGF, and RANTES in a dose-dependent manner. Production of IL-6 from RAW 264.7 cells with RF (25, 50, 100, and 200 μg/mL) were 90.71 ± 2.86%, 86.09 ± 6.48%, 81.58 ± 4.52%, and 79.675% ± 5.9% of the LPS alone, respectively; production of MCP-1 was 77.65 ± 3.81%, 64.67 ± 10.02%, 61.73 ± 8.88%, and 58.47 ± 4.14%, respectively; TNF-α was 87.31 ± 3.81%, 69.78 ± 22.36%, 80.5 ± 14.54%, and 76.73 ± 12.05%, respectively; G-CSF was 95.79 ± 0.45%, 94.92 ± 2.63%, 94.73 ± 2.19%, and 94.03 ± 0.24%, respectively; GM-CSF was 57.76 ± 4.91%, 52.2 ± 8.32%, 57.44 ± 7.98%, and 66.48 ± 8.63%, respectively; LIF was 89.1 ± 5.63%, 72.43 ± 17%, 68.2 ± 5.4%, and 67.06 ± 7.78%, respectively; LIX was 80.23 ± 2.96%, 75.11 ± 3.12%, 70.3 ± 7.42%, and 67.26 ± 4.23%, respectively; M-CSF was 84.55 ± 5.85%, 72.87 ± 8.2%, 76.49 ± 9.85%, and 75.45 ± 4.67%, respectively; MIP-1α was 94.8 ± 1.14%, 93.8 ± 0.75%, 93.12 ± 1.57%, and 92.02 ± 1.21%, respectively; MIP-1β was 97.85 ± 1.2%, 97.42 ± 1.2%, 93.52 ± 3.66%, and 92.93 ± 3.22%, respectively; MIP-2 was 97.37 ± 0.57%, 96.69 ± 0.81%, 93.58 ± 2.42%, and 93.16 ± 2.45%, respectively; VEGF was 85.71 ± 1.25%, 77.54 ± 12.82%, 53.28 ± 16.42%, and 41.97 ± 7.72%, respectively; RANTES was 92.07 ± 13.19%, 89.13 ± 3.04%, 77.7 ± 7.13%, and 71.77 ± 5.62%, respectively; and IP-10 was 84.42 ± 5.19%, 90.04 ± 6.85%, 99.26 ± 7.16%, and 98.33 ± 5%, respectively (Figure 2). These data indicated that RF might alleviate hyper-inflammation leading to excessive production of cytokines, chemokines, and growth factors in LPS-stimulated macrophages.

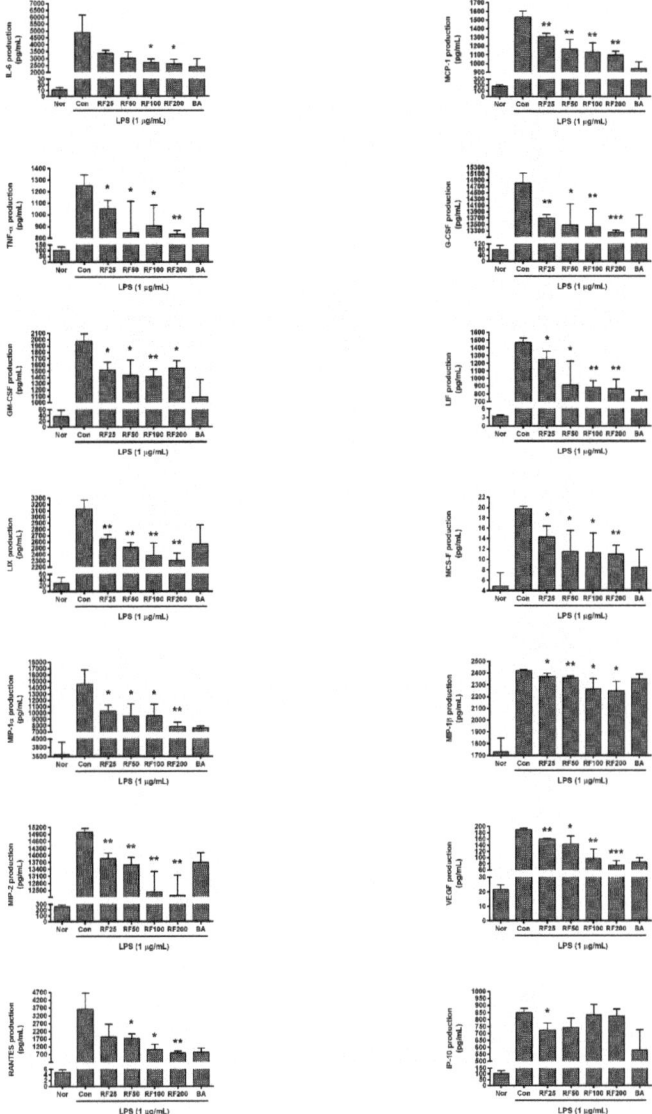

Figure 2. Effects of Rubi Fructus water extract (RF) on the production of interleukin (IL)-6, monocyte chemotactic activating factor (MCP)-1, tumor necrosis factor (TNF)-α, granulocyte-colony stimulating factor (G-CSF), granulocyte macrophage colony-stimulating factor (GM-CSF), leukemia inhibitory factor (LIF), lipopolysaccharide-induced CXC chemokine (LIX), macrophage colony-stimulating factor (M-CSF), macrophage inflammatory protein (MIP)-1α, MIP-1β, MIP-2, vascular endothelial growth factor (VEGF), and regulated on activation, normal T cell expressed and secreted (RANTES), and interferon gamma-induced protein (IP)-10. Cells were treated for 24 h with LPS and RF. "Nor" indicates the group treated with media only. "Con" indicates the group treated with 1 μg/mL of LPS alone. RF25, RF50, RF100, and RF200 indicate 25, 50, 100, and 200 μg/mL of RF, respectively. "BA" indicates treatment with baicalein (25 μM). Values represent means ± SD of three independent experiments (n = 3). Statistical significance was calculated by one-way ANOVA and a Tukey multiple comparison test. * $p < 0.05$ vs. Con; ** $p < 0.01$ vs. Con; *** $p < 0.001$ vs. Con.

3.6. mRNA Expression in RAW 264.7 Cells

RF significantly inhibited the mRNA expression of *Chop, Camk2a, Stat1, Stat3, Jak2, Fas, c-Jun, c-Fos, Nos2,* and *Ptgs2* in RAW 264.7 cells stimulated by LPS (Figure 3). *Chop* expression in RAW 264.7 cells incubated with RF (25, 50, 100, and 200 μg/mL) were 19.35 ± 9.77%, 21.06 ± 7.78%, 33.91 ± 7.73%, and 14.25 ± 5.6% of LPS-treated cells alone, respectively; *Camk2a* expression was 32.76 ± 10.69%, 17.08 ± 8.21%, 33.85 ± 18.44%, and 20.78 ± 15.3% of the LPS group alone; *Stat1* was 19.52 ± 1.36%, 14.73 ± 0.94%, 43.41 ± 7.07%, and 11.36 ± 1.32%, respectively; *Stat3* was 33.76 ± 1.1%, 30.23 ± 16.19%, 54.86 ± 8.74%, and 13.22 ± 5.66%, respectively; *Jak2* was 42.92 ± 23.87%, 21.27 ± 8.54%, 58.1 ± 24.55%, and 30.63 ± 12.68%, respectively; *Fas* was 7.71 ± 0.71%, 7.01 ± 0.55%, 22.49 ± 2.15%, and 6.79 ± 1.15%, respectively; *c-Jun* was 20.29 ± 10.56%, 18.4 ± 6.7%, 32.78 ± 7.4%, and 13.08 ± 2.87%, respectively; *c-Fos* was 45.53 ± 6.31%, 24.94 ± 5.15%, 82.64 ± 8.96%, and 38.25 ± 3.68%, respectively; *Nos2* was 10.44 ± 0.91%, 3.89 ± 0.36%, 28.42 ± 6.43%, and 7.63 ± 0.55%, respectively; and *Ptgs2* was 21.47 ± 0.66%, 13.04 ± 1.17%, 64.17 ± 7.6%, and 2.66 ± 0.82%, respectively. Although RF did not exert a concentration-dependent inhibition of mRNA expression, these data indicate that RF might modulate the expression of inflammatory genes related to ER stress.

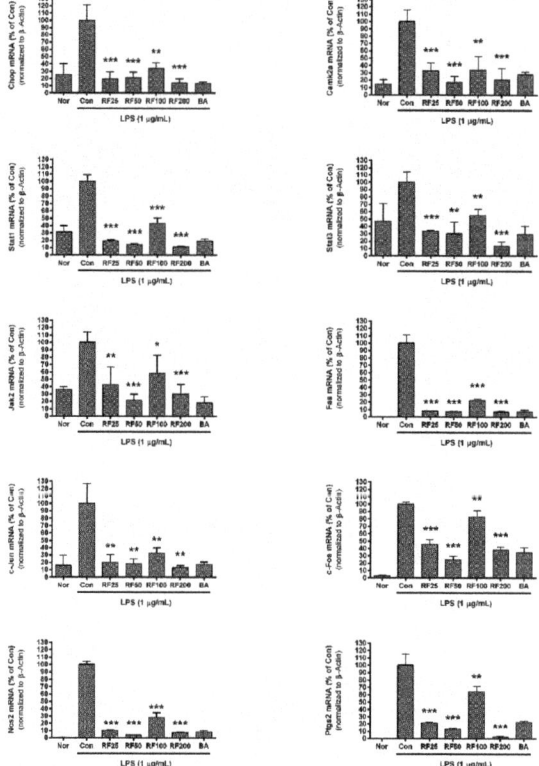

Figure 3. Effects of Rubi Fructus water extract (RF) on mRNA expression of *Chop, Camk2a, Stat1, Stat3, Jak2, Fas, c-Jun, c-Fos, Nos2,* and *Ptgs2*. Cells were treated for 18 h. "Nor" indicates the group treated with media only. "Con" indicates the group treated with 1 μg/mL of LPS alone. RF25, RF50, RF100, and RF200 indicate treatment with 25, 50, 100, and 200 μg/mL of RF, respectively. "BA" indicates treatment with baicalein (25 μM). Values represent means ± SD of three independent experiments ($n = 3$). Statistical significance was calculated by one-way ANOVA and a Tukey multiple comparison test. * $p < 0.05$ vs. Con; ** $p < 0.01$ vs. Con; *** $p < 0.001$ vs. Con.

3.7. Phosphorylation of p38 MAPK in RAW 264.7

Phosphorylation of p38 MAPK was significantly inhibited by RF (Figure 4). p38 MAPK phosphorylation in RAW 264.7 cells incubated with RF (25, 50, 100, and 200 µg/mL) for 30 min was 48.76 ± 3.79%, 39.64 ± 14.53%, 26.11 ± 3.87%, and 38.29 ± 8.46% of that induced by LPS. No non-specific staining was observed with Mouse IgG2b kappa Isotype Control. These data indicated that RF might exert its anti-inflammatory effects via suppressing the activation of p38 MAPK signaling pathway.

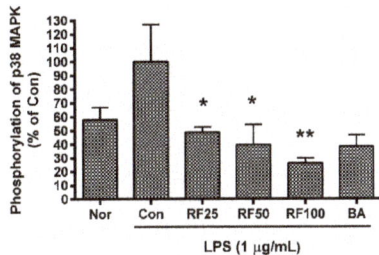

Figure 4. Effects of Rubi Fructus water extract (RF) on phosphorylation of p38 MAPK in RAW 264.7 cells. Cells were treated with LPS and RF for 30 min. "Nor" indicates the group treated with media only. "Con" indicates the group treated with 0.1 µg/mL of LPS alone. RF25, RF50, RF100, and RF200 indicate treatment with 25, 50, 100, and 200 µg/mL of RF, respectively. "BA" indicates treatment with baicalein (25 µM). Values represent means ± SD of three independent experiments ($n = 3$). Statistical significance was calculated by one-way ANOVA and a Tukey multiple comparison test. * $p < 0.05$ vs. Con; ** $p < 0.01$ vs. Con.

4. Discussion

SIRS caused by gram-negative bacteria is known to be a host response to lipopolysaccharide [18,19] and accompanied by increased production of inflammatory mediators such as NO, IL-1, IL-6, and TNF-α resulting in vascular leakage and multiple organ dysfunction syndrome (MODS) [20,21]. Increased endothelial permeability is central to SIRS, leading to MODS and death [22–25]. Indeed, in addition to the cytopathic role in host defense and innate immune functions, NO plays a major role in vasodilation in SIRS [26]. Despite a definitive link between cytokine levels and morbidity/mortality following infection, no effective therapeutic modalities have been developed to subdue the pathology associated with cytokine storm [27]. However, because of the necessary and positive function of cytokines against pathogenic infections, global blunting, rather than ablation, of inflammatory mediators will likely be required to ameliorate pathology associated with cytokine storm [27]. Among immune cells, macrophages are well known to produce many kinds of inflammatory mediators, such as NO and cytokines. Therefore, a drug candidate able to modulate the excessive activation of macrophages stimulated by LPS, including the excessive production of NO and cytokines, might be a beneficial for the regulation of endotoxemia-related inflammatory cascades.

Until recently, many studies have reported on the anti-inflammatory effects of natural products. In the previous study, we reported that *Angelica sinensis* root water extract has an anti-inflammatory effect on LPS-stimulated RAW 264.7 via calcium-mediated JAK-STAT pathway [15]. Since Rubi Fructus has also antioxidative properties like *Angelica sinensis* root, we set the hypothesis that Rubi Fructus inhibits inflammatory reactions in LPS-stimulated macrophages via calcium-STAT signaling pathway. Actually, Rubi Fructus has traditionally been used as a medical drug in East Asia, including Korea and China [8,9]. While the use of Rubi Fructus is indicated in textbooks of traditional medicine such as "Donguibogam (Principles and Practice of Eastern Medicine)" and "Ben Cao Gang Mu (Compendium of Materia Medica)", many researchers are interested in investigating the pharmacological activities of Rubi Fructus [8,9]. A number of studies have reported on the biomedical efficacy of Rubi Fructus, such as its anti-inflammatory effects [12], antioxidative effects [10], improvements in visual sensitivity [28], acetylcholinesterase inhibitory activity [29], improvements in diabetic osteoporosis by simultaneous regulation of osteoblasts and osteoclasts [30], hepatoprotective effects [31], anti-fatigue effects [32], increased hypocholesterolemic activity [33], chemopreventive effects in prostate cancer [34], increased anti-anaphylactic activity [35], and enhanced spermatogenesis [36]. In detail, Seo et al. reported in 2019 that ERF inhibited the production of NO, IL-1β, and IL-6 as well as the activation of inducible nitric oxide synthase (iNOS) and cyclooxygenase 2 (COX-2) via inhibition of the NF-κB signaling pathway in LPS-stimulated RAW 264.7 [12]. Lee et al. reported in 2014 that ERF reduced production of NO, PGE2, TNF-α, IL-1β, and IL-6, and reduced expression of iNOS and COX-2 through suppression of NF-κB activation, as well as phosphorylation of JNK and p38 MAPKs [13]. Kim et al. reported in 2013 that the WRF suppressed NF-κB activation, ROS production, and inflammatory and phase II gene expression in LPS-treated RAW 264.7 cells [14]. Additionally, Park et al. reported in 2006 that ERF exerts anti-inflammatory effects in macrophages via activation of the heme oxygenase-1 signaling pathway [37].

In these experiments, RF significantly inhibited excessive production of NO, IL-6, TNF-α, MCP-1, LIF, LIX, RANTES, MIP-1α, MIP-1β, MIP-2, G-CSF, GM-CSF, VEGF, and M-CSF in RAW 264.7 macrophages stimulated by LPS. The half maximal inhibitory concentration (IC_{50}) of RF in inhibiting expression of these inflammatory markers was 1462.18, 429.54, 570.16, 164.44, 402.72, 2333.46, 121.34, 3749.73, 261.22, 264.24, 364.73, 1733.80, 2167.70, 2167.70, 433.51, and 138.68 µg/mL for NO, intracellular calcium, IL-6, MCP-1, TNF-α, G-CSF, GM-CSF, IP-10, LIF, LIX, M-CSF, MIP-1α, MIP-1β, MIP-2, RANTES, and VEGF, respectively.

Our data indicate that RF may be useful to relieve NO-aggravated vasodilation and cytokine storm in SIRS due to gram-negative bacterial infection. Additionally, RF significantly decreased the release of intracellular calcium, mRNA expression of *Chop*, and phosphorylation of p38 MAPK in LPS-stimulated RAW 264.7 cells, which led to the hypothesis that RF-mediated regulation of inflammatory mediators in LPS-treated RAW 264.7 macrophages might be achieved through ER stress-related CHOP activation.

Many studies have reported ER stress-related calcium release and CHOP expression in stressed cells. In 1996, Wang and Ron reported that CHOP was known to be activated by p38 MAPK in stressed cells [38]. In 2006, Endo et al. reported that LPS stimulation of macrophages causes ER stress and CHOP expression, which initiated inflammasome activation and subsequent macrophage pyroptosis [39]. In 2007, Stout et al. reported that ER calcium stores were reduced and intracellular calcium concentration was initially increased during an inflammatory signaling cascade [40]. Mori also reported that NO depletes ER calcium, causes ER stress-induced CHOP expression, and leads to apoptosis [41]. In 2009, Timmins et al. reported that ER stress-induced calcium release from the ER lumen activates CAMK2a, which might enable macrophage apoptosis via Fas induction and/or activation of Stat1 in macrophages [42]. Tabas et al. also reported that ER-stress-induced CHOP activation, resulting in a release of ER calcium stores into the cytoplasm, and that cytoplasmic calcium activates CAMK2a, which in turn activates a number of pro-apoptotic processes [5]. In 2011, Cho et al. reported that COX-2 is an important mediator of the inflammatory response related to ER stress [43]. In 2017, Lee et al. reported that LPS induces expression of iNOS, COX-2, NO, TNF-α, and IL-6 via p38 MAPK and JAK/STAT signaling pathways in RAW 264.7 macrophages [44]. Guha and Mackman reported that p38 MAPK signaling in LPS-stimulated macrophages can activate a variety of transcription factors, including AP-1 (c-Fos/c-Jun) [45]. In the current study, RF was shown to reduce mRNA expression of *Camk2a*, *Stat1*, *Stat3*, *Jak2*, *Fas*, *c-Jun*, *c-Fos*, *Nos2*, and *Ptgs2* in LPS-stimulated RAW 264.7 macrophages. These results suggest that RF alleviates LPS-stimulated macrophage activation via ER stress-induced calcium/CHOP pathway and the JAK/STAT pathway, resulting in reduced production of inflammatory mediators such as NO, cytokines, chemokines, and growth factors (Figure 5).

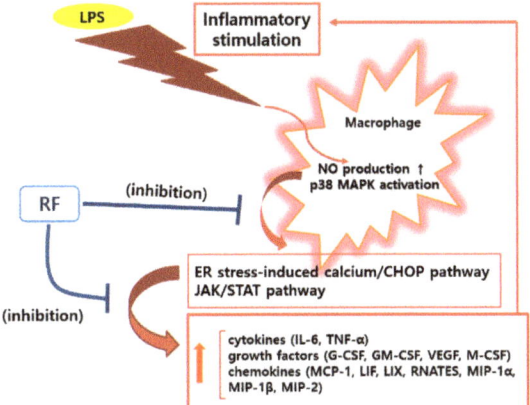

Figure 5. A schematic diagram of the immunoregulatory activity of Rubi Fructus water extract (RF) on lipopolysaccharide (LPS)-stimulated RAW 264.7 macrophages. RF alleviates LPS-stimulated macrophage activation via an ER stress-induced calcium/CHOP signaling pathway and the JAK/STAT pathway.

However, this study could not determine the exact source from which intracellular calcium is released. It remains for future studies to elucidate whether the intracellular calcium level is increased through the influx of extracellular calcium or through depletion of ER calcium stores in LPS-stimulated RAW 264.7 macrophages. Moreover, we could not evaluate effects of RF on IL-1β production, phosphorylation of JNK, NF-κB activation, and ROS production in LPS-stimulated RAW 264.7. More detailed research will clarify the efficacy of RF in treating bacterial infectious diseases.

Author Contributions: Conceptualization, W.P. and D.-H.K.; methodology, W.P. and D.-H.K.; software, W.P.; validation, W.P.; formal analysis, W.P.; investigation, J.-Y.L., Y.-J.K., H.-J.K., and W.P.; resources, W.P.; data curation, W.P.; writing—original draft preparation, W.P.; visualization, W.P.; supervision, W.P.; project administration, W.P.; funding acquisition, W.P. All authors have read and agreed to the published version of the manuscript.

Funding: This research was supported by the Basic Science Research Program through the National Research Foundation of Korea, funded by the Ministry of Science, ICT, and Future Planning (2017R1A2B4004933).

Conflicts of Interest: The authors declare no conflict of interest. The funders had no role in the design of the study, in the collection, analyses, or interpretation of data, in the writing of the manuscript, or in the decision to publish the results.

Abbreviations

RF	Water extract of Rubi Fructus
LPS	Lipopolysaccharide
NO	Nitric Oxide
PGE2	Prostaglandin E2
IL	Interleukin
MCP	Monocyte chemotactic activating factor
TNF	Tumor necrosis factor
IgG2b	Immunoglobulin G2b
OD	Optical density
LIX	Lipopolysaccharide-induced CXC chemokine
LIF	Leukemia inhibitory factor
G-CSF	Granulocyte colony-stimulating factor
GM-CSF	Granulocyte macrophage colony-stimulating factor
VEGF	Vascular endothelial growth factor
M-CSF	Macrophage colony-stimulating factor

MIP	Macrophage inflammatory protein
RANTES	Regulated on activation, normal T cell expressed and secreted
IP	Interferon gamma-induced protein
ER	Endoplasmic reticulum
CHOP	C/EBP homologous protein
CAMK2a	Calcium/calmodulin dependent protein kinase II alpha
MAPK	Mitogen-activated protein kinase
JAK	Janus kinase
STAT	Signal transducers and activators of transcription
FAS	First apoptosis signal receptor
NOS	Nitric oxide synthase
PTGS	Prostaglandin-endoperoxide synthase
SIRS	Systemic inflammatory response syndrome
RE	Rutin equivalents
ERF	Ethanol extract of Rubi Fructus
WRF	Water extract of Rubi Fructus
DMEM	Dulbecco's modified Eagle's medium
HMSB	Handheld Magnetic Separation Block
SB	Staining Buffer
Nor	Normal group
MODS	Multiple organ dysfunction syndrome
JNK	Jun NH2-terminal kinase
NF	Nuclear factor
iNOS	Inducible nitric oxide synthase
COX-2	Cyclooxygenase 2
IC_{50}	Half maximal inhibitory concentration
ROS	Reactive oxygen species

References

1. Si-Tahar, M.; Touqui, L.; Chignard, M. Innate Immunity and Inflammation—Two Facets of the Same Anti-Infectious Reaction. *Clin. Exp. Immunol.* **2009**, *156*, 194–198. [CrossRef]
2. Li, H.S.; Watowich, S.S. Innate Immune Regulation by STAT-Mediated Transcriptional Mechanisms. *Immunol. Rev.* **2014**, *261*, 84–101. [CrossRef] [PubMed]
3. Wang, J.; Nikrad, M.P.; Travanty, E.A.; Zhou, B.; Phang, T.; Gao, B.; Alford, T.; Ito, Y.; Nahreini, P.; Hartshorn, K.; et al. Innate Immune Response of Human Alveolar Macrophages during Influenza A Infection. *PLoS ONE* **2012**, *7*, e29879. [CrossRef] [PubMed]
4. Arango Duque, G.; Descoteaux, A. Macrophage Cytokines: Involvement in Immunity and Infectious Diseases. *Front. Immunol.* **2014**, *5*, 491. [CrossRef] [PubMed]
5. Tabas, I.; Seimon, T.; Timmins, J.; Li, G.; Lim, W. Macrophage Apoptosis in Advanced Atherosclerosis. *Ann. N. Y. Acad. Sci.* **2009**, *1173* (Suppl. 1), E40–E45. [CrossRef]
6. Wang, H.; Ma, S. The Cytokine Storm and Factors Determining the Sequence and Severity of Organ Dysfunction in Multiple Organ Dysfunction Syndrome. *Am. J. Emerg. Med.* **2008**, *26*, 711–715. [CrossRef]
7. Zheng, W.R.; Li, E.C.; Peng, S.; Wang, X.S. Tu Youyou Winning the Nobel Prize: Ethical Research on the Value and Safety of Traditional Chinese Medicine. *Bioethics* **2020**, *34*, 166–171. [CrossRef]
8. Lee, T.; Jung, W.M.; Lee, I.S.; Lee, Y.S.; Lee, H.; Park, H.J.; Kim, N.; Chae, Y. Data Mining of Acupoint Characteristics from the Classical Medical Text: DongUiBoGam of Korean Medicine. *Evid. Based Complement. Altern. Med.* **2014**, *2014*, 329563. [CrossRef]
9. Wang, W.Y.; Zhou, H.; Yang, Y.F.; Sang, B.S.; Liu, L. Current Policies and Measures on the Development of Traditional Chinese Medicine in China. *Pharmacol. Res.* **2020**, 105187. [CrossRef]
10. Bhandary, B.; Lee, H.Y.; Back, H.I.; Park, S.H.; Kim, M.G.; Kwon, J.W.; Song, J.Y.; Lee, H.K.; Kim, H.R.; Chae, S.W.; et al. Immature Rubus Coreanus Shows a Free Radical-Scavenging Effect and Inhibits Cholesterol Synthesis and Secretion in Liver Cells. *Indian J. Pharm. Sci.* **2012**, *74*, 211–216.

11. Lee, J.H.; Bae, S.Y.; Oh, M.; Seok, J.H.; Kim, S.; Chung, Y.B.; Gowda, K.G.; Mun, J.Y.; Chung, M.S.; Kim, K.H. Antiviral Effects of Black Raspberry (*Rubus Coreanus*) Seed Extract and its Polyphenolic Compounds on Norovirus Surrogates. *Biosci. Biotechnol. Biochem.* **2016**, *80*, 1196–1204. [CrossRef] [PubMed]
12. Seo, K.H.; Lee, J.Y.; Park, J.Y.; Jang, G.Y.; Kim, H.D.; Lee, Y.S.; Kim, D.H. Differences in Anti-Inflammatory Effect of Immature and Mature of Rubus Coreanus Fruits on LPS-Induced RAW 264.7 Macrophages Via NF-kappaB Signal Pathways. *BMC Complement. Altern. Med.* **2019**, *19*, 89. [CrossRef] [PubMed]
13. Lee, J.E.; Cho, S.M.; Park, E.; Lee, S.M.; Kim, Y.; Auh, J.H.; Choi, H.K.; Lim, S.; Lee, S.C.; Kim, J.H. Anti-Inflammatory Effects of Rubus Coreanus Miquel through Inhibition of NF-kappaB and MAP Kinase. *Nutr. Res. Pract.* **2014**, *8*, 501–508. [CrossRef] [PubMed]
14. Kim, S.; Kim, C.K.; Lee, K.S.; Kim, J.H.; Hwang, H.; Jeoung, D.; Choe, J.; Won, M.H.; Lee, H.; Ha, K.S.; et al. Aqueous Extract of Unripe Rubus Coreanus Fruit Attenuates Atherosclerosis by Improving Blood Lipid Profile and Inhibiting NF-kappaB Activation Via Phase II Gene Expression. *J. Ethnopharmacol.* **2013**, *146*, 515–524. [CrossRef]
15. Kim, Y.J.; Lee, J.Y.; Kim, H.J.; Kim, D.H.; Lee, T.H.; Kang, M.S.; Park, W. Anti-Inflammatory Effects of Angelica Sinensis (Oliv.) Diels Water Extract on RAW 264.7 Induced with Lipopolysaccharide. *Nutrients* **2018**, *10*. [CrossRef]
16. Mocan, A.; Vlase, L.; Raita, O.; Hanganu, D.; Pǎltinean, R.; Dezsi, Ş.; Gheldiu, A.; Oprean, R.; Crişan, G. Comparative Studies on Antioxidant Activity and Polyphenolic Content of *Lycium Barbarum* L. and *Lycium Chinense* Mill. Leaves. *Pak. J. Pharm. Sci.* **2015**, *28* (Suppl. 4), 1511–1515.
17. Shahidullah, A.; Lee, J.Y.; Kim, Y.J.; Halimi, S.M.A.; Rauf, A.; Kim, H.J.; Park, B.Y.; Kim, D. Anti-Inflammatory Effects of Diospyrin on Lipopolysaccharide-Induced Inflammation using RAW 264.7 Mouse Macrophages. *Biomedicines* **2020**, *8*, 11. [CrossRef]
18. Park, B.S.; Lee, J.O. Recognition of Lipopolysaccharide Pattern by TLR4 Complexes. *Exp. Mol. Med.* **2013**, *45*, e66. [CrossRef]
19. Cross, A.S. Anti-Endotoxin Vaccines: Back to the Future. *Virulence* **2014**, *5*, 219–225. [CrossRef]
20. Deutschman, C.S.; Tracey, K.J. Sepsis: Current Dogma and New Perspectives. *Immunity* **2014**, *40*, 463–475.
21. Tisoncik, J.R.; Korth, M.J.; Simmons, C.P.; Farrar, J.; Martin, T.R.; Katze, M.G. Into the Eye of the Cytokine Storm. *Microbiol. Mol. Biol. Rev.* **2012**, *76*, 16–32. [CrossRef] [PubMed]
22. Fujishima, S. Organ Dysfunction as a New Standard for Defining Sepsis. *Inflamm. Regen.* **2016**, *36*, 24. [CrossRef] [PubMed]
23. Meegan, J.E.; Shaver, C.M.; Putz, N.D.; Jesse, J.J.; Landstreet, S.R.; Lee, H.N.R.; Sidorova, T.N.; McNeil, J.B.; Wynn, J.L.; Cheung-Flynn, J.; et al. Cell-Free Hemoglobin Increases Inflammation, Lung Apoptosis, and Microvascular Permeability in Murine Polymicrobial Sepsis. *PLoS ONE* **2020**, *15*, e0228727. [CrossRef] [PubMed]
24. Hauser, B.; Matejovic, M.; Radermacher, P. Nitric Oxide, Leukocytes and Microvascular Permeability: Causality or Bystanders? *Crit. Care* **2008**, *12*, 104. [CrossRef] [PubMed]
25. Thompson, B.T.; Chambers, R.C.; Liu, K.D. Acute Respiratory Distress Syndrome. *N. Engl. J. Med.* **2017**, *377*, 562–572. [CrossRef]
26. Kilbourn, R.G.; Traber, D.L.; Szabo, C. Nitric Oxide and Shock. *Dis. Mon.* **1997**, *43*, 277–348. [CrossRef]
27. Tejiaro, J.R. Cytokine Storms in Infectious Diseases. *Semin. Immunopathol.* **2017**, *39*, 501–503. [CrossRef]
28. Wahid, F.; Jung, H.; Khan, T.; Hwang, K.H.; Park, J.S.; Chang, S.C.; Khan, M.A.; Kim, Y.Y. Effects of Rubus Coreanus Extract on Visual Processes in Bullfrog's Eye. *J. Ethnopharmacol.* **2011**, *138*, 333–339. [CrossRef]
29. Kim, C.R.; Choi, S.J.; Oh, S.S.; Kwon, Y.K.; Lee, N.y.; Park, G.G.; Kim, Y.J.; Heo, H.J.; Jun, W.J.; Park, C.S.; et al. Rubus Coreanus Miquel Inhibits Acetylcholinesterase Activity and Prevents Cognitive Impairment in a Mouse Model of Dementia. *J. Med. Food* **2013**, *16*, 785–792. [CrossRef]
30. Choi, C.; Lee, H.; Lim, H.; Park, S.; Lee, J.; Do, S. Effect of Rubus Coreanus Extracts on Diabetic Osteoporosis by Simultaneous Regulation of Osteoblasts and Osteoclasts. *Menopause* **2012**, *19*, 1043–1051. [CrossRef]
31. Teng, H.; Lin, Q.; Li, K.; Yuan, B.; Song, H.; Peng, H.; Yi, L.; Wei, M.C.; Yang, Y.C.; Battino, M.; et al. Hepatoprotective Effects of Raspberry (*Rubus Coreanus* Miq.) Seed Oil and its Major Constituents. *Food Chem. Toxicol.* **2017**, *110*, 418–424. [CrossRef] [PubMed]

32. Lee, S.; You, Y.; Yoon, H.G.; Kim, K.; Park, J.; Kim, S.; Ho, J.N.; Lee, J.; Shim, S.; Jun, W. Fatigue-Alleviating Effect on Mice of an Ethanolic Extract from Rubus Coreanus. *Biosci. Biotechnol. Biochem.* **2011**, *75*, 349–351. [CrossRef] [PubMed]
33. Nam, M.K.; Choi, H.R.; Cho, J.S.; Cho, S.M.; Ha, K.C.; Kim, T.H.; Ryu, H.Y.; Lee, Y.I. Inhibitory Effects of Rubi Fructus Extracts on Hepatic Steatosis Development in High-Fat Diet-Induced Obese Mice. *Mol. Med. Rep.* **2014**, *10*, 1821–1827. [CrossRef] [PubMed]
34. Kim, Y.; Kim, J.; Lee, S.M.; Lee, H.A.; Park, S.; Kim, Y.; Kim, J.H. Chemopreventive Effects of Rubus Coreanus Miquel on Prostate Cancer. *Biosci. Biotechnol. Biochem.* **2012**, *76*, 737–744. [CrossRef] [PubMed]
35. Shin, T.Y.; Kim, S.H.; Lee, E.S.; Eom, D.O.; Kim, H.M. Action of Rubus Coreanus Extract on Systemic and Local Anaphylaxis. *Phytother. Res.* **2002**, *16*, 508–513. [CrossRef] [PubMed]
36. Oh, M.S.; Yang, W.M.; Chang, M.S.; Park, W.; Kim, D.R.; Lee, H.K.; Kim, W.N.; Park, S.K. Effects of Rubus Coreanus on Sperm Parameters and cAMP-Responsive Element Modulator (CREM) Expression in Rat Testes. *J. Ethnopharmacol.* **2007**, *114*, 463–467. [CrossRef] [PubMed]
37. Park, J.H.; Oh, S.M.; Lim, S.S.; Lee, Y.S.; Shin, H.K.; Oh, Y.S.; Choe, N.H.; Park, J.H.; Kim, J.K. Induction of Heme Oxygenase-1 Mediates the Anti-Inflammatory Effects of the Ethanol Extract of Rubus Coreanus in Murine Macrophages. *Biochem. Biophys. Res. Commun.* **2006**, *351*, 146–152. [CrossRef]
38. Wang, X.Z.; Ron, D. Stress-Induced Phosphorylation and Activation of the Transcription Factor CHOP (GADD153) by p38 MAP Kinase. *Science* **1996**, *272*, 1347–1349. [CrossRef]
39. Endo, M.; Mori, M.; Akira, S.; Gotoh, T. C/EBP Homologous Protein (CHOP) is Crucial for the Induction of Caspase-11 and the Pathogenesis of Lipopolysaccharide-Induced Inflammation. *J. Immunol.* **2006**, *176*, 6245–6253. [CrossRef]
40. Stout, B.A.; Melendez, K.; Seagrave, J.; Holtzman, M.J.; Wilson, B.; Xiang, J.; Tesfaigzi, Y. STAT1 Activation Causes Translocation of Bax to the Endoplasmic Reticulum during the Resolution of Airway Mucous Cell Hyperplasia by IFN-Gamma. *J. Immunol.* **2007**, *178*, 8107–8116. [CrossRef]
41. Mori, M. Regulation of Nitric Oxide Synthesis and Apoptosis by Arginase and Arginine Recycling. *J. Nutr.* **2007**, *137*, 1616S–1620S. [CrossRef] [PubMed]
42. Timmins, J.M.; Ozcan, L.; Seimon, T.A.; Li, G.; Malagelada, C.; Backs, J.; Backs, T.; Bassel-Duby, R.; Olson, E.N.; Anderson, M.E.; et al. Calcium/calmodulin-Dependent Protein Kinase II Links ER Stress with Fas and Mitochondrial Apoptosis Pathways. *J. Clin. Investig.* **2009**, *119*, 2925–2941. [CrossRef] [PubMed]
43. Cho, H.K.; Cheong, K.J.; Kim, H.Y.; Cheong, J. Endoplasmic Reticulum Stress Induced by Hepatitis B Virus X Protein Enhances Cyclo-Oxygenase 2 Expression Via Activating Transcription Factor 4. *Biochem. J.* **2011**, *435*, 431–439. [CrossRef] [PubMed]
44. Lee, S.B.; Lee, W.S.; Shin, J.S.; Jang, D.S.; Lee, K.T. Xanthotoxin Suppresses LPS-Induced Expression of iNOS, COX-2, TNF-Alpha, and IL-6 Via AP-1, NF-kappaB, and JAK-STAT Inactivation in RAW 264.7 Macrophages. *Int. Immunopharmacol.* **2017**, *49*, 21–29. [CrossRef] [PubMed]
45. Guha, M.; Mackman, N. LPS Induction of Gene Expression in Human Monocytes. *Cell. Signal.* **2001**, *13*, 85–94. [CrossRef]

Publisher's Note: MDPI stays neutral with regard to jurisdictional claims in published maps and institutional affiliations.

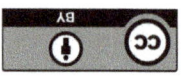

© 2020 by the authors. Licensee MDPI, Basel, Switzerland. This article is an open access article distributed under the terms and conditions of the Creative Commons Attribution (CC BY) license (http://creativecommons.org/licenses/by/4.0/).

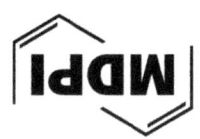

MDPI
St. Alban-Anlage 66
4052 Basel
Switzerland
Tel. +41 61 683 77 34
Fax +41 61 302 89 18
www.mdpi.com

Nutrients Editorial Office
E-mail: nutrients@mdpi.com
www.mdpi.com/journal/nutrients